Overcoming Dyslexia in Children, Adolescents, and Adults

Overcoming Dyslexia in Children, Adolescents, and Adults

Second Edition

DALE R. JORDAN

pro·ed

8700 Shoal Creek Boulevard
Austin, Texas 78757-6897

pro·ed

© 1996, 1989 by PRO-ED, Inc.
8700 Shoal Creek Boulevard
Austin, Texas 78757-6897

Library of Congress Cataloging-in-Publication Data

Jordan, Dale R.
    Overcoming dyslexia in children, adolescents, and adults / Dale R. Jordan.—2nd ed.
        p.   cm.
    Includes bibliographical references and index.
    ISBN 0-89079-642-4 (soft : alk. paper)
    1. Dyslexia—Popular works.   2. Learning disability—Popular works. I. Title.
RC394.W6J67   1996
616.85′53—dc20   95-37940
                                                        CIP

This book is designed in Frutiger Bold and Bookman Light.

Production Manager: Alan Grimes
Production Coordinator: Karen Swain
Managing Editor: Tracy Sergo
Art Director: Thomas Barkley
Reprints Buyer: Alicia Woods
Editor: Lisa Tippett
Editorial Assistant: Claudette Landry
Editorial Assistant: Martin Wilson

Printed in the United States of America

1 2 3 4 5 6 7 8 9 10   00 99 98 97 96

To
Alexandra and William,
my beloved grandchildren
who learn differently.
May the Lord bless you
and keep you
as you grow up
in the new century.

Contents

Preface

Shortly before closing private practice in 1990 to return to teacher education, I met the grandchild of one of the struggling sixth graders I taught to read in 1957 when I was a fledgling classroom teacher. In the 1950s no one knew that deep dyslexia is passed down the family line, usually in males. As a neophyte teacher, I taught Joe to read at a slow, labored rate when he was 12 years old. Eighteen years later I taught his struggling son to read during a summer institute on a university campus. Seventeen years after that I confirmed that Joe's struggling grandson is also dyslexic. Like father, like son, like grandson.

In 1996 I stand atop a divide, looking back upon my 4 decades of experience with three generations of bright learners who struggled with dyslexia and other forms of learning disabilities (LD). From this divide I also look ahead to the 21st century that holds exciting promise for those who learn differently. On looking back, I see several of my early students serving prison sentences. I have lost count of how many became addicted to drugs and alcohol or became mentally ill. Several have committed suicide. I also see the victorious ones who overcame dyslexia well enough to achieve success. Like all committed teachers, my heart is heavy because I did not know what to do for strugglers back in the 1950s.

Ironically, all too few classroom teachers of the 1990s know much more than my generation did about effective accommodations for learners with LD. In spite of our wealth of new knowledge about the causes and characteristics of dyslexia, only a handful of teacher education programs prepare new teachers to recognize and accommodate for LD in their future learners. Here, on this divide, I review the explosion of new knowledge that began during the 1960s. How quickly our understanding of specific learning disabilities expanded! Such memorable leaders as Samuel Kirk and Samuel Clements described specific patterns of learning dysfunction that pointed the way to better education for young strugglers. Following the lead of pioneers such as Samuel T. Orton, Beth Slingerland, and Marianne Frostig, medical scientists began to discover how brain functions affect academic learning. The late Norman Geschwind and his colleagues made astonishing discoveries concerning neurological differences in the brains of struggling learners. The emergence of brain imaging science in the 1980s allowed Martha Denckla, Albert Galaburta, Antonio Damasio, Russell Barkley, Erin Zaidel, and many others to uncover a wealth of new knowledge about brain-based dysfunctions, especially dyslexia and Attention-Deficit Disorders. As we near the end of the 20th century, we have at hand knowledge and technology no one dreamed of when I was Joe's inexperienced teacher 40 years ago.

This book is not intended to be a scientific treatise about dyslexia. The purpose of *Overcoming Dyslexia in Children, Adolescents, and Adults* is to translate the mysteries of specialized clinical data into everyday language for diagnosticians, classroom teachers, counselors, tutors, parents, and anyone else who needs more practical knowledge of this critical issue. This book is intended to interpret research information in a simple, practical form. To paraphrase ancient mythology, my goal is to bring fire down from Olympus for the benefit of those who do not have the time or the background to translate research language for themselves.

Chapter 1

The Nature of Dyslexia

EARLY HISTORY OF DYSLEXIA

The stage was set for the recognition of dyslexia in Europe almost 200 years ago. At the start of the 19th century, a German neurologist, Franz-Joseph Gall, presented the first comprehensive description of how the central nervous system is structured (Gall & Spurzheim, 1809). That neuronal roadmap paved the way for many 19th-century studies of how the brain processes language-based information. In 1861 the French neurologist Pierre Paul Broca explained how changes in regions of the left brain cause loss of speech (cited by Opp, 1994). Seven years later Theodor Meynert, a German physician, demonstrated that certain psychological patterns are associated with specific regions of the left brain. In 1869 English neurologist Henry Charlton Bastian introduced the term *agraphia* to describe unique written language deficits in patients with aphasia. A few years later the German physician Carl Wernicke (1874) presented a map showing where the left brain produces speech. That same year, the British neurologist John Hughlings Jackson (1874) explained that the left brain controls most of the oral communication function in language processing.

The actual term *dyslexia* was introduced in 1884 by German ophthalmologist Reinhold Berlin to describe poor reading ability in persons with normal vision. Just 1 year after that, German neurologist Ludwig Lichteim (1885) reported seven types of speech disturbance caused by interrupted functioning of certain nerve pathways in the left brain. Lichteim introduced the term *alexia* to describe severe reading disability. He also was the first to show a relationship between handwriting and the ability to read printed symbols. The same year, another German neurologist, Hubert Grashey, published evidence of the relationship between certain types of closed head injuries (skull fractures) and loss of memory, visual perception, and language processing (Grashey, 1885). Sir William Broadbent, an English ophthalmologist, followed Berlin's research by describing *word blindness* (discussed later in this chapter) in persons with good vision who had dyslexia (Broadbent, 1872). A Scottish eye surgeon, James Hinshelwood, built upon the work of Berlin and Broadbent by diagnosing a type of reading dysfunction that kept certain readers from recognizing printed symbols on a book page (Berlin, 1887; Hinshelwood, 1900). Using Hinshelwood's model, British educator James Kerr began to identify word blindness in pupils within the British education system (cited in Jordan, 1989a). In 1892 German neurologist J. K. Goldscheider introduced the idea that reading depends upon integration of specific brain regions that process speech sounds, interpret spatial relationships, and comprehend time sequence. These pioneers of the 19th century paved the way for rapid growth during the 20th century in understanding of brain-based learning disabilities.

TWENTIETH-CENTURY DISCOVERIES

During World War I, an American neurologist working with soldiers who had received head injuries became intrigued by language disabilities he discovered in these men. Samuel T. Orton introduced the term *strephosymbolia* to describe what he called "twisted symbol" patterns that appeared following certain types of head injury. In 1925 Orton linked the European concept of word blindness to certain types of left-brain injuries. Orton later described dyslexia as a dysfunction in visual perception and visual memory and speculated that it was caused by deficits in brain structure (Orton, 1937).

During World War II, Stanley Taylor developed a photographic process for studying the eye movement and eye tracking patterns (*saccadic movements*) of persons who struggled to read (Taylor, 1960). Samuel Kirk introduced the term *learning disability* (LD) in 1962, and it rapidly became the universal label for certain types of classroom learning difficulties (cited in Hammill, 1990). A year later, Samuel Clements proposed the concept of *minimal brain dysfunction* (MBD), which widely influenced diagnostic and educational thinking for more than 2 decades (Clements, 1966). Approximately 1 decade after that, Dale Jordan published his study *Dyslexia in the Classroom* (1972), which documented the specific ways that dyslexia interferes with classroom learning for bright students with LD. During the 1960s and 1970s three American neurologists, Norman Geschwind, Walter Levitsky, and Albert Galaburda at Harvard Medical School, conducted the first in-depth anatomical studies of dyslexic brains (Galaburda, 1983; Geschwind, 1984). Those studies made it clear that persons with dyslexia have specific neurological differences in how left-brain pathways are developed.

During the 1980s the new science of brain imaging allowed researchers and physicians to watch the living brain at work. Through such technologies as positron emission tomography (PET), magnetic resonance imaging (MRI), computerized tomography (CT), and brain electrical activity mapping (BEAM), researchers around the world began to map how the left brain learns language skills, then processes those skills in reading, handwriting, spelling, and basic arithmetic (Montgomery, 1989). The regions of the left brain that must be integrated before good literacy skills can be developed are shown in Figure 1.1. The science of brain imaging demonstrated that dyslexia is caused by incomplete neuronal pathways throughout these left-brain language-processing regions and that Attention-Deficit Disorders originate in the limbic system (cerebellum) as well as in certain regions within the left cerebral cortex (Jordan, 1995).

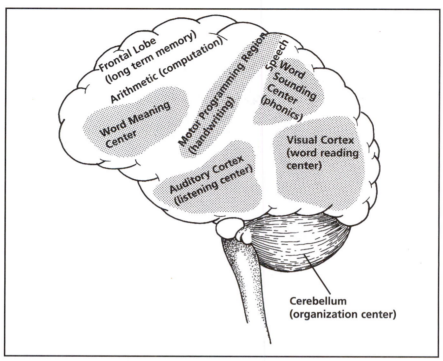

FIGURE 1.1. Regions of the left brain that participate in processing language. These language centers must be well integrated for the learner to develop fluent literacy and arithmetic skills.

Differences in Brain Cell Development

During the early 1990s two important discoveries were made about how brain cell development contributes to the learning struggles called LD. The first discovery concerned the four-step developmental sequence each nerve cell must follow to reach full maturity (see Figure 1.2). To become fully functional, every cell within the central nervous system must pass through these four steps. Throughout the brain pathways of persons with learning disabilities, many cells skip a step in this developmental sequence. This results in incompletely formed cell structures throughout the language-processing regions of the left brain and midbrain. When brain cells are incomplete, it is impossible for synapse pathways to relay neurotransmitter messages successfully. Too

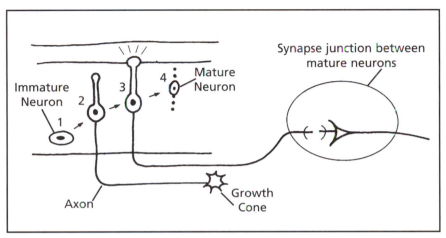

FIGURE 1.2.   Each cell within the central nervous system must go through a 4-step maturation process to become a functional, mature cell. Each newly formed neuron starts to migrate from its place of birth toward its final position within the nervous system. If any developmental steps are skipped, the cell cannot carry out its intended function when it enters the neuronal chain. A learning disability is caused when too many brain cells skip one or more steps of this developmental process.

many "bridges" are out along important information highways to permit fluent language processing. Persons with these neurological differences do not have the neurological talent for fluent reading, spelling, and writing.

A second kind of difference exists within the nerve pathway development of individuals with LD. Figure 1.3 shows the dendrite structure within the brain. All new brain cells put forth many hairlike tendrils called dendrites. These dendrites become the lines of communication between mature clusters of cells that form ganglia centers throughout the brain. As new brain cells finish their development, specialized enzymes dissolve away unnecessary dendrites, leaving only certain ones that are required for mature connecting pathways. This process is called *pruning.* Figure 1.4 shows mature dendrite structure that lets pruned cells communicate without interference. It is now known that brain structures of persons with LD often do not prune away extra dendrites, leaving too many unnecessary nerve pathways. The unfortunate result is thought processing filled with

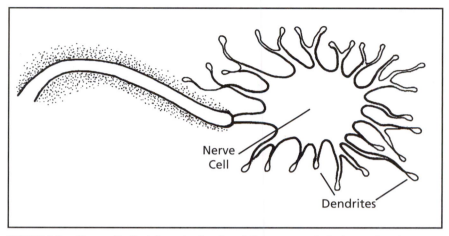

FIGURE 1.3. New cells that have just entered the neuronal chain send out many hairlike tendrils called dendrites. These dendrites become the links between mature cells. At a certain point in nerve cell maturation, the brain produces enzymes that dissolve away the extra dendrites that are not needed; this is called dendrite pruning. In persons who have LD, too many dendrites remain. Unpruned dendrites contribute to short attention span, loose thought patterns, and difficulty developing short-term and long-term memory.

distraction and a type of neurological "static" that keeps brain centers from doing their intended work fluently.

Reading Ability and the U.S. Workplace

The decade of the 1970s in U.S. education started with a bombshell that shattered many assumptions about literacy accomplishments. The National Reading Council reported that 18 million men and women in the United States between the ages of 18 and 55 were illiterate (Harris, 1970, cited in Harris, 1989a). As shall be shown later in this chapter, this shocking figure was a serious undercount of the actual presence of low literacy in the U.S. workforce. A large number of U.S. workers could not read a restaurant menu, successfully follow a road map, interpret street signs, fill out job application forms without help, apply for a Social Security card, fill out applications for government assistance, read a newspaper, or help their children with homework assignments.

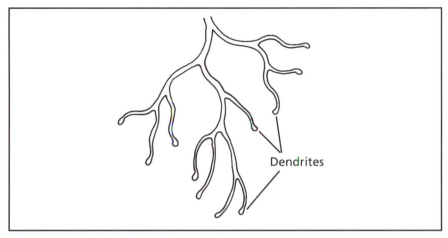

FIGURE 1.4.   When brain enzymes prune away surplus dendrites, the brain pathways have clearly defined routes for sending information. In persons with LD, not enough of these pruned neuronal pathways exist to deliver well-organized information.

Other studies revealed that as many as one third of all public school students dropped out before finishing high school (Jordan, 1989a). Upon checking over school records, several states discovered that from before World War II and on, public high schools had been losing one third of their students before graduation. During the 1970s, more than 70 literacy studies were done with the populations of adjudicated juveniles and adult males serving prison sentences. It was discovered that three out of four adjudicated or incarcerated youths and men could not read, write, or spell above a third-grade level (Jordan, 1974). Not only was the national labor market teeming with illiterate adults, but the prison systems also were crowded by those who could not function in tasks requiring fourth-grade or higher literacy skills. Billions of federal and state dollars were dedicated to remediating this crisis. Adult education became a well-financed enterprise as all levels of government sought to turn back this tide of low literacy that saturated the workforce.

In 1992 the U.S. Department of Labor released a new report on the status of literacy in the workplace (Kirsch, Jungeblut, & Campbell, 1992). Researchers conducted in-depth interviews with a cross-section of adults ages 16 through 65 and discovered that 90 million adults in the workforce are subliterate, having literacy skills below the sixth-grade level. Of these 90 million adults, 50 million have literacy skills at fourth- and fifth-grade levels. This means that if these individuals have enough time, they can read most street signs, order from a simple menu, get essential information from a newspaper, figure out a bus schedule, keep track of simple financial transactions, do basic reading on the job, and fill out simple application forms by themselves. They cannot, however, cope with more difficult literacy tasks. The remaining 40 million adults at the bottom of the labor pool are below a third-grade level in reading ability. They have virtually no independent literacy skills. These persons cannot read a newspaper, interpret street or road signs effectively, fill out application forms without help, interpret a menu, read to their children, or do on-the-job reading or writing without assistance. The stunning fact is that as society nears the end of the 20th century, 45% of the U.S. workforce is functionally illiterate. This vast army of subliterate adults do not have the skills to enter into the technologically challenging workplace of the 21st century.

Learning Disabilities as a Factor in U.S. Literacy Rates

Numerous researchers in learning disabilities have concluded that 8 out of 10 of the nonreading adults in the U.S. workforce have undiagnosed, untreated learning disabilities (Jordan, 1995; Kidder, 1991; Payne, 1994; Pollan & Williams, 1993; Weisel, 1992). According to this estimate, 30 million subliterate adults have LD. Their specific learning differences are lifelong barriers to literacy that have not been recognized or treated during their years in classroom learning.

This stunning discovery that the number of functionally illiterate adults more than quadrupled in 20 years sent shock waves through the U.S. workplace. How could the most productive nation in the world fail to educate such vast numbers of men and women?

No reasonable person would infer that dyslexia is the sole cause for this much illiteracy in U.S. society. Dyslexia is only one of several forms of specific learning disability. Sub-literate persons who have attended school for several years often have a variety of overlapping problems that keep them from mastering literacy skills. Although many illiterate adults do have dyslexia (Jordan, 1995; Kidder, 1991; Payne, 1993; Pollan & Williams, 1993; Rawson, 1989; Weisel, 1992), other disorders that may be involved include residual attention deficit disorder (Barkley, 1990; Copeland, 1991; Hallowell & Ratey, 1994; Jordan, 1992; Weis, 1992) and deficits in central visual perception (word blindness) (Geiger & Letvin, 1987; Irlen, 1991; Jordan, 1995; Lehmkuhle, Garzia, Turner, Hash, & Baro, 1993; Livingstone, Rosen, Drislane, & Galaburda, 1991). It is not known how many persons in the United States have been disabled academically by mental illness. In addition, social and economic deprivation can be major factors in illiteracy. There clearly is no single reason why 50 million adults are subliterate and another 40 million are illiterate in spite of the extraordinary investment of national effort and financial support. However, dyslexia is among the most prevalent of causes for lifelong inability to master the basic skills of reading, spelling, writing, and arithmetic.

THE WORKPLACE OF THE TWENTY-FIRST CENTURY

In pondering the economic and social impact of untreated learning disabilities in adults, Kirsch et al. (1992) described the workplace of the future as one that will overwhelm these unprepared individuals. The workplace of the next century will be built upon the emerging technology often called *cyberspace.* Tomorrow's workers increasingly will have to do all sorts of rapid, computer-based information processing. All jobs will require rapid comparing and contrasting of many types of data on paper, barcodes, computer screens, videotapes, and audiotapes. Workers in the 21st century will be required to generate new information at an incredible pace, be fluent in arithmetic operations, and quick to interpret math-based situations, without calling for help. Those who have dyslexia and those with low literacy skills will be left out of the job market unless each person's specific learning differences are documented and appropriate accommodations are made (Kirsch et al., 1992, cited in Jordan & Stephens, 1995).

DEFINITIONS FOR LEARNING DISABILITIES AND DYSLEXIA

I began my work with struggling learners before U.S. education included the concepts of learning disability and dyslexia. For the past three decades, I have observed and participated in the effort to define language dysfunction in this culture. It has not been easy for professional groups to reach consensus on the definitions of dyslexia and learning disability, although in a general sense, progress has been made. In his landmark review of the effort to define learning disabilities, Donald Hammill (1990) pointed out that there has been more agreement than disagreement among those who have sought to define LD. As Martha Evans (1982) demonstrated in her review of 2,500 studies of dyslexia, more than 200 definitions of this problem were generated by professionals before 1980. However, as we come close to the 21st century, a universally accepted definition has not been developed.

The dominant definitions of LD that have guided professionals' thinking for the past 30 years should be reviewed at this point. In 1962, Samuel Kirk defined learning disabilities as follows:

> A learning disability refers to a retardation, disorder, or delayed development in one or more of the processes of speech, language, reading, writing, arithmetic, or other school subjects resulting from a psychological handicap caused by a possible cerebral dysfunction and/or emotional or behavioral disturbances. It is not the result of mental retardation, sensory deprivation, or cultural and instructional factors. (Kirk, 1962, p. 263; cited in Hammill, 1990, p. 75)

In 1970, Donald Critchley defined dyslexia:

> A disorder manifested by difficulty in learning to read despite conventional instruction, adequate intelligence, and sociocultural opportunity. It is dependent upon fundamental cognitive disabilities which are frequently of constitutional origin. (p. 11)

In sharp contrast to Critchley's simplicity is the definition of dyslexia developed by the International Reading Association:

Dyslexia

> 1.n. A medical term for incomplete alexia; partial but severe inability to read; historically (but less common in current use), word blindness. Note: Dyslexia in this sense applies to persons who ordinarily have adequate vision, hearing, intelligence, and general language functioning. Dyslexia is a rare but definable and diagnosable form of primary reading retardation with some form of central nervous system dysfunction. It is not attributable to environmental causes or other handicapping conditions.
>
> 2.n. A severe reading disability of unexpected origin.
>
> 3.n. A popular term for any difficulty in reading of any intensity and from any cause(s). Note: Dyslexia in this sense is a term which describes a symptom, not a disease. (Harris & Hodges, 1981, p. 95)

The Education for All Handicapped Children Act of 1975 (Public Law 94-142) defined a learning disability as follows:

> The term "specific learning disability" means a disorder in one or more of the basic psychological processes involved in understanding or in using language spoken or written, which may manifest itself in an imperfect ability to listen, think, speak, read, write, spell, or to do mathematical calculations. The term includes such conditions as perceptual handicaps, brain injury, minimal brain dysfunction, dyslexia, and developmental aphasia. The term does not include children who have learning disabilities which are primarily the result of visual, hearing, or motor handicaps, of mental retardation, of emotional disturbance, or of environmental, cultural, or economic disadvantage. (USOE, 1977, p. 65083)

Currently, the most widely accepted definition of LD comes from the report of the National Joint Committee on Learning Disabilities (1988):

> Learning disabilities is a general term that refers to a hetero-geneous group of disorders manifested by significant difficulties in acquisition and use of listening, speaking, reading, writing, reasoning or mathematical abilities. These disorders are intrinsic to the individual, presumed to be due to central nervous dys-function, and may occur across the life span. . . . Although learn-ing disabilities may occur concomitantly with other handicapping conditions (for example, sensory impairment, mental retardation, serious emotional disturbance) or with extrinsic influences (such as cultural differences, insufficient or inappropriate instruction), they are not the result of those conditions or influences. (p. 1)

Score Discrepancy Definition

In 1984, public schools and other agencies that deal with large numbers of struggling learners became obliged to fol-low a new definition of LD based entirely upon scores obtained from standardized tests of intelligence and achieve-ment. To be legally regarded as having a learning disability, a student had to have an arbitrary discrepancy between IQ score, usually the Full Scale IQ from one of the Wechsler intelligence scales, and standard scores from such tests as the *Woodcock–Johnson Psycho-Educational Battery–Revised* (Woodcock, 1991). However, no nationally recognized standard for score discrepancy has ever been set by regulating agen-cies. For more than a decade, public agencies have faced the frustrating facts that the score discrepancy definition of LD varies from state to state, as well as from agency to agency within the same state. For example, Texas might declare that a 14-point discrepancy must exist between IQ and achievement before a person can be considered to have a learning disability. The neighboring state of Oklahoma might establish a 17-point discrepancy as the criterion, whereas Georgia might require a 15-point score discrepancy and Michigan might set a 22-point discrepancy. Furthermore, these score discrepancy standards change from year to year, depending upon funding issues. The situation is especially complicated for mobile families that move from Dallas to Atlanta, then to Flint, then to Oklahoma City, then east to Little Rock. For example, a child with a 16-point score discrepancy would be regarded as having a learning disability in Dallas and Atlanta, but not in Flint or Oklahoma City. That child again would be defined as having LD when his or her family moves to Little Rock. The score discrepancy definition of learning disabilities was an effort to view LD in a scientific way, removing subjective opinions from the process of making a diagnosis of learning difficulty. However, in the eyes of many frustrated parents and professionals who must live with or educate struggling learners, this effort to quantify the struggle to learn has been less than successful. Obviously, there is a long way to go before dyslexia and LD are universally defined and recognized among professionals in the United States.

LEARNING DISABILITIES

In spite of these differences in definition, it is possible to *describe* a learning disability. In the general U.S. culture, a learning disability is a cluster of factors that keeps an intelligent child from learning how to do schoolwork successfully. This special population—persons with learning disabilities—exists in virtually every classroom and community in the United States. Yet, its members have not been identified adequately or treated effectively by our system of education. As such students move upward through the grades, they do not develop fluent skills in reading from printed materials. It is impossible for them to do typical reading assignments expected by adults and they cannot write effectively. Penmanship is poor because fine-motor coordination never becomes smooth in controlling the pencil or pen. Sentence structure is ragged and incomplete. These students usually have trouble copying accurately from the chalkboard or from a book.

Such students seldom do well with basic arithmetic. They must count fingers to add, subtract, multiply, or divide. They usually need to whisper over and over while their fingers touch or handle the page and their work rate usually is very slow. Individuals with LD become intensely frustrated if instructors try to make them work faster.

Vision problems frequently occur because their eyes become overly tired after a few minutes of close work. The ability to see details clearly at desktop level deteriorates and within a few minutes these students who are struggling to learn must look away, rub their eyes, or start using a marker to keep their place on the page. Their attention span is often very short, causing them to dart off on "rabbit trails" instead of being focused fully on the task. They usually listen poorly and cannot keep up with a flow of oral information.

Students with LD seldom can follow directions that involve memory for left and right and also usually are confused by the concepts of north, south, east, and west. They often are much less mature than their same-age peers, which creates conflict with those peers and with instructors. These individuals do very poorly on tests, especially when time is limited. They frequently are misdiagnosed as being borderline mentally retarded or emotionally disturbed because they cannot always give coherent standard responses on diagnostic tests.

Four Concepts of LD

It is easy to describe what a learning disability is; however, developing an acceptable definition is another matter. Four basic, overlapping concepts of what LD means compete for dominance. It is rare to find a struggling learner who demonstrates only one of these manifestations of LD (Jordan, 1995).

1. *LD means learning disability.* Within the central nervous system there are specific differences in how neuronal pathways are developed. These anatomical differences in brain structure disable certain individuals as they struggle to master basic skills in reading, handwriting, spelling, math, oral expression, listening comprehension, and written expression. Dyslexia and other types of learning problems

reflect brain-based disabilities in processing language information.

2. *LD means learning difference.* If information is presented in different ways that fit the unique bent or talent of the student who is struggling to learn, he or she can absorb and retain the same information that is readily learned by others in traditional ways. Learning difference is not the same as learning disability.

3. *LD means learning difficulty.* One who struggles to learn need not have dyslexia or any other form of LD. Learning difficulty may be caused by an unusually slow processing rate. If time limits are removed, the learning difficulty may disappear. As shall be seen in the section on word blindness, learning difficulty may be caused by an inability to decipher black print on white paper. If that visual perception problem is corrected, the learning difficulty may disappear. Those who have difficulty in learning must do multisensory processing that combines several sensory pathways at the same time. The student with a learning difficulty who is given plenty of time while using several sensory pathways together usually learns with much less difficulty.

4. *LD means late development.* Brain pathways may be developmentally "behind schedule" in being ready to learn when certain types of information are presented. Later on, the struggling learner catches up as nerve pathways become fully mature. "Late bloomers" reach breakthrough milestones when hormones start the process of puberty. As puberty advances and young adulthood is achieved, these late bloomers gradually develop the ability to learn quite well later on in life.

Minimal Brain Dysfunction

The present knowledge base regarding specific learning disabilities began to take shape in the 1920s and 1930s when Samuel Orton, Beth Slingerland, Grace Fernald, Marianne Frostig, and other pioneers described their discoveries in working with struggling learners. In the 1960s, Samuel Clements offered a usable paradigm of learning disability when he proposed the concept of minimal brain dysfunction (MBD) (Clements, 1966). Clements described a cluster of behaviors that included hyperactivity, very poor organizational ability, spotty and unpredictable ability to master basic academic skills, and short attention span. MBD also involved soft neurological signs such as poor fine-motor coordination, awkward gross-motor coordination, and an impaired ability of the eyes to team together for accurate focusing and refocusing. Children with MBD often were medicated to reduce hyperactivity and increase attention span. They were regarded as being emotionally volatile and hard to educate, and it was assumed that they would always be that way. As time went by, professionals working with this special population discovered that many youngsters with MBD began to outgrow their earlier patterns of struggle by young adulthood. By the late 1970s, it was clear that this population of struggling learners needed to be redefined.

Attention Deficit Disorder

In 1980 the American Psychiatric Association published the third edition of its *Diagnostic and Statistical Manual of Mental Disorders* (DMS-III). This revision of the guidelines for defining mental health presented a new category of learning difficulty. DSM-III introduced the concept of Attention-Deficit Disorder in three subcategories: (1) Attention-Deficit Disorder with Hyperactivity; (2) Attention-Deficit Disorder Without Hyperactivity; and (3) Attention-Deficit Disorder, Residual Type. This new classification largely replaced the earlier label of MBD. Professionals began referring to ADD or ADD syndrome.

A few years later this clear, easily understood diagnostic guideline was changed by a revision to the DSM-III, commonly referred to as DSM-III-R (American Psychiatric Association, 1987). According to the changes that appeared in the DSM-III-R, the three earlier categories of Attention-Deficit Disorder were lumped together as a single syndrome: Attention-Deficit/Hyperactivity Disorder (ADHD). The editorial board who made that decision held the position that Attention-Deficit Disorder arbitrarily includes hyperactivity. A passive (nonhyperactive) daydreamer with short attention span must have some other type of LD. In 1994, a further revision appeared: DSM-IV (American Psychiatric Association, 1994). To qualify for the new ADHD diagnosis, a person must show 8 of the following 14 behavior patterns for at least 6 months, and the attention deficit patterns must have started before age 7:

1. Often fidgets with hands or feet or squirms in seat (in adolescents [or adults], may be limited to subjective feelings of restlessness)

2. Has difficulty remaining seated when required to do so

3. Is easily distracted by extraneous stimuli

4. Has difficulty awaiting turn in games or group situations

5. Often blurts out answers to questions before they have been completed

6. Has difficulty following through on instructions from others (not due to oppositional behavior or failure of comprehension, e.g., fails to finish chores [or job assignments])

7. Has difficulty sustaining attention in tasks or play activities

8. Often shifts from one uncompleted activity to another

9. Has difficulty playing or working quietly

10. Often talks excessively

11. Often interrupts or intrudes on others (e.g., interrupts other persons' games or conversations)

12. Often does not seem to listen to what is being said

13. Often loses things necessary for tasks or activities at school, at home, or at work (e.g., toys, pencils, books, assignments, tools)

14. Often engages in physically dangerous activities without considering possible consequences (not for the purpose of thrill seeking, e.g., runs into the street without looking, drives wrecklessly without considering traffic conditions)

Three Types of Attention Deficit

As was stated previously, when DSM-III-R became the ruling standard in 1987, the original three subcategories of Attention-Deficit Disorder with Hyperactivity, Attention-Deficit Disorder Without Hyperactivity, and Attention-Deficit Disorder, Residual Type were buried inside new terminology. Regardless of the 1987 changes in diagnostic nomenclature, Attention-Deficit Disorder refers to persons who cannot keep attention focused on an academic or work task. No matter how hard they try, their attention darts or drifts away to other issues instead of staying on the assigned task. This individual may or may not be hyperactive. A common mistake made by many diagnosticians is the assumption that Attention-Deficit Disorder always includes hyperactivity. Many of the attention drifters in the classroom and the workplace are not hyperactive but often are passive and withdrawn (Copeland, 1991; Hallowell & Ratey, 1994; Jordan, 1992; Weis, 1992; Weiss & Hechtman, 1994). Whether hyperactive or passive, Attention-Deficit Disorder is marked by specific behavior patterns: short attention span, cluttered impressions of new information, continual distraction by what is going on nearby, frequent conflict with others, usually messy and cluttered space, inability to remember details or carry out responsibilities, need for constant reminding and job supervision, extremely poor listening comprehension, often good reading ability for short periods of time, usually good phonics skills, and an inability to apply one's knowledge in productive ways.

The person with an attention deficit, whether hyperactive or passive, appears irresponsible, scatterbrained, unreliable, lazy, and unproductive. Most individuals with these patterns are considered to be misfits with immature social skills. If they do not outgrow these patterns during adolescence, they become terribly frustrated, unsuccessful adults who cannot keep a job, hold a marriage together, be good parents, or contribute to society in a productive way. Attention-Deficit Disorder is found in most classrooms and workplaces. The irony is that few definitions of learning disability include this frequently seen problem. Few students with attention deficits are included in special programs for youngsters who are LD.

Disruptive Behavior Disorders

A major change in how our culture thinks about ADHD (Attention-Deficit/Hyperactivity Disorder) was reflected in the way DSM-III-R categorized ADHD as a Disruptive Behavior Disorder. In 1990 two comprehensive research studies defined the complex disruptive components of ADHD. The Canadian team of Russell Schachar and Rod Wachsmuth explored the links between ADHD, Oppositional Defiant Disorder (ODD), and Conduct Disorder (CD) in disruptive children (Schachar & Wachsmuth, 1990). An American team led by Russell Barkley reported that 65% of those who are diagnosed as having ADHD also display a chronic disruptive behavior called Oppositional Defiant Disorder (Barkley, 1990). Its symptoms included the following:

1. Often loses temper
2. Often argues with adults
3. Often actively defies or refuses adult (or authority) requests or rules (e.g., refuses to do chores at home, refuses to obey laws or regulations)
4. Often deliberately does things that annoy other people (e.g., grabs other person's things)
5. Often blames others for his or her own mistakes
6. Often is touchy or easily annoyed by others
7. Often is angry and resentful
8. Often is spiteful or vindictive
9. Often swears or uses obscene language

Barkley's research also indicated that 30% of those diagnosed as having ADHD display the disruptive behaviors known as Conduct Disorder. The symptoms for CD include the following:

1. Has stolen without confrontation of a victim on more then one occasion (including forgery)

2. Has run away from home overnight at least twice while living in parental or surrogate parental home (or once without returning)

3. Often lies (other than to avoid physical or sexual abuse)

4. Has deliberately engaged in setting fires

5. Often skips school (for older person, often absent from work)

6. Has broken into someone else's house, building, or car

7. Has deliberately destroyed others' property (other than by setting fires)

8. Has been physically cruel to animals

9. Has forced someone into sexual activity

10. Has used a weapon in more than one fight

11. Often initiates physical fights

12. Has stolen with confrontation of a victim (e.g., mugging, purse-snatching, extortion, armed robbery)

13. Has been physically cruel to people

Barkley (1990) developed still another category of disruptive LD behavior often linked to ADHD, called Multiplex Developmental Disorder (MDD). This complex syndrome is a mixture of erratic thought patterns and eccentric, disruptive, odd, unpredictable, and often explosive habits and behaviors:

1. Misses the point or main idea in conversations

2. Rambles on in speech with one idea not connected to the next

3. Makes irrelevant comments that have no connection to what is going on in the group

4. Insists on sticking to unusual or odd routines (a great deal of ritual behavior for the sake of doing the same thing over and over)

5. Has strong attachments to inanimate objects (stuffed toys, playthings, collectibles of little or no value)

6. Engages in repetitive or stereotyped behavior (shaking or flapping hands, repeatedly touching or fluffing hair, stroking/touching/smoothing clothes, straightening things)

7. Displays extreme reactions to minor irritations, inconveniences, or changes

8. Has trouble handling changes in daily schedules or routines

9. Shows little concern for personal appearance or grooming

10. Has no tact or social discretion (blurts out criticisms or rude comments without regard for who may overhear or be embarrassed)

11. Is a poor judge of the feelings or reactions of others

12. Shows no interest in peers on a typical socially polite level

13. Has poor eye contact

14. Displays rapid mood changes for no apparent reason

15. Describes details of events but misses the meaning or importance of those events

16. Shows no compassion when others are hurt, or may think it is funny when someone else is hurt (or dies)

17. Laughs or cries for no apparent reason

18. Is drawn to distant or background sounds that others ignore

19. Confuses the causes of events and fails to understand cause-and-effect relationships

20. Speaks in half-thoughts or incomplete phrases without noticing that others cannot understand or follow the fragmented train of thought

21. Flies into angry tantrums for no apparent reason

22. Has unusual fears that are not typical for that age (afraid to take a shower, afraid to put head under water, afraid of blown-up balloons)

23. Hoards worthless objects that have no value or apparent meaning

24. Speaks in an excessively loud or excessively soft voice that is inappropriate for the situation

25. Spends an unusual amount of time fantasizing

26. Is extremely gullible or naive for his or her age (believes everything he or she is told)

27. Continually picks at body parts (nose, skin, eyes, eyebrows, fingernails, genitals, lips, teeth, ears, hair)

28. Habitually makes bizarre, exaggerated, outlandish statements as the truth

29. Lives by rituals, repeats certain actions over and over

30. Lacks the modesty usually found at that age and often has obsessive interest in or curiosity about seeing the genitals of others

Delayed Language Development

Many researchers of learning disabilities have looked for ways to identify predictive patterns of future dyslexia or LD in young children. One of the most helpful models for early identification of LD markers in preschool youngsters was developed by Barbara Wilson and her colleagues in Manhasset, New York (Wilson & Risucci, 1986). Wilson called this early identification paradigm the Delayed Language Development syndrome (DLD syndrome). By following groups of children from infancy to kindergarten, Wilson and her staff developed the following cluster of "red flag" signals. Young children who display these patterns are at very high risk for having dyslexia, a learning disability, and/or disruptive behavior when they enter formal class-room learning.

1. *Poor hearing.* Cannot hear ordinary sounds well.

2. *Atypical (irregular) language development.* Use of words is noticeably different, immature, or abnormal. Does not copy oral language patterns successfully.

3. *Poor auditory perception.* Cannot keep up in listening. Continually loses the flow of what is being said. Does not get the point of what is being said. Responds by saying, "What? Huh? What do you mean?"

4. *Poor auditory cognition.* Cannot comprehend the meaning even though he or she can repeat what was said. Clamors, "What do you mean?" Seldom gets the meaning without hearing the oral message several times.

5. *Poor short-term memory.* Cannot remember new words, names, song lyrics, or rhymes. Usually mixes up words and names.

6. *Poor organizational ability.* Cannot keep things orga-nized. Always losing or misplacing things. Personal space is cluttered and messy. Has poor ability at keeping space organized. Is usually bewildered when told to "clean up your room" or "pick up your things."

7. *Poor phonics.* Cannot hear different sounds in words. Cannot connect sounds to letters. Cannot remember sounds and letters over a period of time. Cannot say certain speech sounds clearly after much practice.

8. *Short attention span in listening.* Does not finish lis-tening. Attention darts away to something else. Has no interest in listening to stories or reading books. Cannot stay still when asked to listen.

9. *Poor naming.* Struggles to remember names of things. Continually loses his or her words. Goes blank while telling or naming. Points to things instead of trying to name them. Becomes frustrated when asked to name or tell. Often knows what things are but cannot think

what to call them. Continually calls familiar people by other names.

10. *Poor word retrieval.* Cannot recall specific words learned earlier. Gets stuck trying to tell, describe, or name. Substitutes other words when the main word will not come. Points a lot. Continually says, "You know." Uses "it" more than saying the names of things. Mixes pronouns: "Him and she did it." Uses wrong structure: "Him gots the candy." Often reverses words: Says "me" when means "you" or "her" when means "him."

11. *Poor visual discrimination.* Has trouble telling how things are alike or different. Does not notice important details. Does not recognize clues and markers that distinguish things from each other.

12. *Poor spatial perception.* Does not notice how things are placed. Does not see space or how things are positioned. Cannot judge distance. Continually knocks things over, bumps into things, spills at the table, misses the edge of furniture when setting things down.

13. *Poor visual cognition.* Cannot interpret what is seen. Sees things clearly, but cannot tell what they are. Does not recognize simple shapes (circle, square, triangle). Cannot distinguish alphabet letters or numerals. Does not see important small details (capital letters, periods, commas, dollar signs, quotation marks). Does not notice when things are moved to different locations.

14. *Poor response to instructions.* Nothing happens after instructions are given. Does not start to do what he or she is told. Does not understand what has just been said. Says "What?" or "What do you mean?" even when instructions are repeated several times.

15. *Poor expressive language.* Words come out in a scrambled way. Talks in bits and pieces that often do not connect. Speech is often a collection of disorganized words and phrases. Cannot tell, describe, or explain in an organized, sequential way. Becomes

frustrated trying to tell things. Bursts into tears, has a tantrum, or gives up trying to talk. Continually loses his or her words or goes blank while talking.

Word Blindness

Earlier in this chapter, the 19th-century concern with word blindness was discussed. Within the British educational system, Hinshelwood (1900) and Kerr (cited in Jordan, 1989a) developed diagnostic procedures for identifying students with word blindness who had normal acuity (20/20 or 20/30) but who could not "see" printed symbols on book pages. In the 1930s Orton brought this European insight to the U.S. education system. During the middle years of the 20th century, both optometrists and ophthalmologists developed eye-training strategies that often reduced word blind patterns somewhat. But it was Helen Irlen in 1976 who made the first breakthrough in effective remediation for a disability that is found in approximately 35% of the LD population (Irlen, 1991; Jordan, 1995). While teaching remedial reading skills in the 1970s to college students with dyslexia, Irlen discovered that placing colored overlays on book pages eliminated the problem for some of her struggling readers. As her research in the use of color progressed, Irlen named this phenomenon Scotopic Sensitivity syndrome. Figures 1.5 through 1.13 show examples of the visual perception distortions seen when readers with word blindness look at black print on white paper under bright overhead light.

Irlen developed the Irlen procedure, a standardized diagnostic system for identifying word blindness and remediation through the application of carefully selected colors that significantly reduce word blind patterns. By the early 1980s this remedial strategy was in use worldwide. Irlen's research led to the technology of applying color to corrective lenses, known as Irlen filters. In 1995 it became possible to apply Irlen procedure color to contact lenses. In 1991 Scotopic Sensitivity syndrome was renamed Irlen syndrome in Irlen's book, *Reading by the Colors.* Irlen syndrome is related to how the central nervous system responds to reflected light.

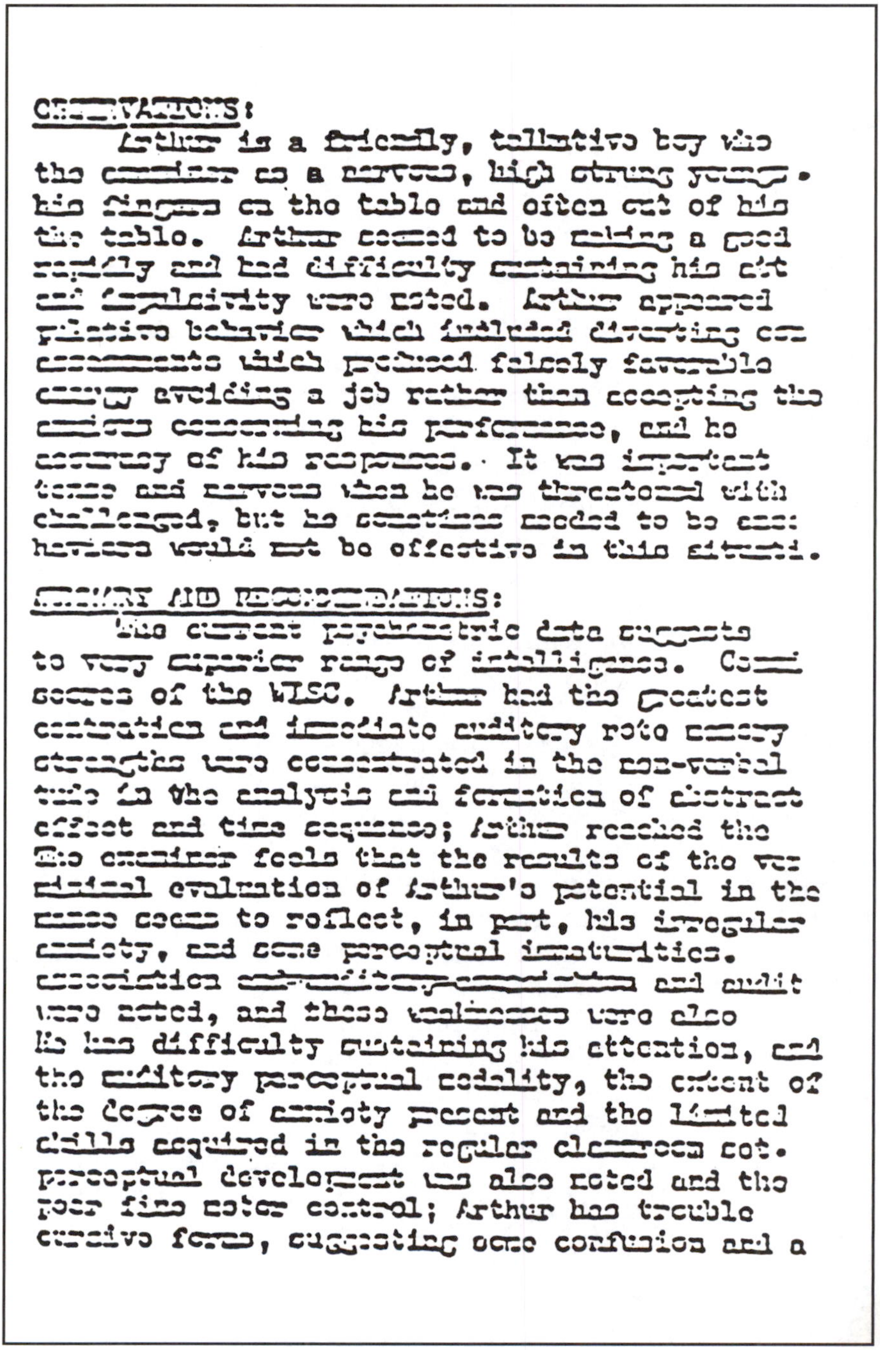

OBSERVATIONS:
Arthur is a friendly, talkative boy who
the examiner as a nervous, high strung young.
his fingers on the table and often out of his
the table. Arthur seemed to be making a good
rapidly and had difficulty sustaining his att
and impulsivity were noted. Arthur appeared
related behavior which included diverting on
assessments which produced falsely favorable
easily avoiding a job rather than accepting the
anxious concerning his performance, and he
accuracy of his responses. It was important
tense and nervous when he was threatened with
challenged, but he sometimes needed to be enc
behaviors would not be effective in this situati.

SUMMARY AND RECOMMENDATIONS:
The current psychometric data suggests
to very superior range of intelligence. Comb
scores of the WISC. Arthur had the greatest
concentration and immediate auditory rote memory
strengths were concentrated in the non-verbal
task in the analysis and formation of abstract
effect and time sequence; Arthur reached the
The examiner feels that the results of the ver
medical evaluation of Arthur's potential in the
cases seem to reflect, in part, his irregular
anxiety, and some perceptual immaturities.
association auditory association and audit
were noted, and these weaknesses were also
He has difficulty sustaining his attention, and
the auditory perceptual modality, the extent of
the degree of anxiety present and the limited
skills acquired in the regular classroom set.
perceptual development was also noted and the
poor fine motor control; Arthur has trouble
cursive forms, suggesting some confusion and a

FIGURE 1.5. The washout effect.

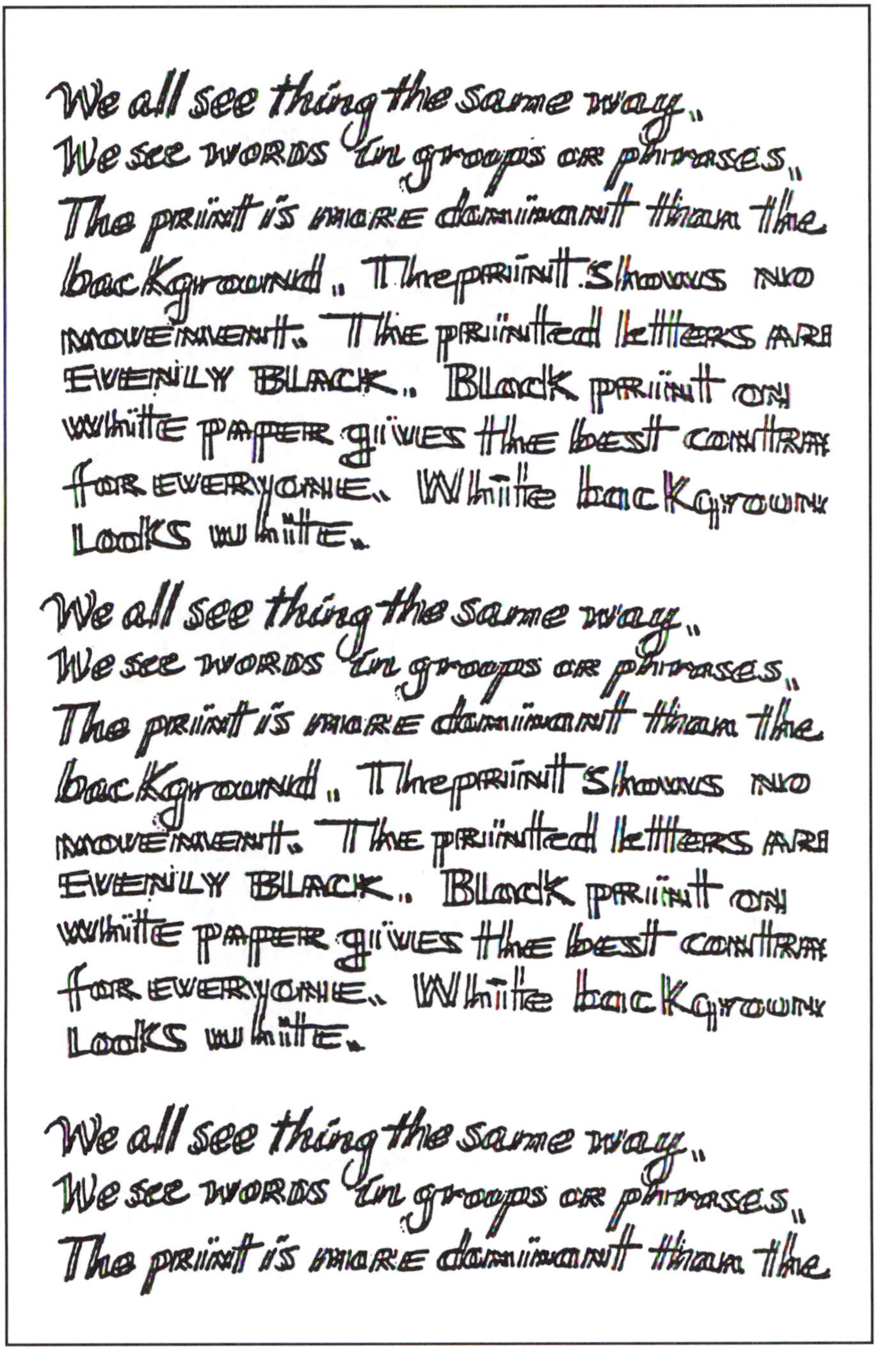

We all see thing the same way.
We see words in groops or phrases.
The print is more dominant than the
background. The print shows no
movement. The printed letters are
evenly black. Black print on
white paper gives the best contrast
for everyone. White backgroun
Looks white.

We all see thing the same way.
We see words in groops or phrases.
The print is more dominant than the
background. The print shows no
movement. The printed letters are
evenly black. Black print on
white paper gives the best contrast
for everyone. White backgroun
Looks white.

We all see thing the same way.
We see words in groops or phrases.
The print is more dominant than the

FIGURE 1.6. The halo effect.

However,bytheend oftheday hehad decidedthat this
schoolwasbetter   than the   last oneeventhough   he
didn'tlikeit.   Nobodyhad   offeredto pullhishead
off,riphiscoat   orthrow   hisshoes   overtheroof.
on theotherhand,   nobody   hadspoken   tohimeither
By Thursdayafter   noon,   nothinghad   changedBill
was notentirely   surprisednoonespoke   tohimbecause
no oneknewhewas   thereeverydayhewas   witanother
group.   Heonly sawhisclasstogether atergistration
after thatthey   weresplitupforall   theirlessons.
Maths   withlx Englishwithlcgames   with2yalesson
which   was   mysteriouslycalled   GSwithlz.Atthe
endof   that   periodhewasnowiser   aboutGSthanhehad
been atthe   beginning,Itseemed   thatthe classwas
on   page135 ofbook2whilethe   teacherwas   onpage
135   ofbook   3asbothbookshad   identical   covers
the lesson   wasoverbeforeany   onenoticed   Billhad
had nobook   anywaybeingadvised   toshare   withaboy
in   apink   shirtwhokepthiselbow   firmly between
Bill and   thebook.Whenthebellrang   Bill   grabbed
the boy   inthepinkshirtbeforehe   could leave.
However,bytheend oftheday hehad decidedthat this
schoolwasbetter   than the   last oneeventhough   he
didn'tlikeit.   Nobodyhad   offeredto pullhishead
off,riphiscoat   orthrow   hisshoes   overtheroof.
on theotherhand,   nobody   hadspoken   tohimeither
By Thursdayafter   noon,   nothinghad   changedBill
was notentirely   surprisednoonespoke   tohimbecause
no oneknewhewas   thereeverydayhewas   witanother
group.   Heonly sawhisclasstogether atergistration
after thatthey   weresplitupforall   theirlessons.
Maths   withlx Englishwithlcgames   with2yalesson
which   was   mysteriouslycalled   GSwithlz.Atthe
endof   that   periodhewasnowiser   aboutGSthanhehad
been atthe   beginning,Itseemed   thatthe classwas
on   page135 ofbook2whilethe   teacherwas   onpage
135   ofbook   3asbothbookshad   identical   covers
the lesson   wasoverbeforeany   onenoticed   Billhad
However,bytheend oftheday hehad decidedthat this
schoolwasbetter   than the   last oneeventhough   he
didn'tlikeit.   Nobodyhad   offeredto pullhishead
off,riphiscoat   orthrow   hisshoes   overtheroof.
on theotherhand,   nobody   hadspoken   tohimeither
By Thursdayafter   noon,   nothinghad   changedBill
was notentirely   surprisednoonespoke   tohimbecause
no oneknewhewas   thereeverydayhewas   witanother
group.   Heonly sawhisclasstogether atergistration

FIGURE 1.7. The rivers effect.

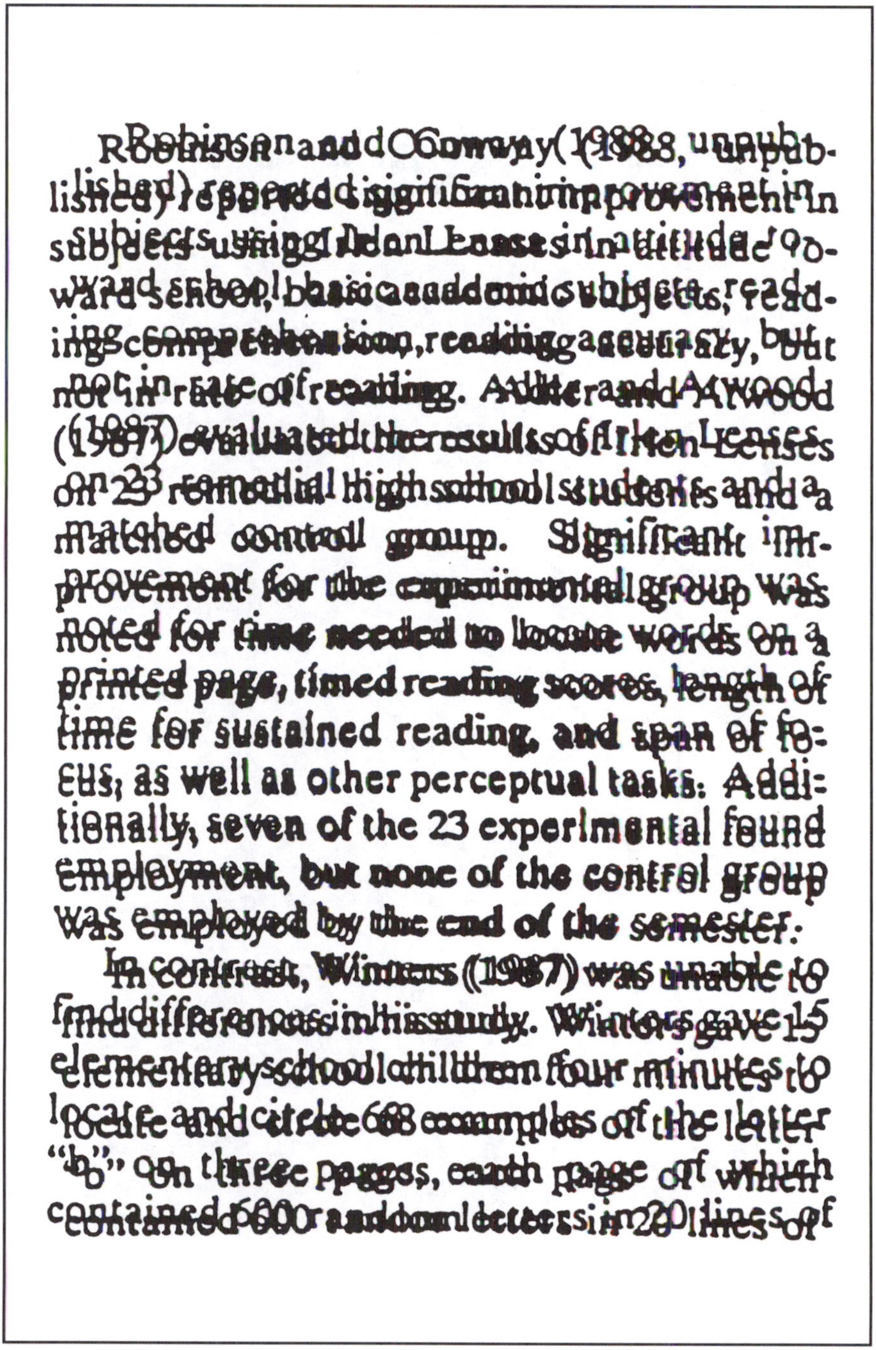

Robinson and Conway (1988, unpublished) reported significant improvement in subjects using Irlen Lenses in attitude toward school, basic academic subjects, reading comprehension, reading accuracy, but not in rate of reading. Adler and Atwood (1987) evaluated the results of Irlen Lenses on 23 remedial high school students and a matched control group. Significant improvement for the experimental group was noted for time needed to locate words on a printed page, timed reading scores, length of time for sustained reading, and span of focus, as well as other perceptual tasks. Additionally, seven of the 23 experimental found employment, but none of the control group was employed by the end of the semester.

In contrast, Winters (1987) was unable to find differences in his study. Winters gave 15 elementary school children four minutes to locate and circle 68 examples of the letter "b" on three pages, each page of which contained 600 random letters in 20 lines of

FIGURE 1.8.   The swirl effect.

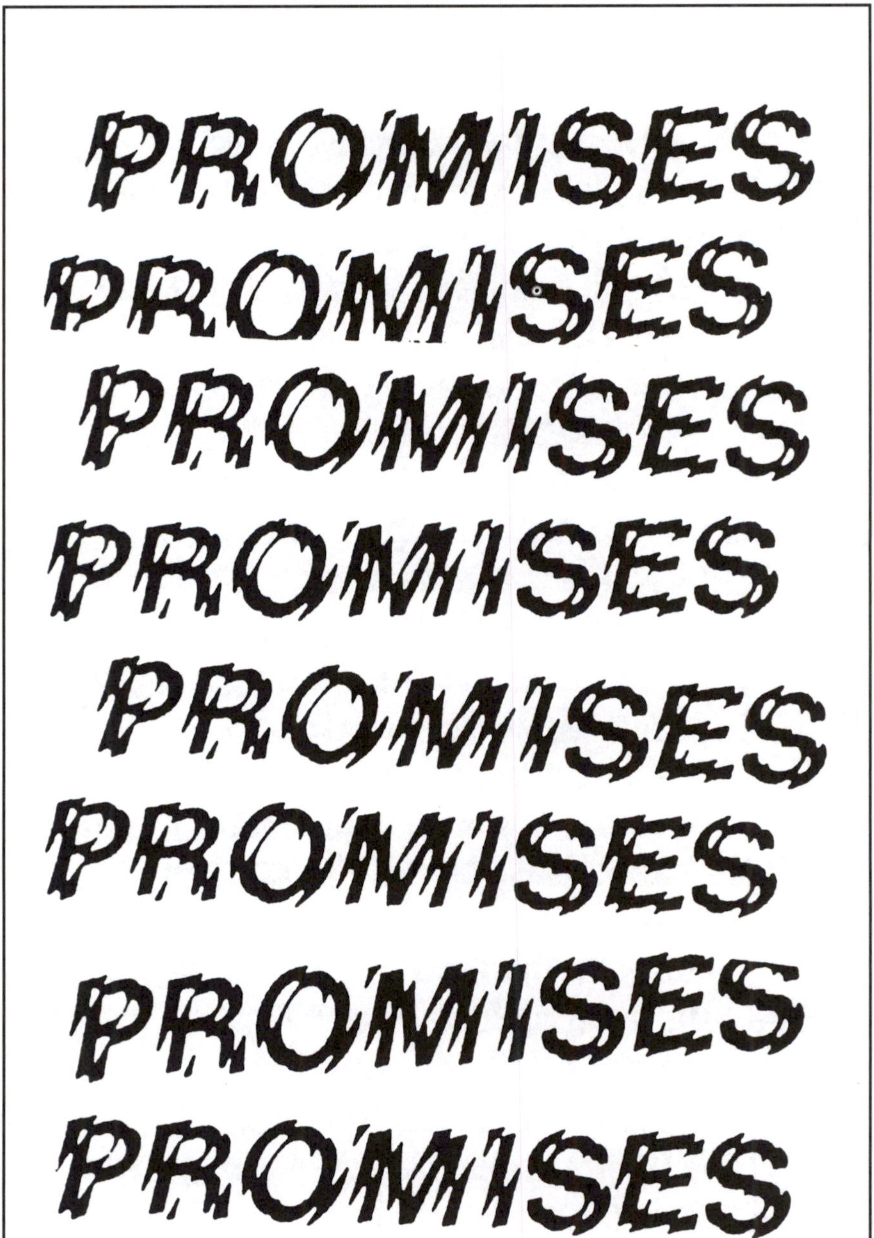

FIGURE 1.9. The shaky effect.

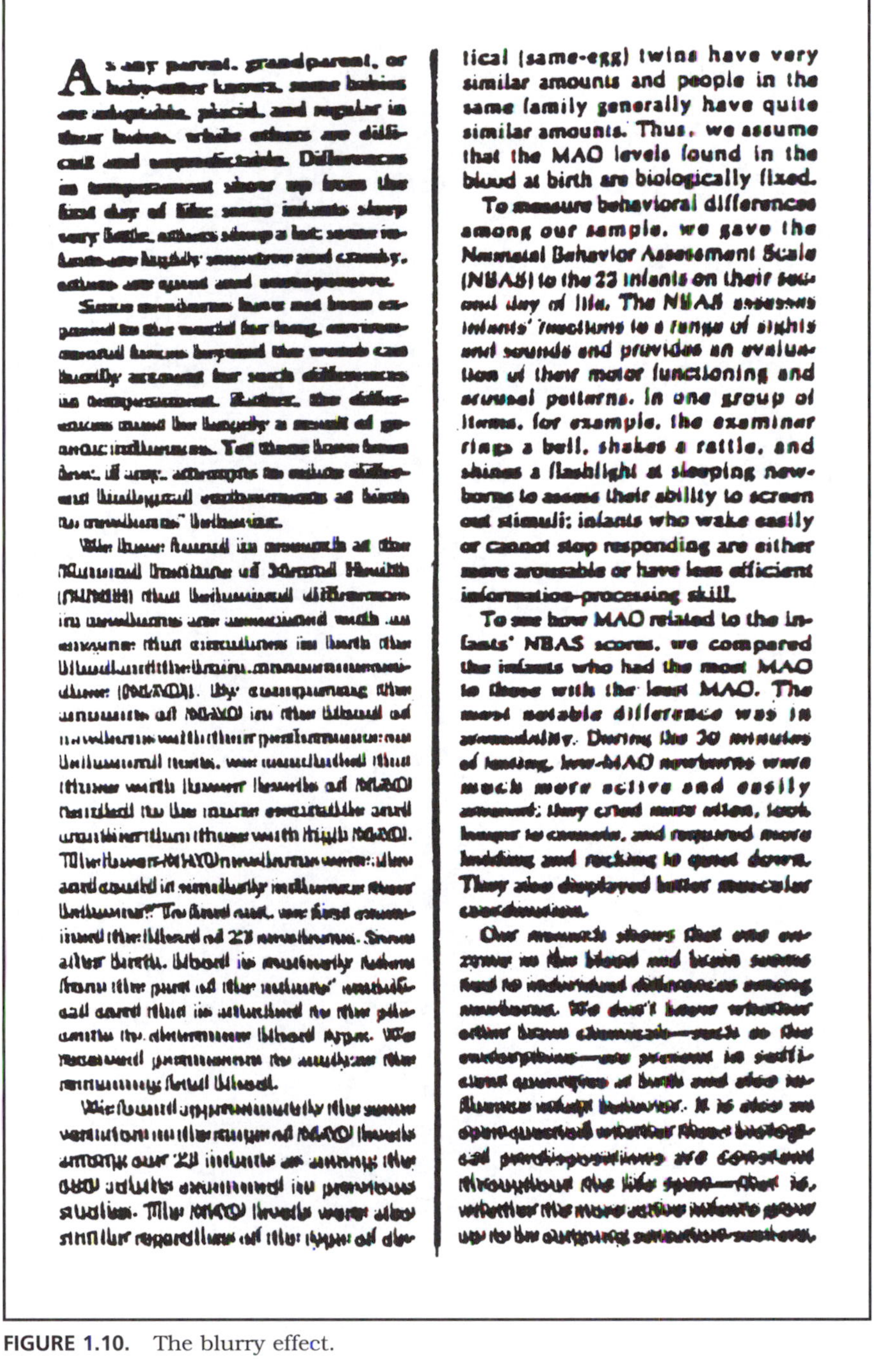

A s any parent, grandparent, or babysitter knows, some babies are adaptable, placid, and regular in their habits, while others are difficult and unpredictable. Differences in temperament show up from the first day of life: some infants sleep very little, others sleep a lot; some relax easily, some are highly sensitive and cranky...

tical (same-egg) twins have very similar amounts and people in the same family generally have quite similar amounts. Thus, we assume that the MAO levels found in the blood at birth are biologically fixed.

To measure behavioral differences among our sample, we gave the Neonatal Behavior Assessment Scale (NBAS) to the 23 infants on their second day of life. The NBAS assesses infants' reactions to a range of sights and sounds and provides an evaluation of their motor functioning and arousal patterns. In one group of items, for example, the examiner rings a bell, shakes a rattle, and shines a flashlight at sleeping newborns to assess their ability to screen out stimuli; infants who wake easily or cannot stop responding are either more arousable or have less efficient information-processing skill.

To see how MAO related to the infants' NBAS scores, we compared the infants who had the most MAO to those with the least MAO. The most notable difference was in arousability. During the 30 minutes of testing, low-MAO newborns were much more active and easily aroused; they cried more often, took longer to console, and required more holding and rocking to quiet down. They also displayed better muscular coordination.

Our research shows that one enzyme in the blood and brain seems tied to individual differences among newborns. We don't know whether other brain chemicals—such as the endorphins—are present in sufficient quantities at birth and also influence behavior. It is also an open question whether these biological predispositions are constant throughout the life span—that is, whether the more active infants grow up to be outgoing, sensation-seeking...

FIGURE 1.10. The blurry effect.

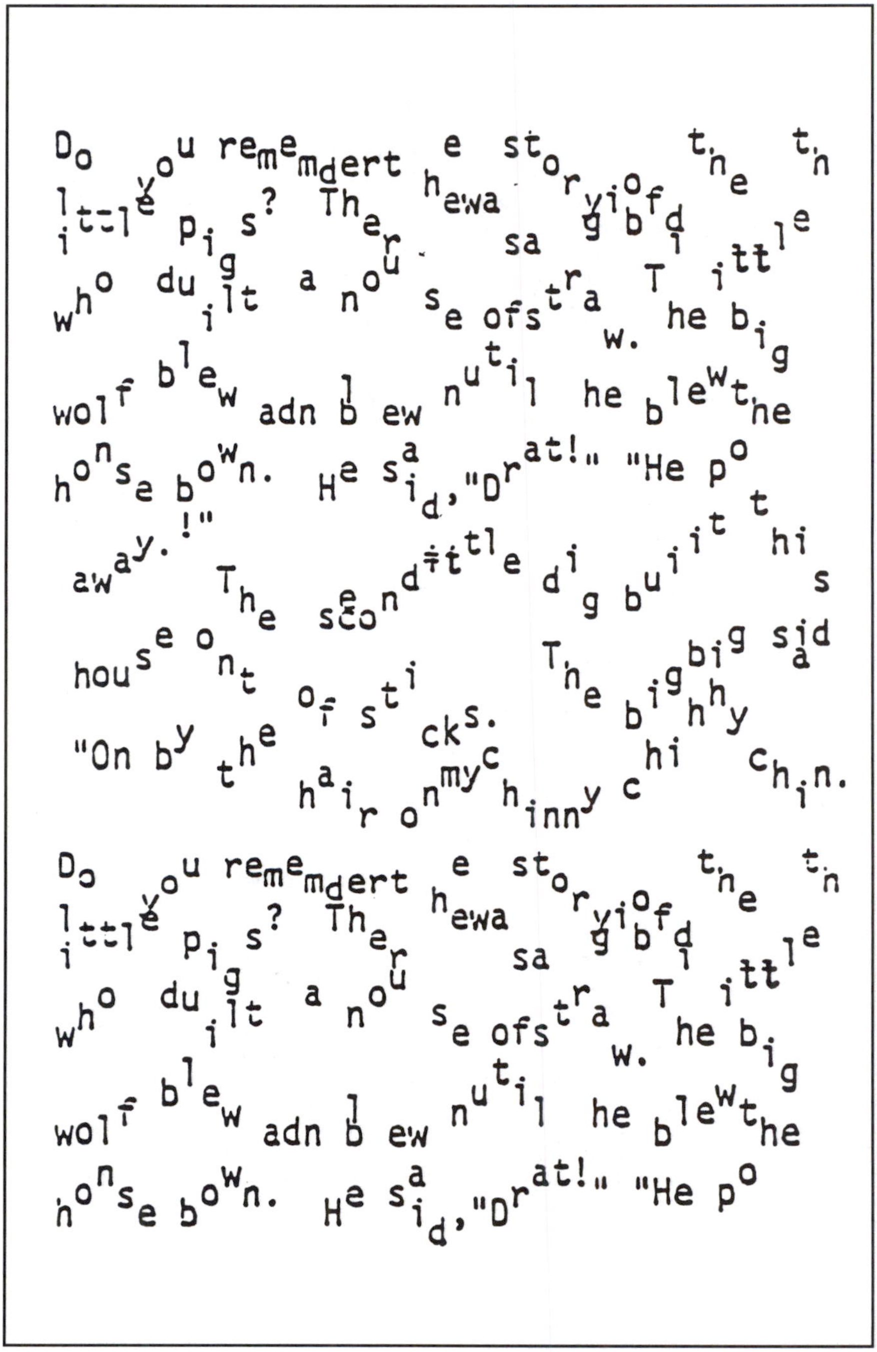

Do you remember the story of the three little pigs? There was a big little pig who built a house of straw. The big wolf blew and blew until he blew the house down. He said, "Drat!" "He po away.!" The second little pig built his house out of sticks. The big big big hhy "On by the hair on my chinny chin chin.

Do you remember the story of the three little pigs? There was a big little pig who built a house of straw. The big wolf blew and blew until he blew the house down. He said, "Drat!" "He po

FIGURE 1.11. The seesaw effect.

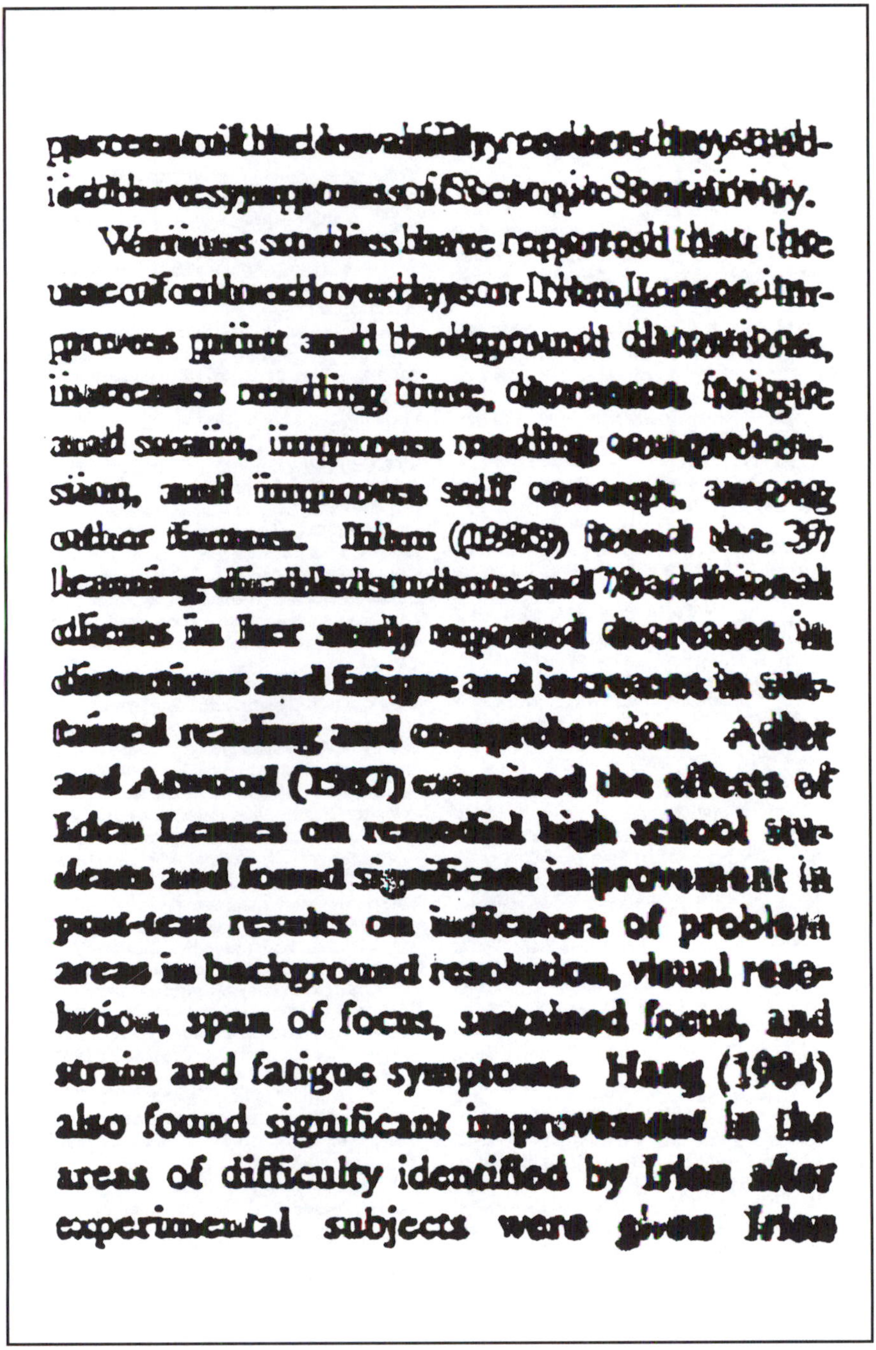

percents it had done initially, reductions in eyestrain, and it has no symptoms of Scotopic Sensitivity.

Various studies have reported that the use of colored overlays or Irlen Lenses improves print and background distortions, increases reading time, decreases fatigue and strain, improves reading comprehension, and improves self concept, among other factors. Irlen (1988) found the 39 learning-disabled students and 76 additional others in her study reported decreases in distortions and fatigue and increases in sustained reading and comprehension. Adler and Atwood (1987) examined the effects of Irlen Lenses on remedial high school students and found significant improvement in post-test results on indicators of problem areas in background resolution, visual resolution, span of focus, sustained focus, and strain and fatigue symptoms. Hang (1984) also found significant improvement in the areas of difficulty identified by Irlen after experimental subjects were given Irlen

FIGURE 1.12.   The smudged effect.

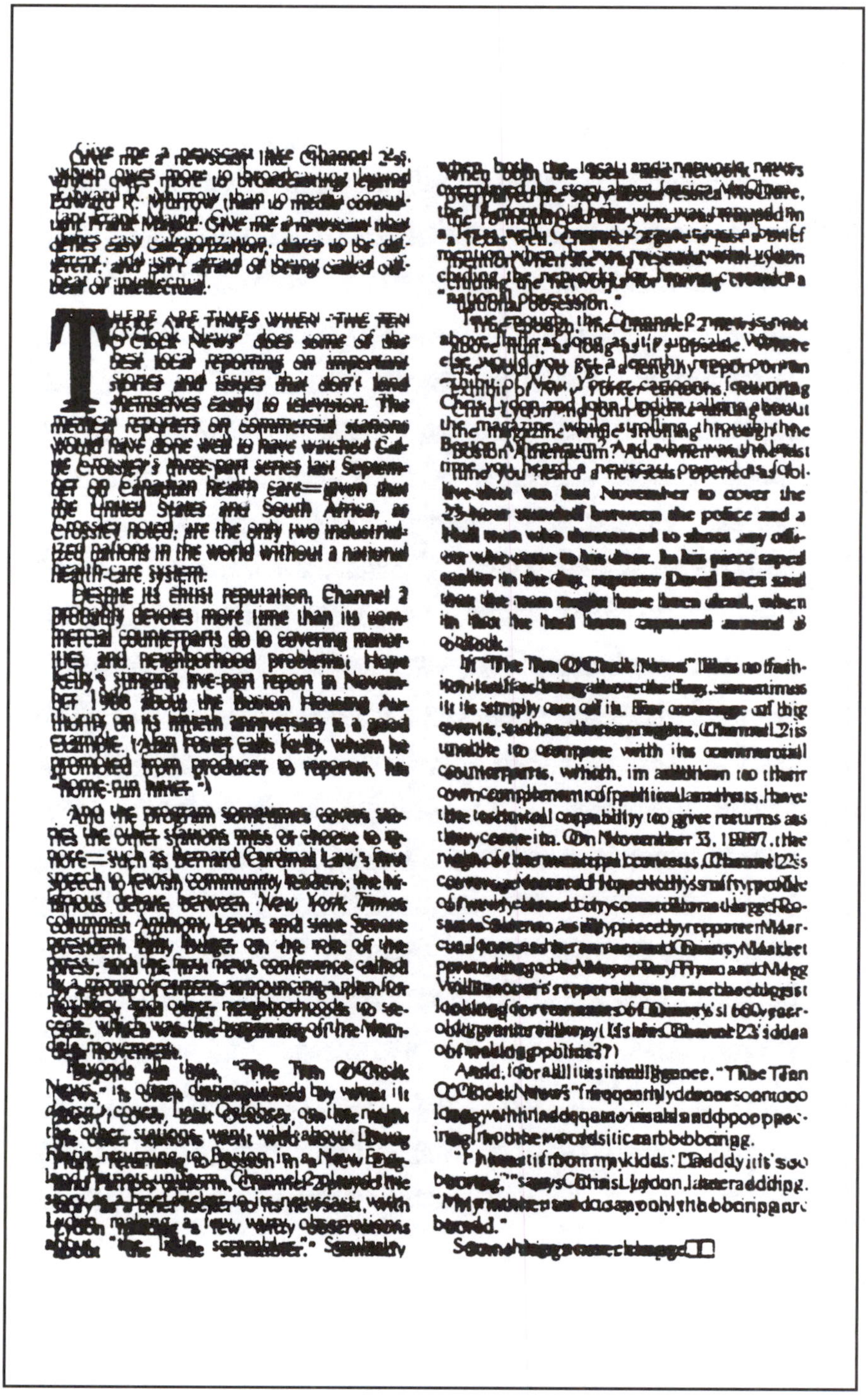

FIGURE 1.13. The overlap effect.

Irlen Syndrome in the Classroom

Instructors can identify rather easily symptoms of word blindness or Irlen syndrome by observing how students react to reading black print on white paper under bright light. The following is a list of typical symptoms:

1. Eyes begin to burn or sting.

2. Eyes start to squint to shut out bright light.

3. Eyes begin to hurt after a few minutes under bright light.

4. Student must shade the page by leaning over it.

5. Student holds a hand above the eyes to shade against the light.

6. Student wants to wear bill cap in the room to shade against overhead light.

7. Print begins to blur under bright light.

8. Letters or words run together on the page.

9. Details start to swirl or move around on the page.

10. Words merge (stack on top of each other), then separate.

11. Lines begin to merge (stack on top of each other), then separate.

12. Rivers of space run down the page, separating words into chunks that don't make sense.

13. Details begin to flicker or blink on and off.

14. Details begin to fade out, then come back.

15. Words seem to fall or slide off the edges of the page.

16. Details become three-dimensional, with some items rising up off the page while other items sink into the background of the page.

17. Print begins to pulse in and out of focus.

18. Student begins to lean down close to page, then stretch back away from the page.

19. Student begins to trombone the page, bringing it close to the face, then pushing it further away.

20. Student begins to turn body, shoulders, and head in different directions to see at different angles.

21. Headache develops—first around the eyes, then across the forehead or over one eye, and finally across the temples and down the back of the neck.

These word blind patterns often diminish or disappear when a certain color is laid on the book page (Appendix A explains how to obtain specially designed colored overlays from the Irlen Institute.) Most students who display some or several of these word blind patterns will respond significantly when the correct color is added to their reading. Persons who respond well to color overlay also will do better with print on softly colored paper.

In addition to color, it is important for students with word blindness to reduce the brightness of light where they study. Overhead lights should be turned off. Low-wattage lamps should be available to let these students work under soft, indirect light as much as possible. Each individual should be free to create his or her most comfortable lighting environment. Some learners with Irlen syndrome prefer a half-dark place for reading. Others want only the light that comes through a window. Still others prefer a low-wattage lamp behind them or off to one side. If parents, teachers, or tutors notice a student displaying the kinds of visual perception struggles mentioned in the list, they should have that student look at Figures 1.5 through 1.13 to see if reading pages ever resemble any of these distortion patterns.

As with most new techniques or strategies, the Irlen procedure has been controversial. Those individuals whose word blindness has been decreased or eliminated through color application credit Irlen's methods, but critics complain that the Irlen procedure has not yet been researched sufficiently or validated scientifically.[1]

---

[1] I have a personal interest in the Irlen procedure because all my life I have struggled with moderate word blindness. Lenses designed to correct my astigmatism and *hyperopia* (farsightedness) did not stop print from swimming and pulsing in and out of focus as I struggled to read. In 1987, I experienced the joy of being rid of word blindness when I received my Irlen filters. The colored lenses I wear have made it possible to be under overhead fluorescent lights for long periods of time without developing headache.

Causes of Word Blindness

In the early 1990s, two research teams discovered the cause of Irlen syndrome. In 1991, Margaret Livingstone and her colleagues at the Harvard Medical School found a certain type of incomplete cell structure within the magnicellular pathway that links the retina of each eye with the visual cortex (Livingstone et al., 1991). Figure 1.14 shows the magno cells (large cells) and parvo cells (small cells) that transfer visual information from the retina to the visual cortex. When the magno cells are incompletely developed, the visual cortex receives a swimming, pulsing, and blurred impression from black print on white paper, especially under bright fluorescent light. This discovery was corroborated by Stephen Lehmkule and his colleagues at the University of Missouri (Lehmkule et al., 1993). Incomplete cell development in the visual pathway between the retina and visual cortex triggers the word blind phenomenon that was first observed more than 100 years ago by European specialists.

Overlap of Behavior Patterns

Martha Denckla, a pioneer in brain imaging studies of Attention-Deficit Disorders, pointed out that only rarely is one form of LD found in a person who is a struggling learner (Denckla, 1985). Denckla's model for defining LD includes the concept of overlap (comorbidity). In most instances of a learning struggle, two or more types of LD occur, overlapping like shingles on a roof. In my personal work with three generations of struggling learners of all ages, I rarely have met a person with dyslexia who does not also display such overlapping, or comorbid, patterns as short attention span, quick distractibility, social immaturity, late development, or poor reading vision that complicate classroom performance and make it hard to build successful relationships.

DYSLEXIA

Brain-Based Talent for Reading

Denckla expressed an interesting point of view when she stated that the ability to read is a specialized neurological

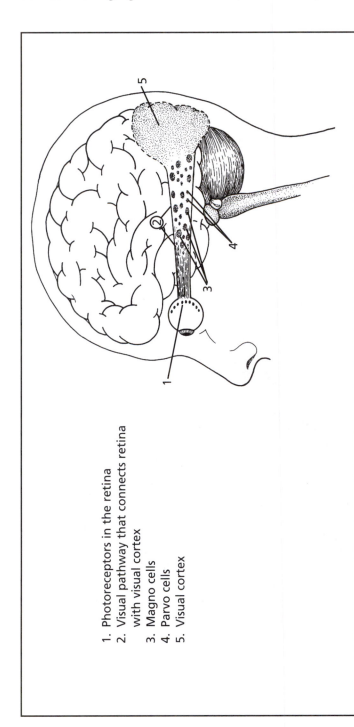

1. Photoreceptors in the retina
2. Visual pathway that connects retina with visual cortex
3. Magno cells
4. Parvo cells
5. Visual cortex

FIGURE 1.14.   Between the retina and visual cortex is a "visual highway" made of two kinds of cells that work as a team in carrying visual impressions to the back of the brain. Large cells called magno cells very rapidly transfer portions of what the eyes see to the visual cortex, where this first information waits. The small cells called parvo cells more slowly transfer the rest of the visual image. The visual cortex blends these fast and slow information chunks into complete visual images. Irlen syndrome is caused by incomplete development of the large magno cells. This deficit in cell development prevents the visual systems from processing the full light spectrum. The visual cortex receives poorly integrated images like those shown in Figures 1.5 through 1.13. By adding the correct color, the brain no longer struggles to process reflected light from book pages.

talent (Denckla, 1993). Individuals with certain types of brain formations have a specialized talent for athletics; some of us do not. Persons who have certain differences in brain structure have the talent to sing grand opera, but most of us do not. Persons with specially developed right-brain structures have the talent for painting or sculpting or doing advanced mathematics. Individuals who have fully developed left-brain language-processing regions have the neurological ability to be talented readers, but persons with differently developed language-processing regions do not. Our culture calls these nontalented readers illiterate, as well as being dyslexic or having a learning disability. Figure 1.1 shows the regions of the left brain that work together as a well-integrated team in persons who have good language-processing skills.

According to what we know about brain structure, it is valid to conclude that not everyone can become a talented reader, speller, or writer, just as not everyone can paint the Sistine Chapel or sing the role of Tosca or play baseball like Babe Ruth. Our body of knowledge about how the brain learns language-based information indicates that 85% of us have the left-brain neurological structure to develop talents in reading, spelling, and writing (Jordan, 1995; Montgomery, 1989). Approximately 15% of us do not. Unfortunately for that 15%, society places a high priority on reading, writing, and spelling; it has not yet learned to value other kinds of talent that enrich our lives and contribute enormously to our social well-being.

Research History

In 1985, Drake Duane, a neuroscientist who has devoted much of his professional life to the study of dyslexia, made a prophetic statement during a symposium at the Menninger Foundation: "Dyslexia is now the most thoroughly researched of all learning disabilities" (cited in Jordan, 1989, p. 6). Many pioneers in neurological research have documented the organic causes of this specific learning disability. As shown earlier in this chapter, European researchers in the 19th century discovered the first proof of brain-based causes for dyslexia and word blindness, and in the early 1920s Orton documented specific patterns in brain-injured adults who at one time could read, spell, and write adequately. After these adults sustained brain injury, they reversed letters, read words backwards, forgot how to spell, stumbled over basic math computation, and lost penmanship skills. Today the Orton Dyslexia Society carries on the research started half a century ago by this insightful neurologist.

In the 1960s, a remarkable neurologist at the Harvard University School of Medicine became deeply interested in the controversial issue of dyslexia. Norman Geschwind began a series of research projects designed to determine whether dyslexia in fact existed. He enlisted the help of several talented colleagues, including Walter Levitsky, Albert Galaburda, and Antonio Damasio. A series of brain autopsies using the brains of men who had been labeled dyslexic proved that certain neuronal structures are different in the brains of persons with dyslexia (Galaburda, 1983). Specific areas of the left brain where language concepts, printed symbols, and arithmetic information are processed do not develop normally. In the dyslexic brain, there are structural differences in those areas that govern the development of literacy skills. The Harvard studies also established the fact that families with several blood relatives who have dyslexia display differences in health patterns and physical characteristics. This research made it clear that dyslexia is a comprehensive syndrome involving a cluster of factors that extend far beyond difficulty with reading and spelling. Having dyslexia involves a great deal more than turning letters backwards or reading poorly.

As these facts of dyslexic brain differences became known, new brain imaging technologies were developed to identify dyslexia according to brain wave patterns. A series of studies demonstrated how specific areas of the brain respond to stimulus. During the 1980s, Sondra Jernigan at the Menninger Foundation in Topeka, Kansas, pioneered evoked potential EEG (electroencephalograph) measurements to identify certain forms of deep dyslexia (Jernigan, 1985). William Deering and Jane Flynn at LaCrosse Lutheran Hospital in Wisconsin developed a system to diagnose dyslexia through patterns in the theta band of an EEG evaluation (Deering & Flynn, 1985). Frank Wood at the Bowman Gray School of Medicine used PET (positron emission tomography) to study left-brain blood flow differences in persons with dyslexia (Wood, 1991). Using MRI (magnetic resonance imaging), Denckla identified immature structures in the cerebellum of persons with attention deficits (Denckla, 1991b). From his PET and MRI research, Alan Zametkin reported irregular glucose metabolism in the left brains of persons with attention deficits (Zametkin et al., 1990). Biochemical research at the Weizmann Institute of Science in Israel, under the direction of Veronika Grimm, determined that body chemistry is an important factor when dyslexia exists (Grimm, 1986). In the mid 1980s, researchers determined that deep dyslexia (discussed later in this chapter) is linked to chromosome 15 (Jordan, 1989a). In 1994, John DeFries at the University of Colorado reported that certain types of dyslexia are linked to chromosome 6 (DeFries, 1994). Today, dyslexia remains the most thoroughly researched of all forms of learning disability.

Family Patterns in Dyslexia

Geschwind's studies yielded a profile of the families of dyslexics (Geschwind, 1984). According to the Harvard studies, left-handedness appears in 13% of the blood relatives of persons with dyslexia, although only 3% of the general population are left-handed. Nine times more men than women have symptoms of deep dyslexia (Jordan, 1995), which will be discussed later in this chapter. The hair of blood relatives of individuals with dyslexia tends to become gray or white starting by the late teens and early 20s.

Numerous problems seem to be associated with families in which dyslexia occurs. For example, environmental allergies (dust, pollen, animal fur) and food allergies (milk, spices, caffeine, salicylic foods) are prevalent. A major family pattern is the tendency for lifelong gastrointestinal problems and digestive sensitivity, such as chronic ache in the lower GI tract, excessive flatulence, and intolerance of milk. These individuals live with chronic sour stomach and lower intestinal discomfort after meals. Families of persons with dyslexia often have a high rate of Crohn's disease (polyps in the small intestine) and a higher than normal level of autoimmune disorders in which the body attacks itself. Female relatives frequently develop lupus. Most individuals with dyslexia and their blood relatives have arthritis along with fibromyalgia that torments the large muscle systems.

The research of Gad Geiger and Jerome Lettvin (1987) at the Massachusetts Institute of Technology added irregular central vision to this profile of individuals and families with deep dyslexia. They discovered off-center foveal vision in many persons with deep dyslexia. In other words, these individuals cannot continue to see clearly by looking straight ahead because the fovia in the retina of each eye is slightly off center. As a result, looking straight ahead triggers blurred visual images. These persons must compensate by quickly glancing from different angles with their peripheral vision.

Definition of Dyslexia

It is currently known beyond doubt that dyslexia is linked to physical patterns within the person's brain as well as to the body chemistry and genetic traits of certain families. Dyslexia is not caused by poor teaching, poor parenting, or lack of cultural opportunity. It has no ethnic or economic preferences and is seen in all cultures where literacy skills are important. Dyslexia is a complex condition. In spite of this vast body of knowledge, popular opinion often holds that dyslexia merely means that a person reverses *b* and *d* and reads words backward (*saw* for *was*). This overly simple understanding of what is actually a complex disorder is misleading. Like any other human condition, there is nothing simple about dyslexia, which occurs in a variety of ways on many levels of severity. Some individuals with dyslexia do reverse letters, numbers, and words, but many do not.

There is no universally accepted definition of this condition; each group with a vested interest in this problem adheres to its own. Based upon my 40 years of one-to-one experience with the dyslexic population, I have developed the following definition:

> Dyslexia is the inability of an intelligent person to become fluent in the basic skills of reading, spelling, and handwriting in spite of prolonged teaching and tutoring. Math computation may also remain at the level of struggle. Dyslexia means that the person will always struggle to some degree with reading printed passages, writing with a pen or pencil, spelling accurately from memory, and developing sentences and paragraphs with correct grammar and punctuation. Dyslexia may also include difficulty telling information orally as well as listening to oral information accurately. No matter how hard the person tries, certain types of errors continue to appear in reading, writing, and spelling. Dyslexia is a brain-based dysfunction that is often genetic. It tends to run in families. Through certain kinds of remedial training, dyslexic patterns can be partly overcome or reduced, but dyslexia cannot be completely eliminated. It is a lifelong, brain-based condition for which individuals with dyslexia can learn successfully to compensate.

Levels of Dyslexia

It is important that a certain point of view be maintained when considering dyslexia. No two persons with dyslexia display exactly the same patterns, and not all these persons show the same level of severity. The cluster of dyslexic patterns must be seen along a continuum from mild to severe. Many persons who are dyslexic show only mild or moderate problems, whereas others are severely disabled. Dyslexia should be seen along the following continuum:

0	1	2	3	4	5	6	7	8	9	10
none		mild			moderate			severe		total

Most adults would show a few dyslexic-like "blips" in their literacy and mathematics skills. In one sense, it would be correct to say that each of us is dyslexic at Levels 1 or 2.

Few persons have perfect literacy skills without some area of deficit. This poses no problem so long as the specific blips do not create costly mistakes on the job. Adults typically choose professions or occupations that permit them to bypass whatever minor deficits exist in spelling, rapid recall of details, rapid mathematics processing, and so forth.

Dyslexia becomes an educational problem when it begins to interfere with classroom performance and academic success. Moderate dyslexia at Level 4 or 5 means continual mistakes in spelling, punctuation, and capital letters; grammar errors; problems with reading comprehension; and many small errors in math computation. A student with moderate dyslexia struggles with every written assignment, but he or she can finally do good work by trying hard enough and rewriting papers several times. With enough effort, persons who have Level 4 or 5 dyslexia can make top grades and be listed on the honor roll; however, they must maintain a high level of self-discipline.

When dyslexia is at Level 6 or Level 7, a major struggle occurs in all areas of academic performance. Spelling is always faulty, and textbook reading is slow and difficult. Much more time than usual is required to finish homework assignments, and a very high level of personal frustration is experienced. Persons at Levels 6 and 7 reach burnout before they can finish assignments. They must continually deal with a sense of failure and discouragement. Occasionally they earn top grades, but they usually show only average or below average performance on grade reports. It is seldom possible for a student with Level 6 or 7 dyslexia to make the school's honor roll or to win praise for academic achievement. It is possible for such a student to finish a college degree, but it requires great effort and courage to do so.

When dyslexia is severe (Level 8 or 9), academic achievement often is impossible unless instructors modify the curriculum. Occasionally the teacher will encounter a Level 10 student whose disability is so severe that academic learning is impossible (*alexia*). A person at Level 8 or 9 remains several years below grade level in skill achievement. Spelling skills remain at a primitive level, reading is a massive struggle, and handwriting is poor and messy. It requires two to three times longer than normal for a person at Level 8 or 9 to finish assignments, and he or she must have continual help to do so. It is virtually impossible for these learners to attain independent study skills. They must have continual tutoring and coaching to prepare for tests, do assignments, master new assignments, and fill in gaps in their skills and knowledge.

If these students are taught to do their writing through a word processor, they can bypass enough problems to turn out good work through the keyboard. In her research that taught students with severe dyslexia to write through word processors, Joyce Steeves developed a model for predicting success through keyboard writing. The students who became skilled at keyboard writing produced 15 times more acceptable written work than they could through handwriting (Steeves, 1987).

With a hand calculator, most learners with dyslexia can do good math. However, it is impossible for learners at the severely dyslexic levels to function academically through the traditional modes of silent reading, production of handwritten papers, and preparation of large quantities of work day after day. Individuals with Level 8 or 9 dyslexia suffer continually from the self-perception that they are "dumb." They rarely win praise for academic work, and they have no good stories to tell about classroom achievement. Unless they excel in athletics or art, these students languish through their school years with intense feelings of failure and low self-worth. Most persons with severe dyslexia drop out without finishing high school. U.S. prison systems are filled with men and women who have severe dyslexia (Jordan, 1995). They could not develop productive literacy or workplace skills, nor could they fit into a society that places top value on the specialized talents of good reading, accurate spelling, rapid math calculation, and fluent writing.

Forms of Dyslexia

Most of the professional controversy about dyslexia is caused by misunderstanding as to which form of this disability one is referring. There are three general forms of dyslexia: acquired, deep, and developmental. It is critically important that these different forms of dyslexia are recognized. If only one form is acknowledged, then it becomes impossible for professionals to discuss the issue effectively.

Acquired Dyslexia

Acquired dyslexia is directly related to brain damage or trauma to specific brain structures. Certain areas of the brain can be irreversibly damaged through experiences that destroy brain tissue, such as a drug overdose, loss of oxygen over a period of time, stroke, debilitating disease that produces senility (such as Alzheimer's), industrial or automobile accidents, athletic accidents, neurological damage at birth, or damage to the developing brain systems in the fetus. These kinds of trauma can produce a dyslexia syndrome (reversal of symbols, loss of phonics, inability to keep details in sequence, inability to connect sounds to letters, loss of reading comprehension, inability to spell).

This form of dyslexia applies only to a small segment of the U.S. population (less than 1%). If this brain-damage model of dyslexia is the only one considered, then there is no explanation for the millions of other individuals with dyslexia who exist within the population but who show no signs of brain damage. A great deal of confusion is generated when the brain-damage model of dyslexia is the only point of reference, because this definition was never intended to address all problems faced by parents and classroom teachers who deal with students with dyslexia.

Deep Dyslexia

A second form of dyslexia runs in families. This is called *deep dyslexia,* or *primary dyslexia,* because the symptoms are so deep-seated they cannot be changed beyond a very limited point. Deep dyslexia is linked to chromosomes 6 and 15 in the genetic chain. It appears nine times more often in men than in women, and from 3% to 5% of the general population have it. The Harvard studies of dyslexic brains found that specific areas of the left cerebral cortex were different from those same areas in nondyslexic brains (Galaburda, 1983; Geschwind, 1984). The term deep dyslexia (or primary dyslexia) refers to deep-seated, lifelong trouble with reading comprehension; sounding out of words; spelling; writing legibly; learning to do arithmetic from memory; pronouncing words without tongue twisting; and creating written material with correct grammar, punctuation, and sentence structure. Deep dyslexia does not improve with age or physical maturity. At age 50 those who have primary dyslexia still struggle to read below 4th-grade level, and spelling from memory is impossible to achieve. This form of dyslexia is seen in other blood relatives, usually males. It can skip a generation if passed along by the mother. A grandfather and his male relatives can be dyslexic but his daughter may not show significant signs. Her son (the third generation) can have severe dyslexia and pass the pattern on down the family line. Relatives of individuals with deep dyslexia have much higher levels of allergies than normal and more digestive problems (duodenal ulcers, colitis, Crohn's disease). Their hair also tends to turn gray or white at an early age. A high percentage of those relatives are left-handed. Yet, persons who have deep dyslexia are above average in intelligence (Jordan, 1995; Pollan & Williams, 1992; Rawson, 1988; Weisel, 1991), which allows them to overcome their disability-related problems in remarkable ways, as shall be shown in Chapter 7.

Developmental Dyslexia

The third form of dyslexia also has two names: *developmental dyslexia* or *secondary dyslexia*. This form also may run in families, although it can appear when no other relatives have the symptoms. Developmental dyslexia is seen in 12% to 15% of the general population, and appears five times more often in males than in females. Research by Geschwind and his colleagues and by Grimm (cited by Jordan, 1989a) indicates that this form of dyslexia is caused early in the development of the fetus. Toward the end of the first trimester of fetal development, the tiny cells that later become the genitals produce a surge of the male hormone testosterone. This occurs long before the baby is physically either male or female. At this stage of fetal development, the brain still has not taken shape. Groups of cells that later become the right-brain and left-brain hemispheres are migrating upward toward the developing head of the fetus. The surge of testosterone temporarily slows down development of the left-brain cells, although the right-brain cells continue to develop on schedule. Figure 1.2 shows the 4-step developmental sequence all nerve cells must take to do their tasks successfully. Developmental dyslexia begins when the testosterone surge slows down this 4-step process in the early stages of fetal development. The left-brain hemisphere catches up later. In fact, in persons with dyslexia, the left-brain hemisphere is the same size as the right-brain hemisphere. In nondyslexic brains, the right-brain hemisphere is somewhat larger.

The result of this developmental imbalance is developmental dyslexia because the language-processing centers of the left-brain hemisphere are late in developing. In this form of dyslexia, the struggle to learn gradually decreases as the child goes through puberty, because the onset of puberty triggers neuronal "catch up." The hormones that bring about body changes during puberty finish "filling in" the language centers of the left brain of students with developmental dyslexia.

As this late maturity of brain tissue takes place, the level of dyslexia drops. Most children with secondary dyslexia begin to break through their learning problems by about age 12, as hormone production gets under way. By age 14, they are usually significantly better able to handle school learning, and by age 16, their academic skills are noticeably better, with math, reading comprehension, and language skills showing much improvement. During their early 20s, these students demonstrate remarkable gains in learning ability, compared with their struggle during the elementary and middle school years. Most individuals with developmental dyslexia are able to do well in college if self-esteem has not been too badly damaged during their early struggles in school.

A Continuum of Dyslexic Symptoms

As noted earlier, dyslexia occurs along a continuum, not on a single level of difficulty. The syndrome ranges widely in complexity from student to student. On the scale of 0 to 10, individuals with deep dyslexia are stuck at the severe level (8, 9, or 10). Their ability to master basic literacy skills is very meager. The struggle to acquire the skills of reading, spelling, and writing soon hits a brick wall, and the skills cannot be developed beyond a certain limited point. Developmental dyslexia falls in the moderate range (4 through 7). Learners with developmental dyslexia have considerable potential to achieve literacy. If a student with secondary dyslexia is identified at Level 7 during the elementary school years, he or she will usually have improved to Level 5 by age 16, and dyslexic symptoms usually will have moved down to Level 4 by age 21. Developmental dyslexia involves progressively less difficulty in learning as the central nervous system finishes maturing during adolescence. As the severity of the syndrome decreases during puberty, academic performance rises, if appropriate remedial training is provided throughout childhood and early adolescence.

How Many Have Dyslexia?

Continual controversy exists as to determining how many individuals with LD or dyslexia there are in the United States. Estimates range from very few to as much as 20% of the population. A consensus has developed among researchers who specialize in dyslexia: They believe that 12% to 15% of the overall population show significant signs of spelling, writing, reading, and math problems attributable to some form of dyslexia (Jordan, 1995; Kidder, 1991; Payne, 1994; Pollan & Williams, 1992; Rawson, 1988; Weisel, 1992). This does not mean that 12 or 15 people out of every 100 are clinically defined as having dyslexia. As Denckla described, much overlapping of problems occurs. It is rare to find a struggling student who manifests only one form of a learning disability. This was well illustrated by Alston and

Taylor, who obtained dyslexic-like handwriting samples of children who were diagnosed as having spina bifida, petit mal epilepsy, spastic quadriplegia, ataxia, cerebellar lesion, Duchenne muscular dystrophy, and osteogenesis imperfecta (Alston & Taylor, 1987). In each of these samples, difficulty with handwriting and poor spelling are seen, which would fit the patterns for individuals with dyslexia.

The difficulty in assigning percentage figures to the prevalence of any form of learning disability lies in not recognizing these overlapping conditions. I have seldom seen a student with dyslexia who was brain injured according to an EEG, CAT, or MRI brain scan. However, I have worked with many brain-injured persons who had dyslexic-like literacy problems.

Characteristics of Dyslexia

Individuals who have dyslexia do not automatically master language symbols, nor do they automatically perceive left to right and top to bottom. Some cannot handle the encoding processes involved in translating oral language into written symbols. These persons cannot transfer what they hear into an accurate written code. Others have difficulty decoding printed symbols into oral language. That is, they do not have the talent to translate what they see in print into a mental voice. Still others cannot express themselves in writing because they cannot remember how to make specific letters correctly. These students cannot control the direction of written symbols. These forms of learning disability are complicated by the tendency to interpret symbols backwards, upside down, and in scrambled sequence.

The major difficulty in the classroom, however, is that few students are handicapped by only one form of dyslexia. Two or more types of this perceptual loss usually exist in a person who has dyslexia, making it all the more difficult for the disability to be corrected. In fact, severe cases of dyslexia (Levels 8, 9, and 10) require special clinical treatment that a mainstream classroom cannot provide adequately. It is essential that teachers know how to screen their pupils in order to make necessary referrals for those who need specialized help. Students with moderate dyslexia (Levels 4 through 7) have enough potential talent for literacy to be taught successfully within the mainstream classroom structure, if teachers make certain adjustments in assignments and learning procedures.

Subtypes of Dyslexia

Visual Dyslexia

The most obvious form of dyslexic handicap is that of visual dyslexia. Visual dyslexia is not caused by poor vision; it is a matter of the brain's visual cortex not interpreting accurately what is seen. Figure 1.1 shows the regions of the left brain where reading occurs. The visual cortex, the part of the left brain where printed symbols are interpreted, has the task of learning the correct *direction* of each symbol. It must be able to recognize symbols instantly, compare them rapidly, and quickly place them in correct sequence. As shall be shown in Chapter 2, the left visual cortex of approximately 15% of the human population does not have the natural talent to do this symbol processing fluently.

Word blindness. Word blindness seldom is identified during typical vision examinations (Geiger & Lettvin, 1987; Irlen, 1991; Jordan, 1995; Lehmkule et al., 1993; Livingstone et al., 1991; Payne, 1993; Pollan & Williams, 1992; Weisel, 1992). Tutors and remedial teachers have long contended that learners with dyslexia have a different way of seeing as they read. However, this point of view is strongly disputed by ophthalmologists and many optometrists because the standard techniques used in vision examination do not identify this irregular visual perception pattern. Figures 1.5 and 1.13 show the kinds of visual perception distortions that can occur because of word blindness. This visual perception anomaly is a constant barrier when students with dyslexia attempt to develop their literacy skills. We do not yet know how many persons have word blindness, but Irlen estimated that 35% of the human population worldwide have this deficit (Irlen, personal communication, June 21, 1995). My personal experience during two decades of private clinical practice has led me to conclude that 65% of those with deep dyslexia are handicapped to some degree by word blindness. I estimate that no more than 20% of those with developmental dyslexia display Irlen Syndrome symptoms. As further research is conducted, we will arrive at a more precise understanding of how prevalent word blindness actually is within the LD population.

Reversing and scrambling details. Most persons with visual dyslexia see certain letters and math numerals backwards or upside down. Reading whole words in sentences is a jumbled process for such an individual. Not only do these readers perceive individual letters incorrectly, they also see parts of words backwards. When these idiosyncracies of dyslexia are at work, the reading experience is disorganized, meaningless, and usually frustrating. Consequently, individuals with visual dyslexia do everything possible to avoid reading. For example, Pete, who has visual dyslexia, is asked to read the following paragraph silently:

> Down the cold, dark stairs crept the man in the black coat. Closer he came, closer and closer. Asleep in their blankets, Dan and Bud were unaware of their danger.

Because of reversals, sequence scrambling, and failure to pick up details the first time Pete reads the paragraph, his perception of it is as follows:

> Now the could, back stars keep the man in the dalk coat. Colser he come, colser and colser sheeping the dantes anD and duB wore nuraw for the bang.

In order to do this reading, Pete touches the words with his finger and whispers each word to himself. The teacher, who is unaware of the nature of Pete's reading disability, has made an issue of his marking with fingers and whispering to himself. The teacher says "Shhhhhh!" when Pete whispers as he reads. His instructor does not realize that by cutting off Pete's speaking and listening channels, she has made it impossible for him to check his visual impressions against what he hears. The result is complete nonsense for Pete. He flunks still another silent reading comprehension quiz because of dyslexic scrambling of what he sees on the page. Had Pete been encouraged to touch the words while whispering them over and over, thus checking them against his listening vocabulary, he could have worked out the meaning of the passage at his usual very slow pace.

Slow visual processing. This kind of scrambled visual perception forces persons with visual dyslexia to work very slowly. Excessive slowness in visual decoding is a factor that is seldom understood by teachers and parents. If most students in Pete's class can digest an assigned reading passage in 3 minutes, it may take him as long as 15 minutes to work out the meaning. Persons with visual dyslexia cannot work rapidly. When they are placed with impatient instructors or tutors who do not understand their need to go slowly while whispering and touching, students like Pete have no way of coping with their assigned reading tasks.

Dyscalculia. Because learners with visual dyslexia have such a constant problem handling information in sequence, they usually have trouble with basic arithmetic. Learning to add, subtract, multiply, and divide involves frequent changes in direction that are opposite from the left-to-right, top-to-bottom orientation stressed in reading and writing. To add, Pete must start at the right side of the problem and work downward, then carry left from bottom to top over to the next column. In simple first-grade work, this orientation is not difficult. However, as more complex addition problems are introduced, Pete becomes confused by this new directionality that is backwards from the direction for reading and writing. To subtract or multiply, Pete must start at the bottom right and think upward. This is exactly opposite from the left-to-right, top-to-bottom orientation for other paper-and-pencil work during the school day. In subtracting and multiplying he must work bottom to top, right to left. Long division involves a complex pattern of beginning left to right, then top to bottom, then bottom to top and right to left, then back to left to right again. If reading this description makes your head swim, you can imagine the confusion Pete faces when he is under pressure to hurry through arithmetic computation. He constantly loses direction and is forced to start over. When he is not given enough time to correct his directionality, he becomes enormously frustrated and confused.

Dyscalculia creates the same confusion with arithmetic symbols that visual dyslexia creates with reading symbols. Dyscalculia is usually a lifelong pattern in persons who have deep dyslexia. Individuals with developmental dyslexia usually become less confused and more successful with mathematics and arithmetic as they move down the severity scale during adolescence.

Poor comprehension of sequence. Persons with visual dyslexia are generally handicapped in any situation that requires them to comprehend sequence. Students like Pete cannot remember the order of the alphabet; months of the year; days of the week; multiplication tables; or even the day, month, and year of their birth. All his life, Pete's parents and teachers have complained about his habit of forgetting to do chores or carry out a set of instructions. The problem is seldom one of laziness or rebellion—Pete simply does not build mental images of things in sequence. His comprehension of household duties and classroom tasks is as scrambled as his perception of printed symbols. Unfortunately, most individuals like Pete are regarded as being irresponsible. In reality, they are confused.

Overcoming visual dyslexia. Of the three forms of dyslexia commonly found in classrooms, visual dyslexia is the most easily corrected. Students such as Pete usually can identify the separate sounds of speech. They usually can learn phonics if it is taught slowly, with plenty of time for review and practice. The major handicap of visual dyslexia is the inability to build mental images of printed symbols in correct sequence or position. Through appropriate drills, Pete can learn to interpret printed symbols accurately, although he will remain a slow reader all of his life. It is critical for instructors to determine if individuals like Pete have word blind tendencies when they look at black print on white paper under bright light.

Pete gradually can learn to identify sequence in his environment, thus reducing his conflict with what adults expect. His greatest enemies will always be pressure to work more rapidly and pressure to produce quantities of written work. If he is given proper allowances for his limitations, Pete can become a strong student. With the right accommodations, he can even achieve advanced scholastic standing. Many adults have gained remarkable success in spite of having visual dyslexia.

Auditory Dyslexia

Tone deafness. The most difficult form of dyslexia to correct is the inability to hear the separate sounds of spoken language. Auditory dyslexia has little to do with hearing ability —most auditory dyslexics have normal hearing. The basic handicap is like being tone deaf to music. In 1993 Paula Tallal, a neurobiologist at Rutgers University, discovered the missing link in the auditory pathways that makes it impossible for certain persons to hear the soft speech sounds that are critical in learning phonics (Tallal, Miller, & Fitch, 1993). Figure 1.15 is a diagram of the neurological pathway that transfers what the ears hear to the auditory cortex, where the brain interprets that oral information. Tallal's research found pairs of specialized nerve cells between the medial geniculate nucleus and the auditory cortex. When these cells are fully developed, they fluently recognize the sequence of the hard and soft speech sounds that make up spoken language. When these cells are incomplete, the person does not hear the soft vowels and softer consonants.

Auditory dyslexia means that the person cannot hear the chain of hard–soft–hard sounds that make up the way we say and spell words in the English language. For example, the word *cat* is formed by hard /k/–soft /a/–hard /t/. A person with auditory dyslexia has no difficulty hearing the first chunk: hard /k/. But the second sound (soft /a/) does not register. This struggling learner may hear the final chunk (hard /t/). Tallal discovered that when the specialized cells along the auditory pathway are incompletely developed, the

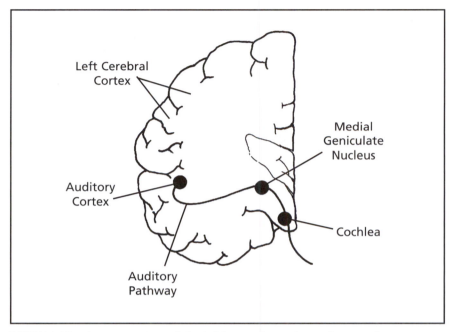

FIGURE 1.15.   A cross-section of the left brain shows the auditory pathway between the ears and the auditory cortex where sound is interpreted. Tallal, Miller, and Fitch (1993) have shown that two types of cells transfer sound patterns from the cochlea (inner ear) through the medial geniculate nucleus to the auditory cortex. Some of these cells send chunks of sound rapidly. Other cells send sound particles more slowly. The auditory cortex assembles these fast and slow particles into complete auditory images. When the fast processing cells are underdeveloped, the person fails to hear all of the fast and slow particle patterns. This produces a "tone deaf" handicap called auditory dyslexia.

listener with dyslexia hears only bits and pieces of oral language, not whole word units.

Poor spelling and word sounding. Because persons with auditory dyslexia cannot distinguish differences between soft vowel and consonant sounds, they cannot connect speech sounds to printed letters. Consequently, these students are very poor at spelling and writing. Traditional phonics instruction is almost meaningless to most persons with auditory dyslexia because they simply cannot hear the variations of softer speech sounds. The rules of phonics and spelling thus do not make sense. These individuals do not hear middle parts of words or soft word endings. As a rule, they fail to hear one third or more of what is said.

For example, Maria displays the problem of tone deafness. The seriousness of her problem is seen most clearly when she must write without help from others. Without being aware of Maria's auditory perception limitations, her teacher has chosen to give a dictation test. Speaking clearly and slowly, the teacher says, "What kind of celebration did the Pilgrims have to show their thankfulness to God?" Maria's task is to encode this sentence with no help from anyone else. As usual, her teacher becomes annoyed when Maria asks for the fifth time that the sentence be repeated. This need for repetition is characteristic of individuals with auditory dyslexia because they never are sure that they have heard correctly. As she struggles to write the sentence, Maria is acutely aware of her teacher's impatient frown. Under these conditions, the best she can do is "What cid selbarshun did the Plegms hev two sho ther takfulnis." At her very best writing speed, Maria requires from 3 to 5 minutes to encode a dictated sentence. Before she can finish one dictated item, her teacher moves on to the next. As usual, Maria completes only 2 or 3 of the 10 dictated sentences. She has met failure again—something she has come to expect.

Poor test taking. Learners like Maria are at a serious disadvantage in standardized testing. The most widely used intelligence tests for certifying that struggling learners need special help are the various Wechsler Intelligence Scales and the *Stanford–Binet Intelligence Scale.* These tests involve careful listening, accurate interpretation of what is heard, quick understanding, then good oral explanation of information requested by the examiner. Individuals with auditory dyslexia seldom score well on these verbal tests, rarely comprehending more than 60% to 70% of what they hear the first time. They also tend to miss one third or more of what is said. If the examiner who administers a standardized test does not repeat instructions or fails to make sure the listener has heard every word fully, these tone deaf listeners are forced to guess, say nothing, or panic, depending upon each person's disposition.

It is incredibly embarrassing to have auditory dyslexia because only part of what the person hears makes sense. Maria almost never gets the point of oral situations as quickly as her peers. She sits isolated inside invisible walls, feeling "dumb." Many individuals with auditory dyslexia develop cover-up behaviors that greatly irritate adults who do not understand the reason why the person acts silly or gives strange or irrelevant responses to oral statements.

Other problems. Persons with auditory dyslexia also have difficulty naming rhyming words, interpreting diacritical markings, applying phonics rules, and pronouncing words accurately. For example, because she does not hear differences between similar vowel sounds, Maria cannot tell the difference between *big* and *beg,* unless she hears the words used in context. She confuses words such as *idea* and *ideal.* She does not know that you put coffee in a *thermos*—she thinks that her dad carries coffee in a *furnace.* Yet, he also lights the furnace when the weather is cold. Children like Maria grow up with hundreds of word misperceptions because they cannot hear the subtle differences in soft speech sound patterns.

One of the earmarks of auditory dyslexia is garbled pronunciation of familiar words. For example, Maria is asked to read aloud the following passage from her science book:

> To test for acidity, place 1 teaspoon of bicarbonate of soda in a beaker. Measure one-fourth cup of vinegar, then pour slowly over the soda. Be sure not to use an aluminum cup.

Because she does not process letter–sound connections accurately, Maria reads aloud:

> To test for a-kye-da-ty, place 1 tee-poon of bi-kair-nate of soda in a braker. May-zer one-for cup vigener, the pore slow over the soda. Be sure not to use alunumum cup.

This tendency toward garbled speech is called *echolalia,* a tongue-twisting speech that constantly is embarrassing to children like Maria. She does not understand why others laugh at her tongue twisters.

Memory strategies. It is extremely difficult to correct the patterns of auditory dyslexia because the person is cut off from hearing the letter–sound connections that constitute literacy. It is possible to devise drills and exercises for students like Maria, but this remedial work requires enormous patience on the part of both teacher and student. As a rule, those who have auditory dyslexia must devise their own sight-memory systems for coping with spelling and writing.

Many intelligent persons with dyslexia have mastered common spelling patterns through *mnemonic* (memory) techniques. For example, Maria has learned to spell *then* and *when* correctly by reciting to herself: "Then is *hen* with *t* in front; when is *hen* with *w* in front." Generally, the most effective teaching procedure for auditory dyslexia is use of word families that are built upon the same internal spelling patterns:

−at	*−ate*	*−ub*	*−ube*	*−it*	*−ite*
rat	rate	cub	cube	sit	site
hat	hate	tub	tube	bit	bite

When similar patterns are studied together, Maria can memorize enough of them to satisfy ordinary writing requirements. However, she always will struggle hard with spelling from memory.

Dysgraphia

A third type of dyslexia, known as dysgraphia, is the inability to coordinate hand and finger muscles to write legibly. Figure 1.1 shows the fine-motor control region (motor programming area) of the left brain, where handwriting control signals originate. When nerve pathways within this fine-motor coordination center are immature or incomplete, the writing fingers receive incomplete signals. The writer cannot make the pencil or pen reproduce the many small strokes, turns, and repeat motions that are required for clear penmanship. Figure 1.16 is an example of dysgraphic penmanship that was done by an intelligent student who had remarkably fluent oral language skills. Many bright students with dyslexia have been seriously misjudged because their teachers could not read their handwriting. The writing of individuals with extreme dysgraphia actually resembles "bird scratching," with few recognizable letters or words. Often

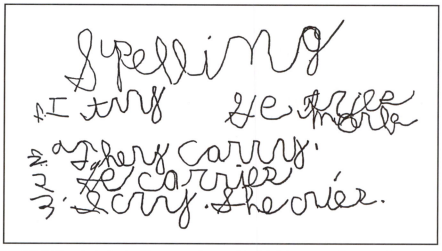

FIGURE 1.16. A student with severe dysgraphia tried to use spelling words in sentences. In numbering the lines, he kept losing the sequence as his pencil inadvertently made backward strokes. He could not fit his pencil strokes between the lines of his work page. He attempted to write:
1. I try. He tries more.
2. They carry.
2. He carries.
3. I cry. She cries.

these struggling students fill page after page with scribbling in order to appear busy. They frequently can read their own writing, although no one else can. It is difficult for persons with this problem to learn to write legibly.

Handwriting training. Specially designed handwriting techniques such as the D'Nealian Handwriting Program can increase the legibility of penmanship for persons with dysgraphia (Thurber, 1993). D'Nealian Handwriting is a continuous-stroke writing system. The pencil seldom leaves the paper, and letters are connected by simple strokes that are difficult to make backwards. Traditional manuscript and cursive writing methods involve too many pencil lifts to let learners who have dyslexia or dysgraphia maintain mental images of left-to-right and top-to-bottom sequences. For sustained writing of longer assignments, students who have dysgraphia do much better in written expression when they are taught how to use a word processor.

The most effective teaching philosophy is to help these individuals strive for legibility, not perfection. As with other persons with types of dyslexia, students who have dysgraphia cannot handle pressure and speed. Any effort to make them hurry triggers intense frustration and often results in painfully poor self-concept. The goal is to help them write as clearly and neatly as they can while giving them all the time they need to do their best.

Dyslexia in the Classroom

As noted previously, rarely does a student exhibit just one form of dyslexia. For example, visual dyslexia is usually accompanied by auditory dyslexia. This obviously complicates the teacher's task. If dyslexia is to be overcome, it must be identified early in a child's school experience. Time is a critical factor in solving perception disabilities. Follow-up studies of students with dyslexia who were diagnosed and treated at the Jordan Diagnostic Center between 1973 and 1990 demonstrate a rather somber pattern. If dyslexia is diagnosed before the child enters third grade, there is an 80% chance that he or she can overcome his or her confusion with language symbols well enough to do satisfactory school work. If the condition is not diagnosed until fifth grade, the possibility of doing well enough to achieve grade-level skills in academic learning drops to 40%. For the individual who reaches seventh grade before treatment is begun, there is only a 5% chance that enough correction can be achieved to enable him or her to attain grade-level skills in writing and reading. Obviously, the hopes for successful remediation when the problem is not found until adulthood are small. When the symptoms are recognized early, much can be done within the mainstream classroom.

Chapter 2

Overcoming Visual Dyslexia

Within the dyslexic struggle to learn to read, spell, write, and do good math computations, a specific type of difficulty is seen in many students. This unique problem, visual dyslexia, is related to interpreting what the student sees in printed or written materials, but it has little to do with the eyes. In fact, most persons with visual dyslexia have normal vision acuity (20/20 to 20/30). In Chapter 1, however, two types of central vision difference were discussed that are found in more than half of those who have visual dyslexia. Word blindness (Irlen syndrome) makes it impossible for the person to see black print on white paper, especially under bright overhead light. Word blindness is linked to incomplete development of the magno cells that are part of the vision pathways connecting the retina to the visual cortex. Off-center central vision also is frequently seen in many struggling readers who have dyslexia. Because the foveal structure of the retina is slightly off center, unstable visual information is sent to the visual cortex and symbol patterns are not processed correctly.

However, these anomalies in visual perception (interpreting what the eyes see on the page) do not *cause* visual dyslexia. The visual dyslexia syndrome discussed in this chapter originates within the visual cortex (see the map of the brain in Figure 2.1). Visual dyslexia involves the chronic tendency to reverse or rotate letters and numbers, as well as to scramble the sequence of printed or written symbols. Having word blindness or off-center foveal visual perception on top of visual dyslexia greatly complicates the struggle to develop fluent literacy skills. But visual dyslexia is not caused by the eyes, nor can it be cured by correcting vision deficits.

VISUAL DYSLEXIA SYNDROME

Since the early 1800s, many theories have emerged to explain this mysterious tendency for intelligent students to reverse letters and numbers, turn them upside down, or scramble the sequence of details. In the early years of the 20th century, a Freudian theory speculated that little boys

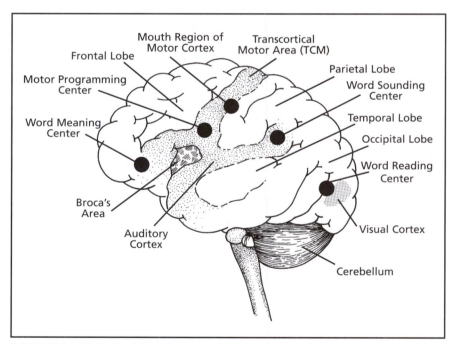

FIGURE 2.1.   Regions of the left brain where language information is processed (based upon brain imaging studies reported by Montgomery, 1989).

who get things backwards are victims of penis envy. For several decades, this bizarre concept influenced certain quarters of education. As is known today, such speculation had little bearing upon the neurological realities of visual processing. A persistent point of view for more than 100 years has blamed poor teaching methods for symbol turning and directional confusion in struggling learners. Ironically, dyslexia is found in certain students no matter what curriculum or teaching strategy is used by instructors. Currently, many concerned educators insist that too much is made of the idea of dyslexia. These earnest instructors believe that if teachers and parents motivate struggling readers more intently, they can overcome their difficulties in mastering basic literacy skills. It is ironic that individuals with dyslexia are often more highly motivated than their peers to become talented readers and spellers. For more than a century, vision specialists guided learners with dyslexia through eye training programs in the belief that poor eye teaming (ocular mobility) was the cause for inaccurate symbol interpretation. This school of thought contended that if eye muscle coordination could be balanced and improved, the reader no longer would stumble over reversed symbols or scrambled visual perception. Practitioners of chiropractic medicine have advanced the theory that manipulation of the skull and certain skeletal systems will adjust the central nervous system so that the visual cortex will no longer get things backward or upside down. Other earnest professionals have developed complex phonics programs that press individuals to memorize hundreds of word-sounding rules in the belief that overteaching will solve the problems of dyslexia. No kind of remedial practice can change the brain structure differences that cause LD or dyslexia.

There is always risk in oversimplifying a complex idea. The human brain is obviously much more complex than a simple diagram or definition can show. But generally speaking, the visual cortex at the back of the brain is the major center where visual information related to reading, writing, copying, and recognizing math symbols is processed. Figure 2.1 shows the regions of the left brain that are involved in visual processing of printed or written information. It is the job of the left brain to master most of the concepts of formal education. The right brain is the picture brain—it processes such functions as space, size, shape, color, form, and texture and recognizes faces and objects and how we represent our world through art, music, and dance. The left brain has the task of learning to read from books, write information on paper, listen to oral information, learn new vocabulary, remember vast quantities of facts over a period of time, and earn educational diplomas and degrees. To become literate, one must have strong enough left-brain talent to allow for the development of the skills required for fluent literacy. Dyslexia is caused by a left-brain difference that makes it difficult or impossible for certain learners to process classroom information. Students who have dyslexia struggle with rapid interpretation of printed symbols, comprehension of oral language, and long-term memory for the myriad facts society regards as important.

Symbol Orientation

In visual dyslexia, the visual cortex cannot learn the correct orientation of printed symbols. Certain symbols appear backwards (*b-d, p-q, 3, 5, 7, Z, S, L*), while other symbols seem upside down (*M-W, N-N, 6-9, p-b*). Frequently parts of words are reversed (*brid/bird, gril/girl, sruprise/surprise*), and occasionally, whole words or number units are read backwards (*on/no, saw/was, 81/18*). This is called *mirror image.* Some persons with visual dyslexia scramble the order of what they see, as when an individual says "four hundred ninety-one" while looking at 941. This kind of printed symbol confusion occurs when the left-brain regions do not communicate (integrate) well enough. The information being processed does not move along the neuronal pathways well enough to produce clear, accurate mental images. Many "glitches" occur along these information highways during processing. Too many details are out of sequence and too many bits of information are mistaken for other bits of information.

No single pattern establishes dyslexia. Most young children go through stages of unstable visual perception before they mature. For example, most preschool youngsters write letters and numbers backwards. Early readers often hold the book upside down before they learn to "turn it over." Before visual dyslexia can be confirmed, a definite set of behaviors (a syndrome) must be identified. Only when an unmistakable cluster of perceptual differences is seen can we safely conclude that a person has dyslexia. The following sections describe the symptoms used to identify visual dyslexia in an individual. (A checklist of visual dyslexic characteristics is presented in Appendix B.)

Confusion with Sequence

The underlying flaw in visual dyslexia is the student's inability to comprehend order or sequence. Few adults realize how much of the school day is devoted to thinking according to the following model:

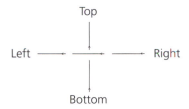

In the English language, all reading must be done left to right, starting at the top of the page or the column. This principle is so commonly taken for granted that parents and teachers seldom mention it to the students above the primary grades. It is assumed that anyone who reads will go automatically left to right and top to bottom. Unfortunately, this is not so for people with dyslexia. The dyslexic orientation is just the opposite, or partly so. The dyslexic tendency is mirror image, meaning that the student's nature is to process symbols backwards (right to left and bottom to top). In fact, one of the developmental milestones looked for in kindergarten pupils is the point at which they "turn it over" and begin to think in terms of left to right and top to bottom. Approximately 80% of the U.S. student population has the neurological talent to learn this standard orientation automatically. Late-maturing children may not do so until the second or third grade. Of the remaining 20% who never fully achieve this automatic orientation, most have dyslexia.

For example, Pete's primary teachers did not understand his difficulty with directionality. When his first-grade teacher introduced the letter *d*, she assumed that all of her pupils perceived it left to right (ball first, then the stick) and top to bottom (stick pointing up from the ball). Pete was completely unaware of his different orientation. He perceived *d* right to left (stick first, then the ball) and bottom to top (stick below the ball). What the teacher perceived as *d*, Pete perceived as *q*. In dyslexia, several critical symbols often are misperceived: *d–b–p–q, M–W, u–n, 7–L, 6–9, h–y*. When students such as Pete only partly rotate symbols, they often confuse *N–Z* and *3–M–W*.

The unfortunate consequence is that Pete is constantly told he is wrong. Unless someone explains how his perception differs, he enters the reading and writing process with no idea that he is heading the wrong direction up a very busy street, which is why he continually "collides with oncoming traffic." His teachers and most of his peers are proceeding in one direction while his perception travels the opposite or partly opposite way. So long as this situation is not recognized and understood, there is no way he can master the symbol system without constant conflict and the put-down of always being wrong.

Trouble with Time and Sequence

Few individuals with visual dyslexia develop automatic or fluent awareness of time, sequence, or details in a certain order. For example, instead of recalling an orderly progression of experiences over a period of time, Pete's memory of early childhood is a jumbled collection of events that do not fall into an orderly time sequence. In his perception of time, a broken arm 2 months ago happened right after he badly bruised his elbow when he was 3 years old. His grandmother's death 5 years ago seems like last month to him. Most children have a confused memory of their early years, but those with normal ability to sequence learn to connect their experiences inside a consistent time frame as they mature. People like Pete seldom do. Because mastery of reading depends upon remembering letters in the right sequence, this learning difference is one of the greatest curriculum obstacles facing individuals with visual dyslexia.

Confusion with time and sequence are major factors in Pete's problem of accepting responsibility. Because of his general frustration with order and sequence, he is continually in conflict with adult demands. At home his parents expect him to carry out the following responsibilities each weekday morning:

1. Make your bed before breakfast.

2. Brush your teeth after breakfast.

3. Feed and water the pets before catching the school bus.

4. Take homework back to school.

They tell him this list over and over, but they have never written it in a visible outline for Pete to see.

In the afternoon Pete faces another set of responsibilities that also have been relayed to him verbally but never put down in a written form:

1. Empty the trash on Monday, Wednesday, and Friday.

2. Feed and water the pets every afternoon.

3. Attend Cub Scouts on Tuesday afternoon.

4. Take a shower by 8:30 P.M. and be ready for bed by 9:00 P.M.

Then there are Pete's weekend chores:

1. Sweep the garage on Saturday.

2. Pick up toys and tools from yard by Saturday evening.

3. Bathe the dog either Saturday or Sunday afternoon.

Pete has never seen a visible outline of any of these adult expectations. In repeating these routines orally, his parents have assumed that Pete perceives time and sequence as clearly as they do. The child's dyslexic tendencies to scramble the order of things leave him with an unstructured mass of responsibilities. In spite of his intentions to obey his parents, Pete finds himself confused and frustrated. When chores remain undone, adults conclude that he is lazy, stubborn, insubordinate, or forgetful. In reality, Pete is filled with dread and self-defeat. He has no way to communicate his dilemma to people who continually are displeased with him. This generates family friction and almost constant misery for Pete. When this kind of confusion with time and sequence goes unrecognized and uncorrected for several years, children like Pete do indeed become insubordinate and hostile. By the time they enter middle school, these dyslexic strugglers are convinced that they are worthless and incapable of success.

DYSLEXIC PATTERNS IN THE CLASSROOM

Similar frustration occurs in the classroom between teachers who do not understand and confused learners like Pete. With many students to care for, the teacher assumes that the oral instructions to Group A have been clear. As he or she turns to Group B, the teacher is annoyed to see that Pete is not following directions. Pete again has failed in his relationships with the adult world. Because he cannot communicate his confusion to any of his teachers, he is always at risk of being judged lazy, careless, or insubordinate. Teachers who make these kinds of conclusions about the surface behaviors of students who are struggling unwittingly set the stage for misbehavior and unhappiness. Pete's failure to follow class instructions is due to perceptual difficulty in comprehending time and sequence, not willful disobedience.

Trouble with Sequence

An alert teacher can identify confusion with sequence as students work on tasks involving series. For example, students such as Pete usually are fluent in giving oral reports and carrying on conversations. Casual listeners are impressed by their stock of information and the concepts they glean through listening and observation. There is, however, a noticeable flaw in this oral performance—difficulty recalling the correct sequence of details when talking.

Many persons with visual dyslexia cannot remember the day, month, and year of their birth. The teacher can check for this tendency through informal conversation in the room. Although he may know reams of statistics about his favorite ball team, Pete will stumble when asked to tell his full birth date.

Learners with visual dyslexia also have trouble naming the days of the week and the months of the year. When asked to write this information, Pete keeps track by tapping his fingers, whispering a rhyme, or humming the alphabet song.

Pete has enormous struggle learning the multiplication tables. He rarely does well with long division, decimals, fractions, or percentages, and usually has difficulty dealing with money and measurement. Surprisingly, Pete often does mental arithmetic better than he can write it on paper.

Figures 2.2 and 2.3 are examples from the *Jordan Written Screening Test for Specific Language Disability* (Jordan, 1989b). This simple test asks the person to write the alphabet, days of the week, and months of the year from memory. The instructor, explaining that this is not a spelling test, gives the student a sheet of lined paper and asks the individual to do this memory writing the best he or she can. Figures 2.2 and 2.3 demonstrate the difficulty in recalling and writing familiar details in sequence. Teachers and parents not only gain quick insight into sequence failure, but they also see evidence of dysgraphia and auditory dyslexia, if these differences also exist.

Another informal estimate of a student's comprehension of sequence is to ask him or her to repeat a series of numbers. For example, the student listens as the teacher says "6–8–7–9." Then the teacher observes the listener's efforts to repeat the numbers in the same sequence. Persons with

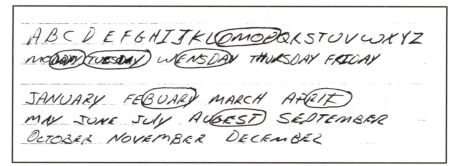

FIGURE 2.2. Student was 19 years old with a high school diploma. Notice the struggle to recall details in sequence as well as difficulty remembering familiar spelling patterns.

dyslexia usually fail this kind of serial task. A similar test would be to ask a student to listen to a sentence and then try to repeat it verbatim: "Three men raced down the hill to their boat in the river." Those who have dyslexia usually omit complete phrases or substitute different words. In fact, they frequently lose the theme of the sentence entirely.

Faulty Reading Comprehension

Faulty perception of sequence is a major reason for poor performance on reading comprehension tests by a student such as Pete. Persons with visual dyslexia are especially poor at retaining information that is presented in sequence. As noted in Chapter 1, they often must also deal with poor central vision. As these students read line after line, several problems begin to interfere with their understanding of what their inner voice is saying about what is on the page.

Awkward, Jerky Oral Reading

Most readers with visual dyslexia cannot maintain a smooth, forward rhythm in sounding out words in sentences. Verbally they take two steps forward, then one step back. It is easy to hear this stumbling decoding pattern when students like Pete read aloud. They start to say the next word,

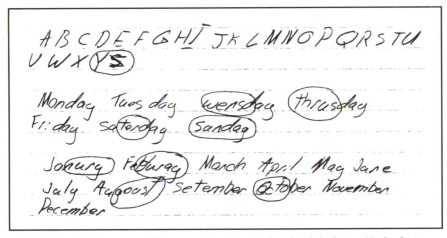

FIGURE 2.3.   Student was 27 years old with a high school diploma. He had attempted several hours of college study before giving up trying to earn a college degree.

stop, get stuck trying to say the sounds in sequence, then back up to try it again. Forward motion in reading is awkward and jerky.

Transposing Words

Individuals with visual dyslexia tend to transpose words as they read. Peripheral vision (described in Chapter 1) causes them to pick up nearby words and insert them in the wrong place. These struggling readers often pull a later word back and insert it earlier in the sentence. As they read, they tend to scramble the sequence of the printed words on the page.

Rapid Burn-out

Individuals with visual dyslexia rapidly reach points of burn-out as they read. Vision becomes overstressed, and the eyes rapidly become too tired to continue focusing clearly. As vision fatigue develops, mental images begin to fade away. At a certain point of perceptual overload, the reader "goes blank" and has to get away from the act of reading. Few individuals with this problem have the stamina to continue to read effectively longer than 3 to 5 minutes without taking a break.

Slow Multisensory Compensation

When all of these factors are considered, it is very difficult for persons with visual dyslexia to read effectively, especially if they must hurry. They are forced to touch the print with a finger or pencil while they whisper to themselves over and over. This slow, tedious, and time-consuming process cannot be speeded up without multiplying errors in decoding and comprehension.

Conservation of Form and Transformation

The pioneering work of Barbël Inhëlder and Jean Piaget into the growth of logic in children has provided a simple yet profound framework that helps us understand how visual dyslexia interferes with language processing (Inhelder & Piaget, 1974). These Swiss researchers introduced the concept of *conservation of form*—the ability of the central nervous system to remember all of the forms humans must recognize and interpret in order to be well educated. For example, we need to remember right-brain forms such as shapes, sizes, distance, colors, and position-in-space relationships. We must remember human faces, animals, buildings, and important community landmarks. Conservation of form also includes our memory for left-brain information such as alphabet letters, mathematics numerals, words, street signs, and word-based labels. Now and in the future, we are and will be required to conserve new forms of barcodes, computer screen information, and electronic signatures on almost everything we buy or sell. Conservation of visual form refers to the ability to see specific forms (letters, numerals, words, or shapes), then hold those mental images intact after the model is taken away.

The act of reading could be described this way. As readers see visual forms on the printed page, memory systems are expected to make lasting impressions that will be used later after the book has been put aside or after the eyes have left a particular point of focus. Readers who have visual dyslexia do not have the ready talent to perform this perceptual act automatically or fluently. Students such as Pete do not conserve the form of what they see on the printed page. Once the visual pattern is no longer in view, the mental image is quickly lost, or parts of it are lost or scrambled. Individuals with dyslexia conserve only bits and pieces of the printed patterns they have seen. In addition, they reverse or scramble the sequence of the parts. People who have severe dyslexia cannot conserve visual form longer than a few seconds. The moment the eyes move away from single words or parts of words, the mental image is lost or scrambled. Reading comprehension is especially difficult and tedious.

In Chapter 1, the severity scale that shows how much struggle is involved in classroom learning was described (see the "Dyslexia" section). Persons who are at Levels 8, 9, and 10 rarely develop conservation of form in reading well enough to achieve comprehension above a third-grade level.

Conservation of form also involves the ability to change forms into new or different patterns. Changing one form into a similar but different form is called *transformation.* For example, in changing a statement into a question, the reader must hold the author's meaning (conserve the form) well enough to restructure the order of the words. Our fictional student, Pete, reads this sentence: "Four boys played ball in the park." His class is asked to change the sentence into a question, but Pete is completely baffled by this task. What does the teacher mean? How can this sentence be anything else than what it is right now? Language-skills teachers can testify how difficult it is to teach students with dyslexia this transformation operation in building variations of sentences. Students who have dyslexia finally manage to understand left-to-right meaning in simple sentences. Transforming left-to-right concepts into a different sequence is more than students like Pete can comprehend. Transformation is also at the heart of arithmetic computation. Students such as Pete finally understand the vertical structure of number problems:

$$9$$
$$+5$$

When the direction of the problem is transformed to a linear form (9 + 5 = _____) these students are confused. The task of transforming one pattern or direction into another often overwhelms the dyslexic learner.

Holding Mental Images

As he reads or listens, Pete does not develop or hold onto complete mental images of what he is reading or hearing. Just as he does not perceive an orderly sequence of time, Pete does not comprehend the organization of an author's writing. When asked specific recall questions about his silent reading, Pete cannot retrieve enough organized information to respond in the expected manner. The constant failure to comprehend creates in Pete a dread of reading early in the school experience. This lack of talent for conservation of form and transformation of form is especially troubling when Pete is asked to draw inferences or arrive at conclusions quickly.

Timed Tests

Standardized reading tests that require the student to read paragraphs quickly, then answer questions within a strict time limit, are almost impossible tasks for individuals with dyslexia. When these struggling persons must also mark bubbles on a separate answer sheet, they give up in frustration and defeat. When given ample time, students like Pete often can arrive at satisfactory answers through trial and error or by logically eliminating wrong answers. Having to hurry only multiplies mistakes in comprehension.

Teachers complain about Pete's tendency to guess on timed tests. However, skipping down the page, marking answers at random, or refusing to check back over his work are perfectly reasonable responses in view of Pete's dyslexia. By this time, he has experienced several years of failure to comprehend what he reads; therefore, there is little else for him to do but guess. This is especially true when Pete is told that no consideration will be made for his slow pace, which is the only speed at which he can succeed.

Struggle with the Alphabet

Teachers are always concerned when any child cannot cope with the alphabet. The unstructured way in which the alphabet is taught to primary pupils is largely to blame for unnecessary visual dyslexic struggle. For the past 50 years, alphabet sequence seldom has been taught to beginner pupils. Young learners with curiosity about letters have discovered the alphabet sequence displayed on wall charts in the classroom. Grandparents and other relatives often teach the alphabet sequence to children before they start to school. It is rare to find classroom teachers presenting the alphabet sequence in an organized, systematic way to beginner pupils. This unstructured approach to knowledge of the alphabet has posed no problem for children without reading problems; however, children who have dyslexia must have a clearly structured, direct encounter with details in sequence. The foundational challenge of visual dyslexia is faulty perception of sequence. Having little or no sequence to follow is disastrous when students such as Pete are confronted with printed symbols. Had Pete been well grounded in the alphabet sequence at the very beginning of his school experience, he could have handled beginning reading tasks more successfully.

As was shown earlier in this chapter, a simple technique for determining a student's perception of the alphabet is for the teacher to watch the student write it on ruled paper. Any dyslexic tendencies will quickly become apparent. Students with no dyslexic tendencies learn to write the alphabet in sequence without hesitation. Those with visual dyslexia cannot.

When asked to write the alphabet, Pete often hesitates, asking whether he should print or "write cursy." When told that it does not matter, he may want to know if he should use big or little letters. Students with dyslexia seldom remember the terms *capital* and *lowercase*. Next, Pete may ask whether he should go across or down the page. The instructor explains that it does not matter, just write it the way that seems comfortable. When finally at work, Pete soon reaches a stalling point, often at the letter *M*. Whenever he bogs down, he goes back to *A* and whispers the letters one by one, trying to remember the whole sequence. Occasionally he hums or sings the alphabet song to remind himself of the alphabet sequence. When he gets stuck, Pete touches each letter with his finger or pencil as he goes back to *A* and reviews what he has written. An observer can easily note the dyslexic problem of synchronizing speech with writing. As he touches the letters while saying them, Pete's voice is usually ahead of his eyes or finger. Consequently, reviewing his written work still does not help him identify errors.

Pete is very slow as he writes or prints the alphabet. The letters *m, n, p, u,* and *v* often are in scrambled positions. In addition to this sequence problem, Pete often confuses similar-looking letters, such as *b–d–p–q, h–u–n, h–y, t–f–j, M–W, N–Z, r–s, v–w–k–y–x,* and *o–e–c*. As he writes, Pete makes circular letters with backward pencil motions. He frequently writes circular parts of letters with a clockwise motion that leaves a small tail or hook at the top of the letter. He makes several letters with a bottom-to-top stroke (*t, f, p, g, b, d*). Unless the teacher carefully observes Pete's pencil at work, she or he might not be aware of this backward motion that is a signpost of dyslexia.

Persons with visual dyslexia often mix capital and lowercase letters when writing the alphabet, as well as mixing manuscript and cursive styles. Pete's reasons for this inconsistent writing are actually quite practical. Because he has not been taught the alphabet sequence, he has never encountered the letters in left-to-right sequential relation to each other. The best he can, he has devised his own system for remembering or recognizing certain letters. Capital *B* and capital *D* are stable in his memory, although they may be written backwards. Capital *B* has two humps. Capital *D* has only one hump. But lowercase *b* is too easily confused with *d, p,* or *q*. So long as Pete continues to deal with isolated letters in manuscript style, there is no dependable left-to-right structure to which he can anchor his perceptions of the alphabet.

Figure 2.3 illustrates the kind of struggle many persons with dyslexia display in writing the alphabet and numbers from memory. It is unfortunate that well-meaning adults often misinterpret this handicapped work as a sign of limited intelligence or laziness. These students struggle very hard to produce even this quality of work. Like Pete, the girl who wrote the copy in Figure 2.3 was doing her best.

Reversal of Symbols

Another clue to visual dyslexia is the student's confusion about which direction certain symbols should face. This faulty conservation of form causes an individual to write or read symbols backwards, upside down, or partially turned over (see the writing examples in Figures 2.4 and 2.5). Persons who have dyslexia generally use capital *B* and capital *D* instead of the lowercase versions. The two humps on capital *B* help them remember which way to turn that letter. It is much easier to remember which way *B* and *D* face than it is to recall the correct direction of *b* and *d*.

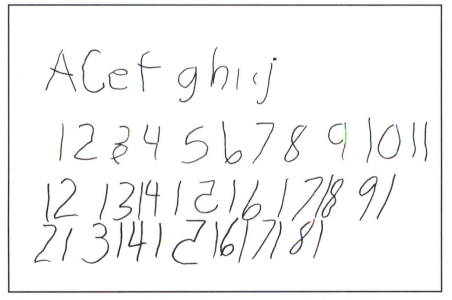

FIGURE 2.4. Writing sample from a female, age 8 years, 7 months. She struggled 15 minutes to write the alphabet and the numbers 1 through 20. As she wrote 19, she completely lost her memory of number sequence. All teen numbers were written with the second numeral first, then 1 placed in front of the second numeral.

Dictated by Teacher		Paul's Dyslexic Responses	
bad		*3 B a b*	lowercase *d* reversed
bag		*4 B ag*	
ball		*5 Ball*	
bed		*6 Be∞*	lowercase *d* reversed on top of unneeded *e*
bell		*7 B ell*	letter *l* made bottom to top
big		*8 Big*	
bill		*9 Bill*	letters *i* and *l* made bottom to top
body		*10 Body*	lowercase *d* reversed
bug		*11 Bug*	letter *g* circled several times with backward strokes
dad	began to write capital *B*	*12 Dab*	lowercase *d* reversed
did	began to write capital *B*	*13 DID*	
dog		*14 Dog*	wrote *o* and *g* with backward strokes
doll		*15 Doll*	wrote o with backward stroke

FIGURE 2.5.   Dyslexic writing with reversed letters, backward strokes, and mixed capital and lowercase letters.

Oral Reading

The tendency to reverse or transpose symbols is a handicap in reading. Students with visual dyslexia often read whole words backwards (*saw* for *was, but* for *tub*). Sometimes only certain kinds of syllables are reversed within words (*bran* for *barn, form* for *from, sliver* for *silver*). Beginning letters, especially lowercase *b, d, p, q, h, r, m, w,* and *u,* are frequently perceived upside down or backwards. This causes the reader to misperceive similar words (*daddy* for *baby, dark* or *park* for *bark*). This results in nonsense, forcing the reader to go back over the context of the sentence to figure out what is wrong. Our student with dyslexia, Pete, usually can learn how to correct these reversal errors when their backward patterns are pointed out over a period of time.

Parents and teachers can detect this reversal tendency by listening as students read aloud. Within a few minutes, the listener hears reversal habits. As the student reads aloud, the adult should make rapid notes of errors. The following oral reading errors often indicate visual dyslexia:

1. Reversal of beginning letters: *dark* or *park* for *bark, dump* or *pump* for *bump;*

2. Transposing blends and digraphs: *preform* for *perform, there* for *three, star* for *stream, porfit* for *profit, frame* for *farmer;*

3. Substituting one letter for another: *sleep* for *sheep, come* for *came, some* for *same;*

4. Transposing letters within words: *vigener* for *vinegar, magilant* for *malignant, macilous* for *malicious;*

5. Reversal of whole words: *on* for *no, saw* for *was, but* for *tub;*

6. Failure to see small details (including a habitual failure to see punctuation marks): *house* for *horse, with* for *wish, butter* for *better, hungry* for *hunger;*

7. Omission of endings: *ever* for *every, her* for *here, happen* for *happening;*

8. Telescoping: *standarize* for *standardized, consently* for *consequently, sudly* for *suddenly;*

9. Perseveration: *hopenen* for *hope, farmerer* for *farmer, sudendely* for *suddenly.*

Dyslexia is suspected only when several of these symptoms exist in the student's oral reading. Teachers must be careful to distinguish between dyslexia and the word-blind or off-center visual patterns described in Chapter 1.

Errors in Copying

It is especially hard for students like Pete to copy from the chalkboard or from a projection screen. Success at copying (also called *vision-to-motor transfer*) involves a high-level talent for conservation of form. Successful copying involves at least six complex steps that must be done in a given sequence:

1. See the forms clearly;

2. Hold these mental images intact (conserve the form);

3. Refocus to the writing space without getting lost;

4. Transform mental images into handwriting (fine-motor coordination);

5. Space the symbols properly on the writing paper (figure-ground control);

6. End up with a legible resemblance to what was on the chalkboard or in the textbook.

Adults who write well often forget what a complex task copying really is. It is a monumental one for students such as Pete, who cannot conserve form without enormous concentration and effort. The use of overhead projectors increases the pressure on many such students to take notes while the teacher lectures. Chronic confusion with symbols forces them to work slowly. If they try to hurry, they quickly become frustrated trying to keep details in correct sequence.

Instructors easily can identify learners who have copying problems. When students are asked to copy a paragraph from the chalkboard or from a projection screen, the teacher should watch for the following tendencies:

1. Losing the place on the board;

2. Erasing frequently;

3. Overprinting to correct mistakes on paper;

4. Misspelling on paper;

5. Failing to observe capital letters;

6. Failing to observe punctuation marks;

7. Failing to space properly on paper;

8. Reversing letters;

9. Reversing whole words;

10. Working unusually slowly.

As with oral reading, observers must be careful not to mistake word blindness or off-center central vision for dyslexia. An example of copying errors often seen when students with dyslexia copy from the board or from textbooks is shown in Figure 2.6. (The story is from the *Jordan Written Screening Test* [Jordan, 1989b].)

Errors in Spelling

There is a unique pattern of spelling errors that distinguishes visual dyslexia from auditory dyslexia (which will be discussed in Chapter 3). The primary disability in visual dyslexia is failure to process details in sequence. Persons with visual dyslexia cannot recall a clear mental image of whole words. They can hear and identify most of the sounds within common words, but the letters will be in scrambled order as the word is written. The following errors illustrate visual dyslexia in spelling from memory:

Word in Pete's Mind	His Written Response
rode	roed
ate	aet
goes	gose
heaven	haveen
marriage	mirarage

> Bob and Dan
>
> Bob and Dan saw Sam Watts on the dock. The three men stopped. "See the big ship?" asked Sam.
> "Sure did," Dan and Bob said. "Must be a mile long."
> Bob and Dan saw Sam was in a hurry. "Got to run," Sam said. "See you."
> "Sure," said Bob and Dan. "See you, Sam."
>
> *[handwritten copy of the above story]*
> Bob and Dan
> Bob and Dan saw Sam Watts on the desk The three men stopped See the big ship?" asked Son.
> Sure did "Dan and Bob said.
> "Must be a mile long."
> Bob and Dan saw Son was in a hurry. "Got to run" Son said.
> See you."
> "Sure," said Bob. "See goy Son"

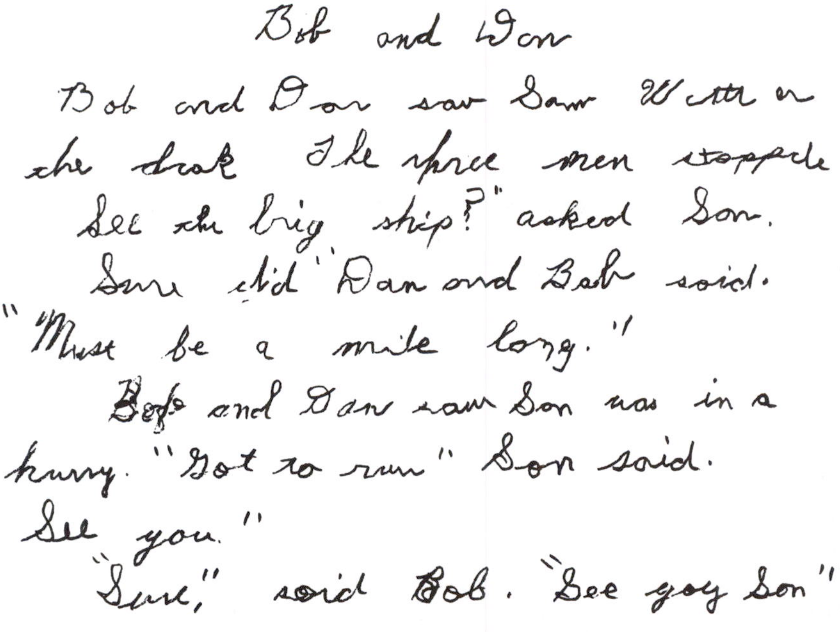

FIGURE 2.6. Student was 14 years old. He needed 37 minutes to copy this story.

ACTIVITIES FOR OVERCOMING VISUAL DYSLEXIA

As every adult who has dyslexia will verify, it is not possible to overcome this disability completely. Persons with developmental or secondary dyslexia gradually do outgrow enough of the patterns to become comfortable students by their late teens or early twenties. On the other hand, individuals with deep, or primary, dyslexia do not outgrow their patterns, even as adults. All persons with some form of dyslexia can master techniques to help them reduce their frustration level and increase success with reading, writing, and math computation. New technologies provide remarkable ways for most of these individuals to work around handicaps in spelling and writing.

For example, Franklin Learning Resources (122 Burrs Road, Mt. Holly, NJ 08060; 800/525-9673) markets a new generation of talking computers called Bookman™. These state-of-the-art miniaturized computers fit into a pocket or purse. Some models fit into a bookbag like a small book. Bookman computers are multisensory. They display information on a screen while they say the information aloud in a clearly legible synthetic voice. A wide range of dictionaries and encyclopedias, a thesaurus, foreign language guides, the complete Bible in two versions, and many other reference books are available for the Bookman series. This remarkable multisensory technology costs less than $200.00.

In addition to the Bookman series, Franklin Learning Resources offers the popular Language Master™ talking pocket computers that have helped thousands of students with dyslexia since the late 1970s. For example, when Pete uses this technology, he types in the word he wishes to spell. Soon he sees the correct spelling on a screen while he hears a voice spell and pronounce the word correctly. Pete thus gets immediate multisensory feedback as he does keyboard writing.

The rest of this chapter presents concepts and strategies that are essential if students with dyslexia are to develop even minimal literacy skills. If these are taught carefully over an extended period of time, it is possible for most persons who have dyslexia to overcome enough of their disability to succeed in formal education.

Teaching Time Sequence

Persons who struggle with visual dyslexia at Level 5 or higher have difficulty with time concepts. They do not automatically perceive how time passes in a given sequence. They live from moment to moment, day to day, week to week, and so on without developing an overall view of how time passes in their lives. It is possible to teach these individuals to think in terms of linear time if this training combines visual guidelines with continual verbal reinforcement.

Visible Reminders

The first step in establishing awareness of time sequence is to provide visible, tangible right-brain reminder systems that show chronological order. In primary grades, this is done with calendars and notebook organizers that show the days of the week within the month. Children who display dyslexic tendencies must be drilled in the basic units of time: seconds and minutes, minutes and hours, hours and days, days and weeks, and so forth. Busy adults usually bypass steps in this continuum, hopping from minutes and hours to days and weeks, omitting years, decades, and centuries altogether.

The usual activities involving time concepts seldom build an unbroken, sequential awareness of time. Youngsters with dyslexia seldom see the continuum from the smallest units (seconds) to the largest (centuries), whereas youngsters without dyslexic tendencies soon figure out this time structure. The former do not conserve the form of time when they only hear about it in bits and pieces. This deficit has crippling effects in social studies (historical sequence), math (lapse of time), and science (seasonal change, geological classification), and it leaves students like Pete unable to cope with myriad time situations that adults take for granted.

Wall Charts and Calendars

Any classroom in which there is a child with dyslexia, and his or her room at home, should have wall charts and calendars showing how time units move forward in relation to each other. These time flowcharts should be displayed in sequence all year long. Students who have dyslexia must be involved continually in a review of basic time units. Gradually, this basic knowledge of time sequence begins to fall into place for them.

At the start of school in the fall, teachers should begin with a visual model of how summer has merged into fall. Day by day, children should see a visual progression of such concepts as *during last summer, this fall, when winter comes, last week, now, next week, last month, this month, next month, how long until Thanksgiving* (November), *how long until Hanukkah or Christmas* (December), and so forth. This permanent visual display should leave nothing to chance.

When this sort of carefully structured visual time sequence is taught and displayed for a long period, adults will see youngsters with dyslexia beginning to grasp the concepts of chronological order. Birthdays, family events, and personal activities are good candidates also for these charts and calendars.

Teaching Alphabet Sequence

For half a century, U.S. education has concealed the alphabet sequence until after children have learned to read. For most children, this has done no harm, largely because youngsters who have a talent for reading learn the alphabet from what they see in the classroom. Children who have dyslexia do not absorb the alphabet because they do not comprehend sequence presented in an indirect way. They are stymied when called upon to alphabetize words, find entries in the dictionary, or locate material in reference books. When the alphabet letters are doled out in random order, there is no left-to-right point of reference by which these children can visualize where letters are within the alphabet sequence. This deficiency obviously poses serious problems in upper grades.

By virtue of their perception differences, students who have dyslexia must memorize cultural and literacy landmarks. If the alphabet sequence is to be mastered, it must be done through memory drill and multisensory practice. Day after day, youngsters like Pete must practice arranging movable letters in correct order, copying from models, and writing the sequence from memory while they say it, hear it, and feel it happen. Children who are just starting school should begin learning the alphabet sequence by handling cutout, three-dimensional letter forms. Creative teachers can devise their own alphabet models using clay, pipe cleaners, or hand-cut paper forms. It is unnecessary to spend meager supply funds on expensive materials to teach alphabet sequence. In fact, the simpler the models, the better they usually are for teaching purposes.

In order to master the alphabet, children with visual dyslexia must learn only one major concept at a time. It confuses them if the instructor introduces phonic principles at the same time that letter shapes are being mastered. Children who have dyslexia must not be expected to manipulate two forms of information during the initial stages of learning a new concept. For example, Pete should begin his literacy training by associating the names of the letters with their shapes. He should not begin by connecting phonic sounds to letter shapes. Pete should match the letter *A* with the name of the letter until he has automatic, fluent talent in knowing that the shape *A* is called "aye." He should not be exposed to phonics until he has first learned the names of all the letters in alphabetic sequence. Sounds for letters should come after the sequence and shapes of the letters have been mastered.

Alert teachers and parents can tell when a child is ready for a more advanced level of handling alphabet sequence. The following learning sequence shows the kinds of activities a student like Pete should do:

Step 1. Master the alphabet sequence with movable letters. Practice finding alphabet sequence on a keyboard.

Step 2. Trace over the alphabet sequence on a chalkboard. Practice typing alphabet sequence on a keyboard.

Step 3. Trace over the alphabet sequence on paper or plastic wipe-off sheets. Practice typing the alphabet sequence.

Step 4. Copy the alphabet sequence at the chalkboard as the student looks at model cards or the teacher's written model. Copy the alphabet sequence on a keyboard by looking at a printed or written alphabet sequence chart.

Step 5. Copy the alphabet sequence on lined paper as the student looks at an alphabet chart or teacher's written model. Practice copying the alphabet sequence on a keyboard.

Step 6. Practice writing the alphabet sequence with a model nearby so the student can see it if he or she forgets. Practice typing the alphabet on a keyboard.

Step 7. Write and type the alphabet sequence from memory with no reversals, rotations, or letters out of sequence.

Adults have made the mistake of rushing students with LD too rapidly through this developmental sequence. Today's kindergarten programs usually introduce Steps 1 through 3. Most schools assume that primary pupils have mastered all seven steps by the time they begin second grade. This is not the case, as has been discovered in millions of adolescents and adults who are illiterate. The most urgent literacy need of students with dyslexia is to master alphabet sequence, no matter how old the student is when the deficiency is discovered. It obviously is irrelevant for them to struggle with book reports or themes until they have mastered the alphabet sequence.

Cursive Writing

Traditionally, cursive writing style has been postponed until third grade, on the assumption that children in elementary grades need to learn the finger dexterity skills of manuscript print before advancing to the more complicated fine-motor requirements of cursive style. This assumption has never been supported by research evidence (Jordan, 1993; Thurber, 1993). As shall be shown in Chapter 4, children who begin handwriting with cursive style seldom show disabling dysgraphic tendencies later in writing activities. Largely because of the consistent, flowing motor patterns established through cursive writing, alphabet sequence is quickly established when cursive style is introduced. For example, the D'Nealian Handwriting Program (Thurber, 1993) is excellent for children who struggle with traditional "ball-and-stick" manuscript printing. This simplified method of beginning writing is based upon continuous stroke penmanship. Only occasionally does the pencil lift from the paper to make the next letter. The first letters the child learns to write are transformed into cursive writing by adding one small stroke.

The traditional method of practicing manuscript print techniques during the child's first 2 years of school, then laying that knowledge aside to learn a different method of handwriting (cursive) in third grade, is far too overwhelming for learners like Pete. Starting the handwriting experience with a unified continuous stroke method such as the D'Nealian helps many struggling learners produce legible penmanship.

Comprehending Instructions

One of Pete's most frustrating experiences is his trouble building complete mental images through listening to a flow of oral information. He almost never escapes criticism from adults who give him verbal instructions. No matter how carefully he tries to listen, Pete does not build a full mental image of the sequence of what is being said. When the speaker stops talking, Pete has only bits and pieces that are seldom in the same sequence as what the speaker said. This inability to comprehend instructions brings Pete into frequent conflict with classmates and family members.

Written Outlines

Helping students such as Pete pay attention to sequential steps in carrying out instructions is actually rather simple. Instead of forcing them to depend upon memory, the parent or teacher should provide a simple, written outline of what is expected. If the student can read, he or she can use an outline listing each step or responsibility. This technique is especially suitable for routine work such as daily chores or work schedules that stay the same from day to day.

When clearly written instructions are given in textbooks or workbooks, the teacher has a ready-made visual aid in teaching how to follow sequence in interpreting instructions. Otherwise the instructor must make new daily lists and outlines for the student to see. Kindergarten and elementary education teachers often solve the problem by creating right-brain picture codes, such as using animal pictures, colored shapes, or other easily interpreted markers as cues. Children who easily lose track can refer back to the chart to see what to do next.

Listening to Instructions

Older students like Pete have the same needs for quick sequence reminders. As they listen to a series of directions, these students start to lose the sequence of what is expected. Most adults are unaware of how complicated their oral directions are. For example, in getting her math class under way, a fourth-grade teacher will usually make 20 or more short statements. Children are adept at "tuning in" and "tuning out"—they seldom pay attention to everything the teacher says. We expect listeners to filter this flow of information. For example, the teacher's instructions might sound like this:

> Now class, it's time for arithmetic. Put away your social studies books and get out your math books. Tom, sit down. Yes, Mary? No, you don't need two pencils. Now, class, be sure you have your pencils ready. Open your workbooks to today's lesson. Yes, Joe? No, I didn't say get them out, but you know I meant for you to. Now, children, open your books to page 25. What, Sue? Yes, you may get a drink for your hiccups. Now, on page 25 we are ready to review short division. . . .

This steady flow of speech is supplemented by "para-language": the unspoken gestures, facial expressions, variations of tone, and other nonverbal ingredients of group communication. Most children edit the running instructions, tuning in only when the teacher or a fellow student says something important that must be remembered. A student without a listening handicap might monitor the teacher's discussion in the following way:

> . . . It's time for arithmetic. . . . Put away social studies books . . . . get out math books. . . . don't need two pencils. . . . open workbooks to today's lesson. . . . open books to page 25. . . . ready to review short division.

Students with dyslexia cannot do this kind of editing. They cannot determine what the teacher thinks is essential because they cannot filter out unnecessary information that bombards them from all sides. Without a visual outline that shows each essential step, Pete is lost. However, if the teacher provides a written list for later reference, he has a chance to go through it again at his own pace and build a mental image of the sequence of important details. When Pete's teacher learned of his special need for a visual point of reference, she began to write a chalkboard outline of her comments:

Today's Math

1. Have one pencil ready.

2. Open textbook to page 25.

3. Open workbook to page 97.

4. For tomorrow: 15 problems on workbook page 97.

Tape-Recording Instructions

Many teachers have learned to help students like Pete by making a tape recording of their daily instructions. After the class has begun to work, those who did not understand the instructions can put on headphones and listen to the assignment again in private. Pete can listen to the instructions as many times as he needs. If the written outlines and tape recording are still not enough, students may go individually to the teacher. When this kind of face-saving safety net is provided for students with dyslexia, the class group is spared the arguments that are triggered when the same few students disrupt the learning atmosphere every day by clamoring for repeated explanations.

Failure to comprehend sequence in instructions is the primary cause for confusion with arithmetic story problems, science experiments, and chronological order in social studies. Although outlining is often introduced in elementary grades, the purpose for making brief outlines frequently is not clear to the students. Pete must know why making lists and outlines is important for his success. Providing lists of instructions or tape recording directions is one way of outlining what the adult expects of the child. However, leaving the interpretation of instructions to the student is not fair, unless the teacher has taken great pains to make things clear.

Correcting Reversals and Rotations

Teaching students like Pete not to turn things upside down or backwards is not always possible in a mainstream classroom setting. This dyslexic pattern often requires a one-to-one tutorial relationship that few teachers can provide during the school day. However, certain remedial steps can be taken regardless of the instructor's time limitations.

Begin with Openness

Remediation of learning differences must begin with openness. Adults rarely deal openly with situations involving a learning disability. If a student is to find relief from the frustrations and defeat fostered by LD or dyslexia, the conflicting patterns must be dealt with openly. However, an adult never should humiliate a student by candid remarks before the class. The approach for successful remedial work requires that the adult privately explain the kinds of mistakes the student makes. Once the student knows what to correct in writing, spelling, copying, or arithmetic, the teacher can develop a reminder system to help that student monitor his or her own work.

For example, in a quiet conference away from the prying eyes and ears of classmates, the teacher explains how Pete's work has been analyzed for certain things that need to be corrected. This might include showing him a checklist of visual dyslexia characteristics (see Appendix B). This list gives specific points of stumbling, such as seeing letters backward or upside down, turning numerals backward, and interpreting words differently. The teacher must carefully explain that these differences have nothing to do with intelligence. The use of words such as "dumb" or "stupid" should never be condoned when students who are struggling to learn compare themselves with more talented classmates who seem to have it much easier. The teacher should emphasize the concept of individual difference and explain why there is nothing wrong with being different. For example, the teacher might explain that the goal now is to learn to be an editor, a specialist who looks for things that are different, and that sometimes differences cause incorrect answers or misspelled words. If so, Pete can learn to be an editor to spot such differences and correct them.

Teachers and parents sometimes recoil from this sort of frankness on the grounds that it is cruel and risky to expose a young person to such self-knowledge. In actuality, it is cruel not to explain to Pete exactly what it is that produces conflict in his learning situation. Of course it might be foolish to tell an overly fearful child that he or she has dyslexia. But if the student is mature enough to wonder what the problem is, he or she should be told. Half of the success of remediating these tendencies depends upon the student's full cooperation. It is impossible to enlist Pete's full cooperation if he never is informed of the nature of the problems he is supposed to be correcting.

Adults might understand more readily the need for openness by recalling how they feel when physicians withhold information about patients' illnesses. We instantly become anxious when an examining physician mutters "Hmmm!" or "Aha!" but does not explain those vocal reactions. If teachers and parents can realize that children have the same need to know what is happening and why, remedial work often will be much more effective.

Quietly, unemotionally, and openly, the instructor sits down with Pete and points to specific examples of dyslexic confusion in his work. The teacher explains that these differences are the reasons for low grades or criticism. The instructor points out examples in assignments where Pete wrote or saw *beb* for *bed* or *mnst* for *must*. Or the teacher might play part of a tape to let Pete hear his own voice invert syllables (*gril* for *girl*, *on* for *no*). The teacher should show examples and explain them in whatever detail the student requests. The instructor should not be judgmental or condescending. If the conference is conducted as a conversation between an interested adult and an intelligent learner with a specific need, the result will be relief and a sense of understanding on the student's part. After all, Pete has known for a long time that something has not been right. At last somebody is explaining it all in simple language.

As this kind of openness occurs, the instructor must encourage the student to suggest ways for correcting the problem. Intelligent students like Pete, even in the primary grades, are able to help in planning their remedial activities. The teacher must make it clear what his or her expectations are. This is often done in the form of a simple contract stating the specific dyslexic patterns (backward letters, transposed syllables, reversed numbers) and what the student promises to do each day to overcome them. The teacher makes it clear how much one-to-one time he or she can give to Pete during the school day. If the teacher can manage three 5-minute periods during recess or the lunch hour, this needs to be specified. The important thing is that Pete knows how much individual attention he can expect.

Study Buddy Helpers

It is usually possible to pair Pete with a classmate who is mature enough to guide him through some practice in those skills that he still has not mastered. Students with dyslexia need personal feedback that comes from working with a partner. The "study buddy" *does not* teach new skills, but rather walks through familiar tasks with Pete. They talk about where he gets stuck. They practice together doing it again until he feels sure of himself. The study buddy becomes a reading partner when Pete needs to read a story or a textbook assignment for tomorrow. This classmate helps Pete edit his writing so that all of his differences are spotted and corrected before he turns in his paper to the teacher.

Older Students as Learning Partners

A promising source of help for one-to-one tutoring during the school day is older students who can fit into the school routine without disrupting classroom procedures. Older students are especially effective as tutors, provided there is no clash between them and the child with dyslexia. A small amount of personal attention from an older learner goes a long way in building self-confidence in this youngster, especially if the older student has overcome learning difficulties. Two or three 30-minute sessions during the school week often are enough to unlock the perceptual block, allowing the younger student to make significant progress in overcoming a specific challenge.

Arithmetic

In Chapter 1, the perceptual dilemma that students with dyslexia face in mastering arithmetic skills was reviewed. Pete's major problem in arithmetic is his frustration in having to change direction in every addition, subtraction, multiplication, and division problem he works. Arithmetic computation above the primary level involves countless transformations as numerals and number units change position inside the problem. Arithmetic symbols are a highly condensed kind of decoding in which a single symbol often stands for a complex abstract concept. It would take many lines of writing to express clearly the memory factors involved in most math problems and equations. Students who tend to scramble sequence, lose direction, or reverse and transpose details find it very difficult to master the countless variations they encounter in advanced arithmetic and mathematics.

The foremost consideration for adults to remember in working with students such as Pete is to keep the structure as nearly the same as possible. It is distressing for Pete to have to shift back and forth from linear form (7 + 13) to vertical form:

$$\begin{array}{r} 7 \\ +13 \\ \hline \end{array}$$

Lessons requiring students to transform frequently on the same page impose enormous memory stress. These students quickly become agitated, overly frustrated, or even rebellious. Thus, keeping the form of problems the same is a good idea. Most students who have dyslexia can learn both vertical and linear formats; however, they cannot rapidly change back and forth on the same page because they need structure that stays the same as much as possible. Whenever teachers have to vary the problem format, these individuals must be given all the time and help they need in making the perceptual shifts. Some students never learn to do so. For them, the standard vertical problem format is the only arithmetic style they can comprehend safely.

Pocket calculators. As today's students move into the 21st century, they must be fluent in using a variety of electronic technology in the workplace. No curriculum should put off the use of pocket calculators beyond primary grades. Students who are gifted in arithmetic and mathematics should be taught calculator usage along with beginning reading skills. Students like Pete need to use pocket calculators to give them the opportunity to find success in the classroom. This does not mean that they will skip a functional knowledge of paper-and-pencil computing, but it is imperative that they be taught to compensate for their math limitations by using modern technology. When using paper and pencil to do math, Pete is forced to plod along at a snail's pace as he struggles to transfer mental images of number information into writing. A pocket calculator gives him an instant means of speeding up his work and increasing his self-confidence because he now can keep up with the fastest pencil performers in the class. What a boost to his morale it is to hold his own after so much embarrassment and sense of failure when he works math problems with a pencil. High school and college math instructors require the use of pocket calculators; therefore, forcing students who have LD to labor with traditional paper-and-pencil computation is as obsolete as requiring math students to use a slide rule.

Finger touching. Students with loose sensory integration have to do something physical to keep all their memory circuits integrated. They cannot develop or hold onto complete mental images just by thinking about numbers—they must touch, say, see, and hear all at the same time. Students with dyslexia cannot do arithmetic without whispering and counting their fingers. They are immediately disabled in most math assignments if adults demand that they work silently with no finger involvement.

Visible and tactile structure. Instructors must keep two cardinal rules in mind when teaching arithmetic skills to dyslexic learners like Pete:

1. *Keep the structure constant.* Because conservation of form is so difficult for individuals who have dyslexia, arithmetic structure must remain the same from day to day. Frequent changes in work-page format and directionality that changes too often are devastating to confused students like Pete, who cannot handle rapid shifts in form.

2. *Keep the pace slow.* Learners who have dyslexia must not be pressured to hurry in doing arithmetic computation. If quantity is important, they must be given alternatives or options, such as using a pocket calculator in order to equalize the situation—making up the vast difference between the perceptual talents of rapid learners and the limited math talent over which the student with dyslexia has little control. If paper-and-pencil routines are essential, then the rate must be slow.

Reading and Writing

Reading orally. Reading aloud is essential for correcting reversals and rotations. As the student with dyslexia reads slowly from a text, the tutor or teacher monitors from another copy. As mistakes occur, the monitor quietly says, "Look at that word again, Pete. How is it spelled?" This sort of cueing is low-key and does not embarrass Pete by calling attention to his errors. By immediately pinpointing error patterns, the tutor reinforces accurate symbol perception on a one-to-one basis. Pete soon begins to catch his own errors by coordinating what he sees, says, hears, and touches as he reads.

Keyboard writing. Most students who have dyslexia can develop satisfactory writing skills through a word-processor system that has self-correcting spelling and grammar features. In Chapter 1, Steeves's research with boys with severe dyslexia was discussed (Steeves, 1987). When these boys learned a simple touch-typing technique using Apple computers, their writing skills became 15 times more efficient than when they used a pencil. As technology continues to develop, Pete and students like him will have access to a variety of talk-back computers that will tell him when he has made errors in writing and math, allowing Pete to bypass most of his problems in producing written work. The goal should be for students with dyslexia to do most of their necessary school writing using a word processor by the time they enter fourth grade. Many schools encourage learners in elementary grades to use laptop computers in the classroom, which is especially important for dysgraphic students, who cannot produce large quantities of written material in a legible form.

Keyboard writing sets the student free to put thoughts and information onto paper without "shorting out" and losing so much of the mental image. The physical act of pinching the pencil (tactile pressure) "shorts out" the mental image, but the quick act of tapping keys does not cause this problem. Keyboard writing for students like Pete sets the mind free for much more fluent expression of ideas and information. Once parents and teachers have accepted keyboard writing as a legitimate alternative for doing school-work, much of the conflict over dyslexic writing disappears. An editor or study buddy must still look over Pete's finished writing to help him spot mistakes, but keyboard writing has allowed him to become skilled with encoding far beyond the level he could achieve with pencil or pen.

Matching word forms. Daily practice activities can be devised by parents, teachers, or study partners to develop greater accuracy in word discrimination. A word is presented on a card and the student tries to find a matching word within a line of similar words. The following examples from the *Jordan Written Screening Test* (Jordan, 1989b) show how this activity is done:

Word on Card	Choices on the Worksheet
barn	barn pran puar buar narb uarp barn
spot	spot tobs tops stop stob sbot tobs
silver	sliver silver vilser rivils revlis selvir

Reading with a marker. Chapter 1 includes a discussion of off-center vision that occurs in many persons with dyslexia. For a majority of individuals with visual dyslexia symptoms, it is essential that they use some kind of marker in order to read paragraphs, stories, and pages of print. Some individuals must use a card with a slot cut out so that only one or two words are seen at one time. Others need a card marker held just below each line as the eyes work across the line of print. Some readers with visual dyslexia can get by without a card by brushing a finger or a pencil beneath each word as the eyes refocus from place to place along the line of print. Others must hold a marker below the line while the left thumb punches each word above the line. Still other students need to use two fingers to frame each word or isolate chunks within words. It does not matter what the student uses as a marker. Educators who have taught literacy skills in storefront classrooms or prison facilities have seen adults use cigarettes, pocket combs, sticks of gum, and other kinds of unusual markers. The point is that most persons with dyslexia must develop some kind of marking system to hold their focus steady. Without marking, their eyes soon lose the place and they no longer see printed details clearly. Reading with a marker usually doubles or triples the length of time a person who has dyslexia can read before he or she must rest from visual burnout.

Keeping Track of Progress

Parents, teachers, and study partners who help students like Pete overcome dyslexia need to keep track of progress. This should be a simple procedure requiring a minimal amount of bookkeeping. Older students can be taught to record their own progress, as they do in other individualized study programs.

The initial task is for the instructor to use checklists like the ones in this book to prepare a *Progress Profile* that outlines all of a student's dyslexic tendencies. For example, in Chapter 1 the patterns of word blindness are listed (see the "Word Blindness" section). If Pete displays any of those difficulties, his Progress Profile lists these visual perception stumbling blocks. If he responds to reduced light, colored page overlays, or reading from colored paper, those facts are noted along with his word blind symptoms. Appendix B lists the characteristics of visual dyslexia (letters reversed or rotated, numbers reversed, words read backward, and so forth). Appendix C lists the symptoms of auditory dyslexia, Appendix D lists symptoms of dysgraphia, and Appendix E outlines dyscalculia. Once Pete's Progress Profile is prepared, the instructor discusses this project with him. He understands that the goal is to eliminate these stumbling blocks one by one. As Pete conquers his dyslexic patterns, brief comments are recorded to indicate improvement. The final entry beside each dyslexic characteristic is the date when Pete and his instructors agree that this specific stumbling block has come under his control. As Pete, his instructors, and his parents compile this record of improvement, his self-confidence and self-esteem grow by leaps and bounds.

The Progress Profile offers two advantages for remedial work at home and in the classroom. First, prescriptive teaching is straightforward, once the specific stumbling blocks are identified on the checklist. Pete's teachers and tutors pace his progress from one skill level to the next without too much confusion. Until the Progress Profile shows that a specific problem has been cleared up, instructors know not to push Pete on to a more frustrating activity level. Second, the Progress Profile forms the basis for a reasonable work contract between Pete and his instructors. At all times Pete knows exactly how much remains to be overcome in his learning behavior. Without this kind of simple record and the open communication it fosters between teachers and learners, everyone involved continues to wallow in frustration and failure.

The most reliable index of how successful Pete's remedial program is will be his frustration level. So long as adults observe tension, frustration, anxiety, dread, avoidance tactics, disruptive behavior, or other symptoms of learning difficulty, they know that Pete's disability continues to overwhelm him. Regardless of the age of the student or the lateness in the school year, it is useless and dangerous to push overly frustrated learners further and further through the books when they clearly are too overwhelmed to succeed. Instructors will know when the perceptual foundation has taken hold. Pete begins to exhibit longer stamina without becoming upset, compared with his former quick frustration during study activities. When he can work rather calmly for half an hour with tasks that used to trigger emotional outbursts within a few minutes, his teachers know that remediation has been effective. Then it is time to take Pete to the next step in perceptual development.

Making Referrals

Four out of five individuals with dyslexia can respond to the techniques suggested in this chapter and remain in a mainstream classroom environment; however, some cannot. One in five will require specialized remedial therapy away from a group environment. Parents and teachers should call for special help when a student like Pete has reached the end of his tolerance. When continuing with his educational program triggers more emotionally charged conflict than growth in learning, it is time for special intervention to take place. A rule of thumb for referral to other agencies might be this:

> So long as the student is making some progress, I will keep up my efforts to cope with his or her special needs. When behavior becomes too disruptive, or when the student becomes so frustrated that he or she cannot continue to learn in the situation, then I will refer that learner to another agency for special help.

In Chapter 1, the dilemma of determining the presence of a learning disability through score-discrepancy testing was described. Most states have firm legal guidelines regarding who is qualified to administer diagnostic tests and who may determine which persons have a learning disability. Some states forbid use of such labels as dyslexia and Attention-Deficit Disorder when school-related psychologists or psychometrists do the evaluation. It is not unusual for parents to be told that a child has a disability according to test-score profiles. But if parents ask whether the child is dyslexic or has Attention-Deficit Disorder, the examiner may not be permitted by law or regulation to use those clinical designations. Nor is it unusual for teachers to see massive symptoms of dyslexia and Attention-Deficit Disorder in daily classroom behavior, yet for that child not to be identified by score-discrepancy evaluation. If Pete fails to show a wide enough discrepancy between his Full Scale IQ score and his standard scores in reading, language skills, and math, he may not be identified as LD in spite of poor reading, very poor spelling, and total frustration with arithmetic.

Appendix F lists a variety of useful publications and support groups that are prepared to advise parents how to obtain special help for a child who needs it. There is no nationwide standard policy for finding appropriate special help for students with LD. Dyslexia is recognized in federal law (Education for All Handicapped Children Act of 1975, P.L. 94-142) as being a specific learning disorder that shall be treated in the least restrictive and most appropriate manner by each school, but each state has different policies for implementing that mandate. Attention-Deficit Disorder is not yet a mandated form of learning disability in most school districts. Appendix F provides sources for finding out how dyslexia, Attention-Deficit Disorder, and other types of LD are treated in the local school district.

WHAT IS REQUIRED TO OVERCOME VISUAL DYSLEXIA

No book can include all of the techniques for overcoming visual dyslexia. Parents, tutors, and teachers must tailor corrective techniques to fit the specific needs of each student. A Progress Profile that shows specifically and clearly what must be done to overcome dyslexia in each learner was described previously. Regardless of what remedial techniques are used, some fundamental principles must be observed in working with students with dyslexia.

Principle 1: Positive Self-Fulfilling Prophecy

Much attention has been drawn to the power that adult attitudes hold over the success or failure of struggling students such as Pete. A general principle can be stated: *Learners tend to behave as teachers and parents expect them to behave.* In other words, students tend to return the feelings and attitudes they sense in their leaders. If the adults in Pete's life believe that he can succeed with their help, he will do his best to do so. Positive teachers who respect their students are usually respected in return. Negative teachers who regard them as failures with little hope for success find these pupils failing while displaying negative, disrespectful attitudes that disrupt the class. What a struggling student achieves is closely tied to teacher attitudes and expectations.

The attitude of the leader is a critical factor for students like Pete. Some instructors are not temperamentally suited for working with students who have dyslexia. They are put off by the struggles they witness when their students do not have talent for reading, spelling, writing, or math. If working with these students is offensive or uncomfortable for an educator, it will be impossible for a warm, accepting relationship to be established. Students with learning differences do not respond positively to uncomfortable or overly critical leaders. More harm than good comes from forced associations between educators who dread dealing with these students and students who are apprehensive toward teachers who feel that way. It is essential that instructors have positive expectations and affection for learners who are struggling.

Principle 2: Work on What the Learner Needs

Unless teaching techniques actually meet the learner's needs, valuable time and energy are wasted and no educational growth is achieved. This principle can be expressed in a practical 3-point guide:

1. What does the student need?
2. What would be nice for the student to know?
3. What is irrelevant at this time?

In overcoming dyslexia, answers to these questions are of great importance. If Pete does not know the alphabet, then learning the alphabet is his need of the moment. It would be nice for him to read 25 books this year, but not essential. It would be totally irrelevant for him to attempt to write book reports. In other words, if the foundation has never been laid, it is foolish to attempt to build the upper floors. If the student needs the foundation, regardless of age or number of years in school, then the foundation is where instruction must begin. Because students with dyslexia do not fit the standard academic mold, they are termed disabled, which is a heavily loaded negative label. A more positive point of view was presented in Chapter 1 in the section on the four current meanings of LD. Regarding dyslexia as a *learning difference* takes away much of the sting and hurt that wrap around the label *disabled.* When parents and teachers discover each student's need, as differentiated from what would be nice and what is irrelevant, a teaching plan can be developed specifying exact skills the student has not yet learned. This practical approach is simple, direct, and nonthreatening. By filling Pete's urgent needs, the instructor enables him to build the foundation that will later let him move on to things it would be nice for him to know. As needs are fulfilled, what was irrelevant becomes increasingly more relevant. The instructors will see Pete working toward higher-level skills surprisingly soon, once a solid foundation has been laid.

Principle 3: Relax the Pressure

Students with dyslexia have two mortal enemies: *a work rate that goes too fast* and *pressure to produce more quantity than limited skills make possible.* They must work slowly as they write and read because there is no way to make the left-brain language centers speed up the process of translating language symbols that reverse, turn upside down, or scramble. The most threatening experience for someone like Pete is to be forced to hurry in reading, spelling, writing, or arithmetic tasks. The result is panic. Timed standardized tests are especially threatening to students with dyslexia. The click of a stopwatch or the starting whir of a timing clock are sounds of failure. Time penalties are as cruel for one who has dyslexia as being forced to run in a track meet would be for a person with a broken leg. Educators who are unaware of this panic reaction to time pressure can inflict deep emotional anguish in students whose thought patterns are slow in processing symbols.

Pressure to produce quantities of written work is equally devastating. When confronted by assignments that demand large quantities of work within a limited amount of time, Pete panics and gives up. A major cause of disruptive behavior is demanding too much quantity from individuals who run out of time or cannot do assignments without help. A rule of thumb should be to expect students with dyslexia to work three times more slowly than classmates who have no perceptual limitations. If classmates who are talented in written language skills can write 20 sentences in half an hour, Pete will struggle to complete 5 or 6 in the same length of time. If most students in the class can handle five pages of silent reading during a study period, the reader who is dyslexic may barely finish one without help.

When adults allow for these very real limitations in work rate, struggling students are usually willing to do their best. If the purpose of assignments is to strengthen skills, then it does not matter whether Pete finishes 5 or 20 items, so long as he does his best. Educators set struggling learners up for failure when quantity in a hurry rather than quality becomes the goal.

WHAT IS FAIR?

In relaxing time pressure and tailoring quantity to fit Pete's special learning needs, instructors may be placed on the defensive by critics who say that it is not fair to let students with dyslexia get out of doing all the work the other students are required to do. There is an answer for this point of view. When educators truly believe that every person is entitled to an education according to his or her needs, ways can be found to fill those needs. Relaxing pressure for speed and quantity is a sensible educational objective, especially for students who do not have the neurological talent for traditional language-based expectations. If dyslexia were a visible difference that required life-support equipment, this complaint would not occur. In Chapter 1, ample evidence was presented that having dyslexia is beyond the control of the individual. Fairness must be pegged to personal limitations. Those who complain about unfairness when accommodations are made for specific differences are speaking out of a lack of knowledge.

Principle 4: Keep It Simple

There is nothing simple about today's school curriculum. Brilliant adults who delight in manipulating complicated theory have designed dozens of advanced programs for elementary and middle schools. Each new textbook adoption startles parents and teachers who see advanced abstract concepts being brought into kindergarten and primary education. All kinds of pressures are exerted by special interest groups for cramming more and more into the already complex curricula of most children. This buildup of high expectations is overwhelming for students with dyslexia, who are confused by the bombardment of new information at every turn. Even fun time is so overorganized in many schools that sensitive children dread recess.

Dyslexia involves the inability to sort out sensory impressions rapidly enough to stay on group schedules. Classroom success is not a matter of learning how to react appropriately to the flow of new information. Instead, academic achievement is the result of learning how not to react to the overload of irrelevant stimuli that bombards students from every side. Those who have dyslexia cannot tune out irrelevant information well enough to keep up with the central data flow. They cannot edit their environment quickly enough to identify what is relevant. The result is a mass of inaccurate, too cluttered, or incomplete mental images that leaves the student unable to cope.

Dyslexia can be remediated only when outside stimulus factors are carefully controlled. Teaching students like Pete requires clearly stated step-by-step routines that expose them only to the amount of stimuli they can handle at a given time. For example, when lessons include several concepts, Pete cannot cope with a variety of expectations at the same time and flounders in a sea of expectations he does not understand clearly. The result is either no gain in learning or loss of learning through frustration and sense of failure. However, if Pete is guided from one skill to the next at a pace he can handle, eventually he will learn to cope with complicated tasks.

Because the principle of simplicity has always been at the heart of good teaching, curriculum materials usually are programmed to introduce new facts step-by-step. The problem is not so much with materials or with curriculum goals, but with trying to accomplish too much too quickly. It is imperative that educators keep instruction simple until perceptual foundations are firmly established.

Principle 5: Keep It Structured

In Chapter 1, Denckla's concept that reading, spelling, language skills, and math are specialized talents fostered by how brain pathways are developed was described (Denckla, 1993). A prominent concept in today's curriculum is that good teaching guides learners to discover essential information rather than being told about it. Denckla's research has convinced many educators that the ability to discover is also a specialized talent not shared by everyone. In every classroom, some students are talented discoverers. No one has estimated the ratio of discoverers to nondiscoverers in our population. Classroom teachers often are confronted by curriculum goals based on the premise that all students will discover fundamental concepts if they explore enough. However, the fact is that millions of students have not acquired basic skills in math, spelling, grammar, science, and reading in spite of attractive materials designed to let students explore and discover for themselves.

A cardinal truth regarding LD and dyslexia is that learning new skills must be highly structured. This principle does not contradict theories of self-discovery. Persons with dyslexia cannot cope with loosely structured situations, and discovery learning is not possible for most individuals until they have experienced specific, structured drill in foundation skills. For example, Pete cannot assemble parts into coherent wholes unless there is a clearly defined model to show him how. Abstract reasoning without visible structure is a major stumbling block.

Parents and teachers must provide clearly structured, familiar teaching routines upon which students with dyslexia can depend. This rules out certain kinds of multiple-stimulus activities specified in teachers' manuals and guidebooks. Words with multiple meanings, variant spellings of vowel or consonant sounds, open-ended grammar or punctuation rules, and indefinite elements of math, science, and

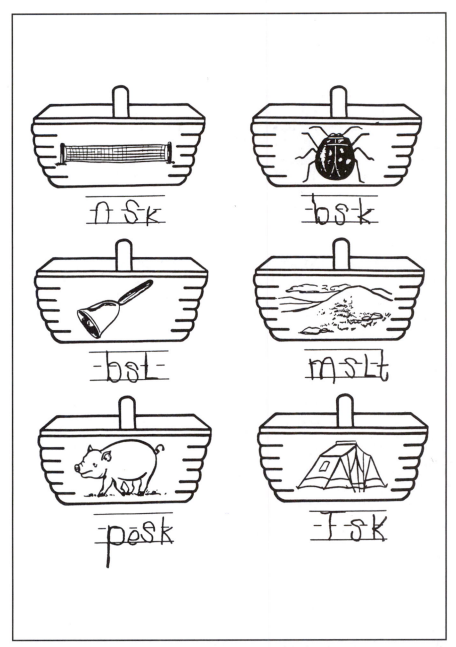

FIGURE 2.7. The instructions were: "Write the word for each picture." Pete saw two pictures. His mental images crossed over and produced mixed images. Every time he wrote the first letter of the *inside picture,* his mental image finished the *outside picture* (basket).

social studies are highly threatening to students who cannot function when things change too much from lesson to lesson.

Figure 2.7 shows what happens when a student like Pete is expected to do more than one task at a time on a page. The teacher decided to make a phonics page more interesting by showing each picture task inside a basket. Pete's task was to write the name of each picture he saw inside each basket. Figure 2.7 shows the phenomenon of *perceptual cross-over.* What Pete saw (visual perception) crossed over into what he heard (auditory perception) as he said each picture name to himself. In each instance, he correctly wrote the first letter/sound for each picture. But the predominant hard consonant cluster /sk/ in *basket* crowded out his perception of the rest of each word. When Pete looked at the visual image of a basket, he could no longer concentrate on the auditory image of the object name. Instructors must not pile perceptual tasks on top of each other on work pages.

Overcoming Auditory Dyslexia

Within the dyslexic population is another specific pattern called auditory dyslexia, which actually has nothing to do with hearing as such. Most of the individuals with auditory dyslexia have excellent hearing ability, but what they hear others say is not interpreted correctly by the language-processing centers of the left brain. In Chapter 1, Tallal, Miller, and Fitch's (1993) discovery that auditory dyslexia is caused by deficits in cell structure within the auditory pathway that links the middle ear with the auditory cortex was discussed. Figure 3.1 shows the listening highway that must function fluently in translating what the ears hear into language information within the auditory cortex. Tallal discovered a double cell structure along the auditory pathway shown in Figure 3.1. One set of cells delivers the fast, hard speech sounds that arrive first in the auditory cortex. The other set of cells delivers the softer, slower speech sounds that arrive somewhat later. When this brain structure is mature, the person has no trouble hearing all of the hard and soft speech sounds in the right sequence. A mature listening brain structure blends all of these chunks of speech into language patterns that make sense. When some of these sound processing cells are incomplete, however, the listener is tone deaf to many of the softer, slower chunks of sound that make up spoken language.

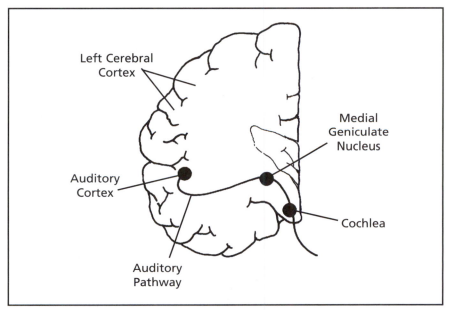

FIGURE 3.1. In 1993, Tallal discovered how the left brain processes oral language. We identify the sounds of our language in a 3-step process. *Step 1:* The inner ear (cochlea) gathers in the sound waves of spoken language. *Step 2:* This sound energy is sent to a portion of the midbrain (medial geniculate nucleus). Here the fast and slow chunks of human speech are organized. *Step 3:* The organized fast and slow sound chunks are sent on to the auditory cortex where the brain recognizes the speech code. Auditory dyslexia is caused by incomplete cell development along the auditory pathway between the cochlea (inner ear) and medial geniculate nucleus (midbrain). This incomplete cell formation makes it impossible for the person to hear the strings of fast and slow sound chunks correctly. This individual is tone deaf to speech sounds.

The spoken English language is built from chunks of sound called *phonemes.* Each syllable, word, phrase, or sentence we speak consists of chains of fast/slow/fast/slow phoneme chunks. Infants and toddlers whose brain pathways are developing on schedule begin to mimic and repeat these chunks or patterns they hear. As youngsters mature, they become increasingly skilled at repeating the phoneme patterns of whatever language they hear in their families and communities. In Chapter 1, Delayed Language Development (DLD) syndrome was described (Wilson & Risucci, 1986). The heart of DLD syndrome is the child's inability to hear oral language correctly. These tone deaf youngsters are locked out of normal language usage. Because they do not hear phoneme chunks clearly, they cannot mimic or reproduce the oral language their culture speaks fluently.

Particular attention should be paid to physical patterns that signal tone deafness in certain children. Those who are born into families in which dyslexia occurs are at a high risk for being tone deaf to the hard/soft/hard/soft chains of sound that make up oral communication. Children who have chronic ear infections (otitis media) during the first 18 months also are at very high risk for being tone deaf when they are exposed to formal phonics instruction. Otitis media in early childhood damages the delicate middle ear systems (hammer, anvil, stirrup, and cilia) so that it is physically impossible for the ears to gather complete sound patterns.

Tallal's research has focused attention upon the structure of oral language. For example, the word *cat* is made of three sound chunks: hard /k/–soft /a/–hard /t/. Persons who have no cell structure deficits along the auditory pathway instantly recognize these three sound chunks in correct sequence. Tone deaf individuals do not. For example, Maria's teacher says, "Listen as I say *cat* . . . *cat*. Maria, tell me the sound of the vowel in *cat*." Maria, who is tone deaf, is bewildered. She does not hear the soft /a/ vowel in the word *cat*. What is the teacher talking about? Maria hears the hard /k/ at the beginning of *cat*. She sort of hears the hard /t/ at the end of *cat*. She has no idea that there is a soft /a/ sound in the middle of *cat*.

Maria faces growing auditory perception problems when she is required to listen to complete sentences. For example, her teacher says, "Get out your blue notebook." This simple oral sentence is made from a chain of hard/fast and slow/soft sound chunks:

/g/e/t/ou/t/yuh/oo/r/b/l/oo/n/o/t/b/oo/k/

Maria's tone deafness blocks several of the slower, softer sound chunks. She hears only part of this string of speech sounds:

/g/–/t/–/oo/r–/b/l/–/o/–/b/–/k/

Maria hears a variation of what the teacher said: "Go tour blow book." This makes no sense. Her first impulse is to blurt out "Huh? What? What do you mean?" But being scolded for interrupting and not trying to listen has taught her not to ask these listening questions. The teacher notices that Maria has not responded to the instructions. "Didn't you hear what I said, Maria?" the teacher asks impatiently. "I said get out your blue notebook." Still the oral message is not clear. She quickly glances around to see what her classmates are doing. Maria gets through the school day by gleaning clues from her neighbors more than from understanding what her teacher says.

Learners such as Maria who have auditory dyslexia struggle with the consequences of not hearing all the chunks of oral language. They cannot rhyme words successfully, do not understand the words in songs, cannot hear rhyming words in poetry, misunderstand conversations and what is said on television or the radio, and have great difficulty connecting sounds to letters from memory. This makes it impossible for them to become good at spelling or word sounding. Children such as Maria are forever in conflict with adults because they do not interpret oral instructions correctly. We can understand the mystery of auditory dyslexia more clearly if we think of individuals who are deaf to the differences in musical tones. Music is processed by the right brain in the same way oral language is processed by the left brain. One of the most painful experiences for sensitive music teachers and vocal coaches is the monotone student who cannot carry a tune. No matter how much musical drill this person receives, he or she never learns vocal music skills. Persons like Maria are tone deaf to sounds of speech the way that other individuals cannot hear notes and tones of music.

AUDITORY DYSLEXIA SYNDROME

At the beginning of the 20th century, U.S. educators had a simple concept of oral language learning. The standard for spoken language was General American English. Those who were coached in singing or in public speaking were drilled in correct articulation of the oral language patterns that set the standard for that day. As radio broadcasting developed following World War I, increasing emphasis was placed upon correct enunciation of General American English. One's cultural status and educational progress were judged by how clearly one spoke the dialect. Of course, there always have been regional speech differences—persons reared and educated in Boston have never been mistaken for individuals from west Texas or Alabama. Immigrants who brought other languages into the United States were largely judged by how quickly they became literate in General American English. Reading, spelling, and written language skills were modeled after this single standard of correctness. The oral language standard for the first part of the 20th century assumed that everyone, regardless of region or origin, had the ability to master the fundamental oral language patterns of that day.

World War II radically changed all that. As U.S. society recovered from that war experience, old standards of correct language usage dramatically changed. Multicultural standards rapidly took the place of the earlier single standard for language development. By the 1960s, federal law mandated that metropolitan schools provide instruction in a variety of languages to meet the communication needs of many U.S. citizens who had come from other countries and cultures. Learning English as a second language (ESL) became a major educational enterprise as millions of non–English speaking children and adults entered the schools and the workforce. Today, U.S. society is quite unsure as to what the standard should be for teaching language usage skills.

Since the 1940s, several valuable lessons about teaching and learning language skills have been learned. First, this great mixing of cultures in the United States has revealed the extent of LD and dyslexic patterns throughout the human race. Regardless of national or cultural origin, dyslexia is a universal presence among children, adolescents, and adults. Second, few persons master all of the letter–sound relationships of their speech culture. There is worldwide evidence to support Denckla's concept that some of us are neurologically talented to become good readers, spellers, writers, or mathematicians. Many of us are not, no matter what our language background, and most of us have certain areas of phonetic weakness.

RECOGNIZING AUDITORY DYSLEXIA

Appendix C provides a list of the characteristics of auditory dyslexia. This checklist permits parents and teachers to make an inventory of the specific points in language processing where struggling students bog down. By identifying specific stumbling blocks in language processing, adults can develop remedial programs designed to remove auditory dyslexic patterns step-by-step. The following descriptions also pinpoint the patterns of auditory dyslexia in the classroom.

Print Does Not Match Speech

It is not difficult to identify tone deaf persons like Maria who struggle to convert oral language into writing or printed language into speech. When trying to write original sentences or paragraphs, Maria cannot think of what to put on her paper. Even when she says good sentences orally, she does not realize that she can write those same words to make sentences. When trying to read, Maria does not recognize that written words stand for oral words she uses in daily speech. Even though Maria has fluent oral speaking skills, she often cannot make the connection between what she or others say and what she sees in print. An observer will notice that these individuals struggle to connect what they see on the page with their own oral language. For them, reading and writing are foreign languages even though the words are pronounced the same. Auditory dyslexia is like a bridge that is out between the form of the words on paper and the meaning of those words in speech.

Tone Deaf to Phoneme Chunks

A primary characteristic of auditory dyslexia is the inability to hear variations of vowel sounds. Most reading programs emphasize the long and short sounds of five vowels: *a, e, i, o, u.* Although *w* and *y* are also vowels (called *semivowels*), teachers do not always teach specific sounds for *w* and *y.* Educators have assumed that students who have clear speech should have no trouble telling the difference between long vowel and short vowel sounds. This is not true for students with auditory dyslexia. They have great difficulty distinguishing such close-sounding words as *big* and *beg* or *cat* and *cot.* For them, subtle distinctions in speech sounds do not exist.

A similar problem exists when they encounter consonant clusters (also called blends and digraphs). Few students with auditory dyslexia can hear the separate consonant sounds in such clusters as *st, sp, gr,* or *pl.* For example, Maria usually can hear the first consonant letter sound in familiar words; however, frequently it is impossible for her to hear the second or third sound in clusters such as *str, spl,* or *shr.*

Auditory dyslexia often remains undetected during the primary grades, particularly when formal phonics and spelling instruction are postponed until late second grade or early third grade. Most beginner pupils stumble in their first encounters with organized reading and writing instruction. When the whole word (sight memory) approach or whole language method is used in primary grades, teachers can remain unaware that certain pupils are not hearing sounds accurately.

Confusion with Words: Alike or Different?

One of the earmarks of auditory dyslexia is the student's inability to tell whether words are the same or different. Maria is typical of an individual who struggles with auditory dyslexia. Her teacher has begun to suspect that she does not hear sounds accurately and uses the *Jordan Auditory Screening Test* (Jordan, 1972; see Appendix C). This structured listening test identifies the accuracy of Maria's auditory perception of the phoneme chunks of oral language. The following is a sample of her performance:

"Maria, listen carefully as I say each set of words. Tell me *Alike* if the two words are exactly the same. Tell me *Different* if the two words are not exactly the same."

Pronounced by Teacher	Maria's Responses
"bed–dead"	Different
"dime–time"	Alike
"back–pack"	Alike
"look–look"	Alike
"tam–dam"	Alike
"pane–bane"	Alike
"dill–bill"	Different
"say–say"	Alike
"fat–vat"	Alike
"no–no"	Alike
"hot–what"	Alike
"vetch–fetch"	Alike
"mile–Nile"	Different
"where–hare"	Alike
"got–got"	Alike

Many students with dyslexia do not follow instructions well enough to give the standard answers a teacher expects. Instead of saying "Alike" or "Different," Maria might say "Yes" or "No" or "Same" and "Not Same." Such responses should not be regarded as incorrect. The point is to find out whether Maria hears sounds accurately, not whether she can parrot back stereotyped answers. Much of the conflict in the classroom between teachers and students with auditory dyslexia is triggered when the adult fails to interpret correctly the student's confusion with signals.

This kind of informal listening evaluation reveals some significant deficiencies in Maria's auditory perception ability. The teacher now has definite guidelines for corrective teaching. This brief activity has revealed Maria's confusion with four sets of similar sound chunks: /d/ and /t/, /b/ and /p/, /f/ and /v/, /h/ and /hw/. The teacher now will be alert for other areas of faulty auditory perception as she guides Maria's reading and spelling growth. One caveat must be mentioned regarding the results of tests such as the *Jordan Auditory Screening Test:* Occasionally, a student with auditory dyslexia can make a perfect score when only single words are said in pairs. The score from an auditory discrimination test neither establishes nor eliminates dyslexia until other kinds of auditory dyslexic symptoms also are identified.

Mishearing Words

Mishearing words creates continual problems for students who have auditory dyslexia as they respond to what goes on around them. For example, Maria's teacher kept a record of the misunderstandings that occurred in the girl's listening during 1 day at school.

Teacher Said	Maria Heard
leopard	leprosy
pity	picky
curiosity	cures
grief	grease
compare	repair
rose	roll
gulf stream	gull stream (later, golf stream)
defends	difference

This kind of record of a student's auditory misperception helps parents and teachers understand much of the conflict that flares in the student's relationships with others. Every time Maria misunderstood what her teacher said, an argument followed. Because she is bright, Maria wanted to tell what she knew as the words were used by the teacher.

Students with this faulty auditory perception are forever "darting off on rabbit trails." Because she misheard *grief* as *grease,* Maria mentally darted away to think about an experience involving grease while everyone else was thinking about the issue of grief. It is hard for adults and classmates to realize that Maria is not just being stubborn or difficult, but that she responds to what she "hears." This sets Maria apart when it comes to fitting into her environment.

Confusion with Spelling

Auditory dyslexia is a primary cause for habitually poor spelling. Because Maria does not hear separate sounds accurately, there is no way for her to remember how to spell. Traditional spelling instruction is filled with frustration for children with auditory dyslexia. When an arbitrary list of unrelated words is assigned on Monday to be memorized by the student for Friday's dictation test, the child with dyslexia faces a frustrating predicament. Creative students often devise their own memory systems for remembering spelling patterns ("when" is *h-e-n* with *w* in front; "mother" is *t-h-e* with *mo* in front and *r* at the end). Today's curriculum involving thousands of words presented at an even faster pace soon produces impossible demands for these students—few of them are clever enough to figure out memory devices for all the words they must write.

Frequent Erasing

One of the surest symptoms of auditory dyslexia is chronic erasing, crossing out, and marking over on paper to correct written mistakes. A careful observer soon understands why students with dyslexia struggle through writing activities so nervously. They usually "think out loud" as they work, whispering over and over, trying it several ways, erasing, then writing another combination of letters. They never are sure they have spelled a word correctly. Handwriting is a very personal picture of any writer's self, but especially so for the insecure student who never has been able to please teachers or parents. Every word committed to paper exposes the insecure speller to probable failure. These students erase again and again, desperately trying to "luck out" with the correct combinations of letters, hoping to please critics but not really expecting to succeed. Many students who have dyslexia try to hide their work as they write, a further indication of their dread of failure.

Spelling Mistake Patterns

Certain mistake patterns are seen in the spelling efforts of persons with auditory dyslexia. Four basic patterns of error will be apparent, regardless of the source of the dictation.

Transposed consonants. Writers with dyslexia habitually change consonant patterns. *Barn* becomes *bran, play* becomes *paly, girl* becomes *gril.* The student seldom recognizes these transpositions because of the underlying difficulty connecting sounds to letters in the right sequence.

Phonetic spelling. It is almost impossible for learners with auditory dyslexia to apply phonics rules to spelling. When attempting to write what she hears, Maria gropes for literal translations. Teachers can spot this tendency if the student's garbled writing is read phonetically. In her attempts to write familiar words, Maria may write *reefews* for *refuse* or *gard* for *guard.* The old cliche that a child cannot spell *cat* is sometimes true: Persons with deep dyslexia often write *kat* for *cat* and *cind* for *kind.*

Sound chunks omitted. The most significant indicator in spelling of auditory dyslexia is the habit of leaving out sound chunks within longer words. This problem is sometimes called *telescoping.* The following examples illustrate this tendency:

Dictated by Teacher	Student's Written Response
remember	rember
extravagance	exstragunce
tuberculosis	toberkulous
candidacy	candiace
indefinitely	endefinely

Sound chunks added. A further characteristic of auditory dyslexia is the tendency to add unnecessary sound chunks when writing words, called *perseveration*. This tendency is illustrated below.

Dictated by Teacher	Student's Written Response
duck	dukey
pretty	patting
party	paturing
doll	dalken
blizzard	blizzered
successful	sucessiful
immediate	immediant
intimate	intament
legitimate	lagetiment
zephyr	zesphir

Figure 3.2 shows an effective 15-word dictation test devised by Ernest Jones. This simple evaluation instrument allows an instructor to detect auditory dyslexic symptoms quickly. A more complete diagnostic picture for older students can be obtained from dictated word lists that include longer words. Figure 3.3 shows the attempt by a 21-year-old man to write from dictation. He had graduated from high school after spending 13 years trying to master basic literacy skills. Figures 3.4 and 3.5 show another simple spelling test from the Jordan Written Screening Test (see Chapter 2). This is a carefully arranged group of words that students with dyslexia commonly misspell. Within a few minutes of watching how students encode these words, the teacher can identify dyslexic tendencies without causing embarrassment. These examples illustrate how a dictation test reveals tone deaf confusion with sounds and letters, as well as dyslexic tendencies to reverse, rotate, and transpose letters.

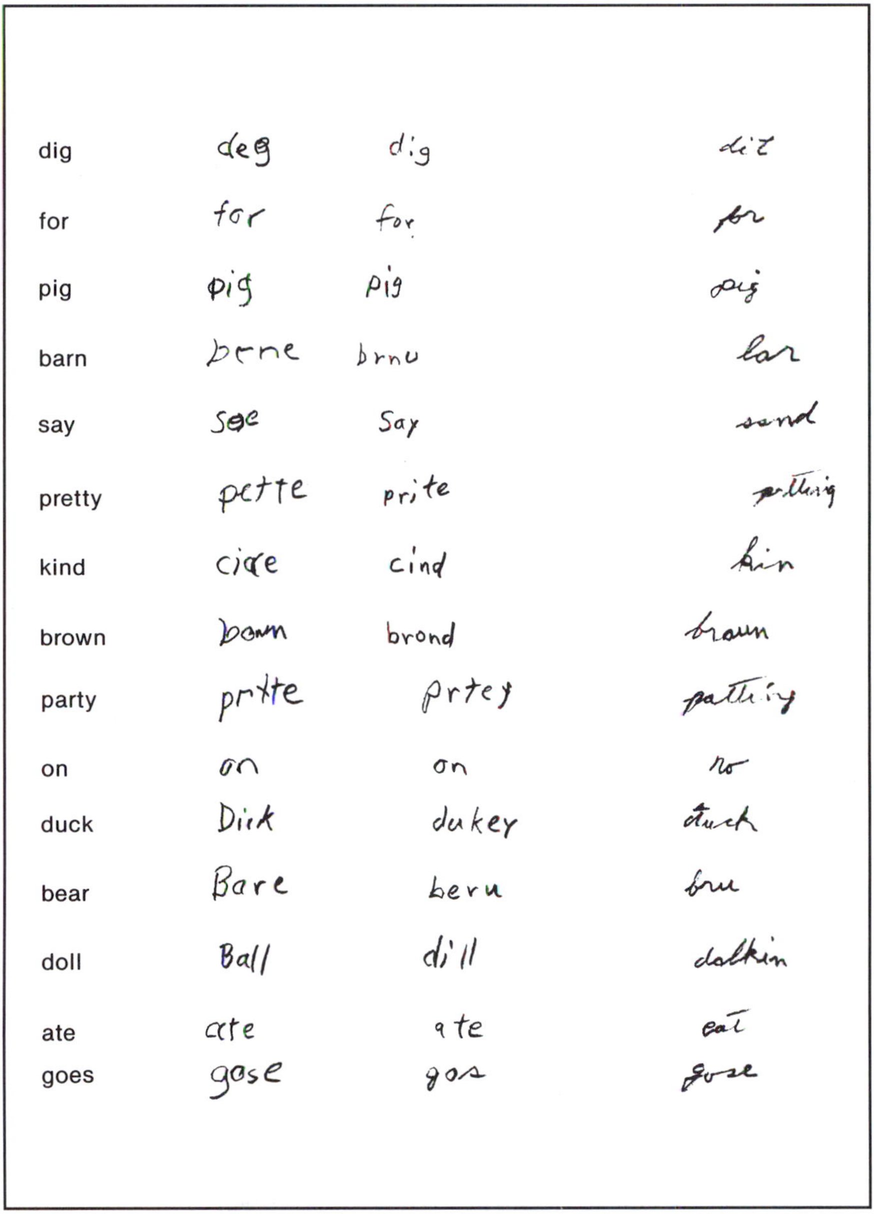

dig	deg	dig	dit
for	for	for	for
pig	pig	pig	pig
barn	bene	brnu	lan
say	see	Say	sand
pretty	pette	prite	pelling
kind	ciqe	cind	hin
brown	bown	brond	braun
party	prtte	prtey	pathiy
on	on	on	no
duck	Dirk	dukey	duch
bear	Bare	beru	bru
doll	Ball	dill	dolkin
ate	arte	a te	eat
goes	gose	gos	gose

FIGURE 3.2.   This dictation test was devised by Ernest Jones to identify dyslexic writing and spelling patterns in students of all ages. Here is the work of three students with dyslexia. The first writer was in third grade, the second writer in fifth grade, and the third in ninth grade.

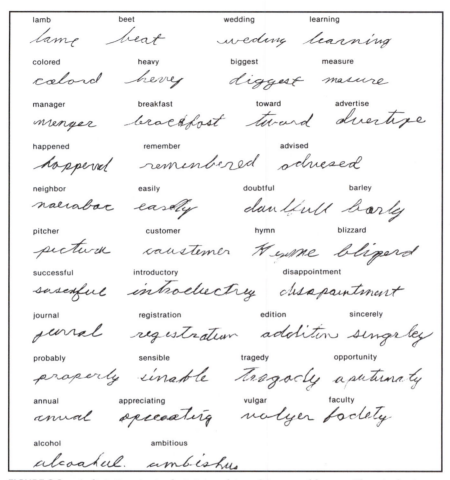

lamb	beet	wedding	learning
lame	*beat*	*weding*	*learning*

colored	heavy	biggest	measure
colord	*hevey*	*diggest*	*masure*

manager	breakfast	toward	advertise
menger	*brackfost*	*tuward*	*dvertize*

happened	remember	advised
doppevd	*remenbered*	*odvesed*

neighbor	easily	doubtful	barley
naeaboc	*easlly*	*danlfull*	*barly*

pitcher	customer	hymn	blizzard
pictude	*caustemer*	*Hyone*	*bliperd*

successful	introductory	disappointment
sasedful	*introeluctry*	*chsapauntment*

journal	registration	edition	sincerely
jurral	*regustratum*	*addtion*	*sengrley*

probably	sensible	tragedy	opportunity
praperly	*sinable*	*Tragody*	*aputunaty*

annual	appreciating	vulgar	faculty
annual	*apecoating*	*volyer*	*foclety*

alcohol	ambitious
alcoakul	*ambishu*

FIGURE 3.3. A dictation test administered to a 21-year-old man. The student required more than 30 minutes to write these words. He had to whisper over and over with frequent erasing. He was exhausted when he finished this dictated spelling test.

Writing Problems

Auditory dyslexia is a major handicap when students like Maria try to write essay answers or produce original stories or themes. Dyslexic spelling frequently is associated with dysgraphia, as will be discussed in Chapter 4. It is not difficult to see the symptoms of auditory dyslexia in a student's

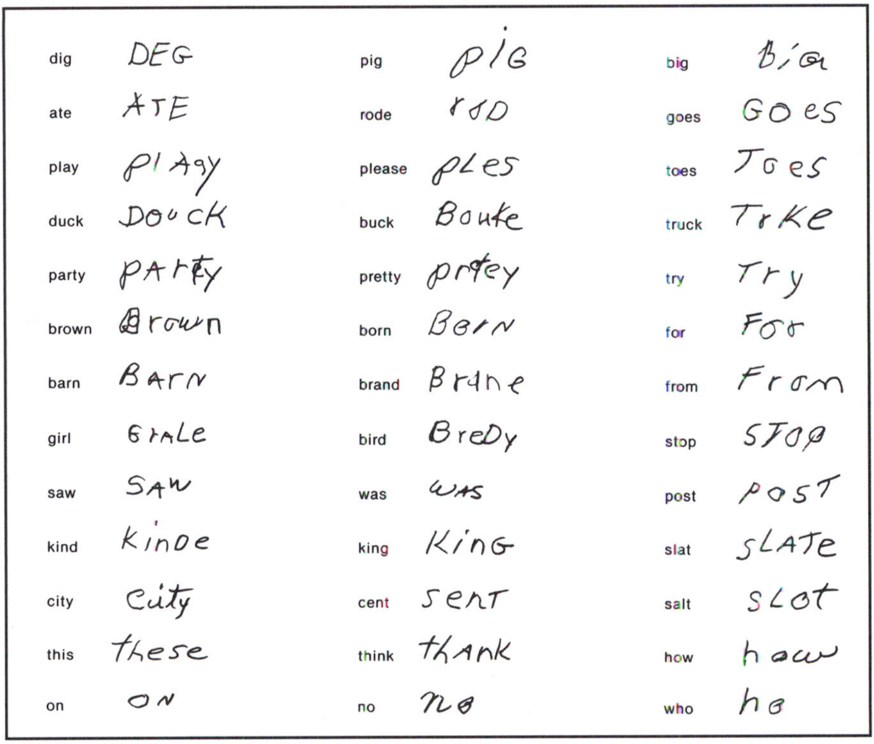

dig	DEG	pig	PIG	big	BIG
ate	ATE	rode	rod	goes	GOes
play	PlAgy	please	PLes	toes	Toes
duck	DOuCK	buck	Bouke	truck	TrKe
party	PArty	pretty	prtey	try	Try
brown	Brown	born	BorN	for	Foor
barn	BArN	brand	Brdne	from	From
girl	GrnLe	bird	BreDy	stop	STop
saw	SAw	was	wAs	post	POST
kind	KinOe	king	KinG	slat	sLATe
city	City	cent	seNT	salt	sLot
this	these	think	thAnk	how	haw
on	ON	no	no	who	ho

FIGURE 3.4. A spelling test from the Jordan Written Screening Test.

written work if instructors carefully study handwritten papers.

Figure 3.6 shows dyslexic writing by a fourth-grade student. Her autobiography was brushed aside as the work of a child with mental retardation until her teachers discovered that the girl had dyslexia. This example illustrates a combination of auditory dyslexia (faulty letter–sound connecting) and dysgraphia (inability to write legibly). Below the writing sample is a typed translation that reveals the auditory dyslexic spelling flaws more clearly.

Figure 3.7 shows extremely dyslexic writing by a 20-year-old college student. She was enrolled in teacher education as a special education major, hoping to become certified to teach children with learning disabilities. A sympathetic professor recognized this student's dyslexic patterns and began working with her one-to-one. She developed word

dig	*dig*	pig	*pige*	big	*big*
ate	*ate*	rode	*rod*	goes	*gos*
play	*gla*	please	*ples*	toes	*toce*
duck	*dog*	buck	*bog*	track	*troc*
party	*prte*	pretty	*pretoj*	try	*tria*
brown	*bron*	born	*brne*	for	*fore*
barn	*brna*	brand	*brand*	from	*fom*
girl	*grle*	bird	*brd*	stop	*stop*
saw	*soe*	was	*wos*	post	*post*
kind	*kind*	king	*ben*	slat	*slet*
city	*cite*	cent	*sint*	salt	*solt*
this	*thes*	think	*thac*	how	*haw*
on	*on*	no	*no*	who	*hoh*

FIGURE 3.5. A spelling test. This student with dyslexia learned cursive writing, which is unusual for someone who has this much struggle in encoding. Notice that most of the circular letters are made with backward strokes.

processor skills that allowed her to bypass her dyslexic writing problems.

No one knows how many intelligent, creative students have been written off as academic failures because instructors have not known how to identify dyslexia. Figure 3.8 shows part of an original story a boy named Larry wrote when he was 15 years old. A poorly administered intelligence test had labeled him borderline retarded with an IQ of 72. When his dyslexic patterns were diagnosed, his mental ability was correctly measured as well above average. He sent five original manuscripts to a publisher of paperback mystery stories. To Larry's astonishment, an alert editor deciphered the poor handwriting as dysgraphia and discovered the story lines that Larry had created. This editor returned the manuscripts with a lengthy critique, advising the boy on how to improve his stories. He encouraged Larry to keep

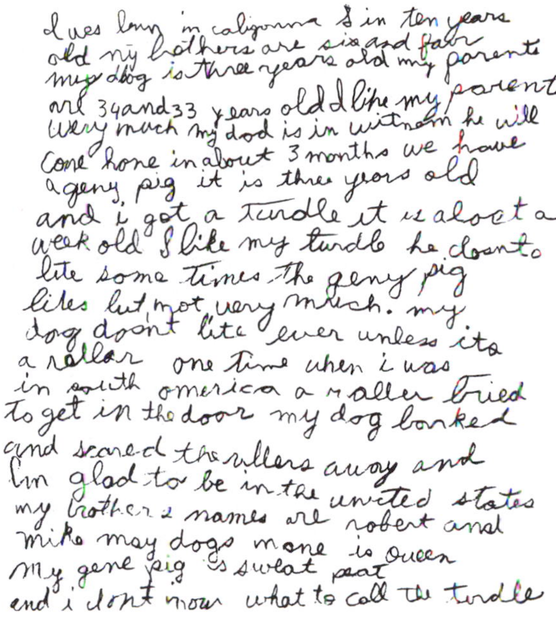

I was born in califarna (California) S (I) in (am) ten years old my
brothers are six and four my dog is three years old my parents are 34
and 33 years old I like my parents wery (very) much my dad is in
watnam (Vietnam) he will come home in about 3 months we have a geny
(Guinea) pig it is three years old and i got a turdle (turtle) it is
aloud (about) a week old S (I) like my turdle he dosnt (doesn't) lite
(bite) some times the geny pig lites (bites) but mot (not) very much.
my dog doesn't bite ever unless its a rolber (robber). one tine
(time) vhen (when) i was in south america a ruller (robber) tried to
get in the door my dog barked and scared the rillers (robbers) away
and Im (I'm) glad to be in the united states, my brothers names are
robert and Mike may (my) dogs (dog's) name is Oueen (Queen) my gene
pig is sweat peat (Sweet Pete) and i dont now (know) what to call the
turdle.

FIGURE 3.6.   A writing sample produced by a 9-year-old girl. Later she developed
excellent writing skills with a word processor that helped her find misspelled
words.

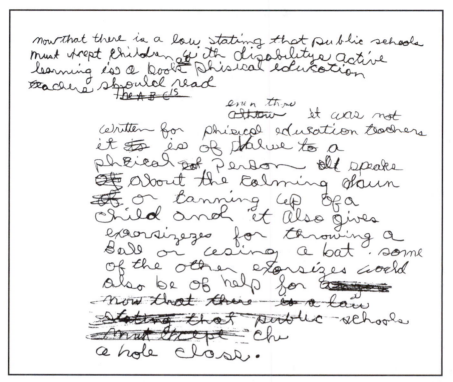

FIGURE 3.7. A sample of dyslexic writing. This 20-year-old student finally earned a special education teaching certificate and became an excellent teacher of youngsters with learning disabilities.

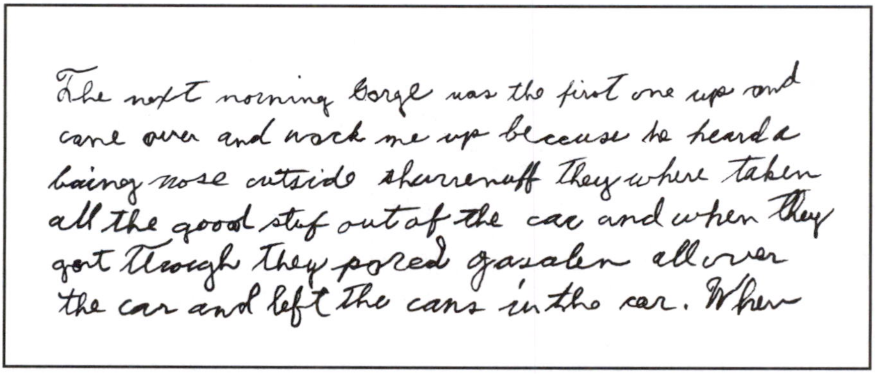

FIGURE 3.8. Notice the extremely small handwriting of this student with dyslexia. Occasionally a person who has severe dyslexia develops tiny writing partly to hide mistakes in spelling. Larry filled several notebooks with this kind of creative story writing.

sending story ideas, pointing out that the publisher was interested in purchasing fresh story material. With this unique incentive, Larry became interested in school achievement for the first time in his life. He quickly developed good writing ability through the use of a word processor. It is a sobering thought that this bright young man had been labeled hopeless by teachers who had not recognized his talent for language usage hidden beneath his dysgraphic penmanship and dyslexic spelling.

Confusion with Rhyming

An easily detected characteristic of auditory dyslexia is difficulty with rhyme. As a standard practice in literacy instruction, teachers often dwell on rhyming words to reinforce pupil awareness of sounds in words. Students handicapped by auditory dyslexia have great difficulty hearing likenesses and differences in words. Awkwardness in hearing or saying rhymes is a major symptom of this disability.

Educators probably make too great an issue of faulty rhyming ability. Aside from providing a convenient vehicle for phonics drills, rhyming skill actually is of little practical importance in overall reading ability, although it does help many individuals master writing and spelling. It is unfortunate that persons with poor rhyming skill often are penalized. Instructors should remember that some students who do well in oral rhyming activities cannot do the same in writing. To determine the extent of this auditory deficit, teachers must use both oral and written activities to evaluate talent for rhyming.

An example of this informal procedure would be to ask Maria to name all the words she can rhyme with *car*. A person with normal auditory perception responds quickly with such words as *jar, far, star, bar*. Because of her auditory dyslexia, Maria needs a lot of time to ponder through each word before saying it. This is particularly evident when she names nonsense words instead of true rhyming words (*dar, sar, nar, har, zar*). Individuals such as Maria also often name words that begin alike but do not rhyme, such as *car, care, core, cure*. If the student cannot match printed rhyming words, or if he or she cannot write familiar rhyming words by substituting beginning consonants, the teacher can be reasonably sure that an auditory dyslexic condition exists.

Need for Speaker to Repeat

An especially irritating characteristic for many instructors is the need for listeners with auditory dyslexia to hear it again. Students like Maria are very insecure, especially in the classroom, where they feel ill at ease because they cannot make accurate letter–sound connections. When writing from dictation or following a series of oral instructions, these students cannot cope with a sustained flow of oral material. Because of their extremely slow rate in changing speech into writing, they lose the sequence of what they hear. Because they are seldom sure that they have heard accurately, they continuously ask the speaker to repeat statements.

This habit produces friction in many learning situations. As learners like Maria fall behind the group, they tend to become disruptive. Discipline problems often stem from the subtle, invisible presence of tone deaf listening. It is not unusual for these individuals to be shunned by their peers, who are annoyed by the "weird" behavior and disruptive habits. Struggling to hold the social position creates friction, which triggers a lot of conflict with other students, instructors, and other adults, such as teacher's aides. What begins as a dyslexic difference often leads to social problems and public embarrassment. Little of this poor behavior, however, is deliberate.

Vocalizing During Silent Reading

A stereotypical image many of us have carried from childhood is of classroom teachers snapping fingers and warning, "Shhh!" For many years, students have been taught that making vocal sounds during silent reading time is forbidden, but students with dyslexia must vocalize if they are to succeed in translating written words into meaningful thought.

Because of the underlying problem in connecting sounds to letters, dyslexic readers must use several brain pathways to verify their impressions. This frustrating need to reinforce seeing with saying, along with touching words with a finger, should not upset teachers. It is not difficult to let these students use their unorthodox ways if the instructor is aware of the problem. The important thing is that they respond to reading in a variety of ways to check their impressions for accuracy. If an instructor snaps fingers and hisses, "Shhh!" an essential learning channel is shut off. The result is increased frustration and failure.

This need to reinforce seeing with voice and touch also appears when students with auditory dyslexia do written assignments, because they must whisper during spelling tests and while writing stories or essays. If these students are allowed to cross-check their impressions by vocalizing as they write, they can learn to correct many of their spelling mistakes. If they are allowed to touch their words and whisper, they can learn to read more fluently.

Struggle to Blend Word Chunks into Whole Words

In Chapter 1, Maria's attempt to read aloud from a science textbook was described. The heart of her reading handicap is faulty blending, which greatly reduces her talent for learning one of the major skills of word analysis. The entire auditory dyslexic syndrome seems to focus upon her problems in "sounding out" words as she reads. For example, a familiar word like *bug* can become a major hurdle for the dyslexic reader. With great effort Maria breaks the word apart: "buh-uh-guh." As this effort illustrates, she has never learned the right way to sound the consonants *b* and *g*. When she feels somewhat confident that she has the separate sound chunks in mind, Maria takes the blending plunge: *blug.* Again she has failed. *Yellow* comes out *yelelow. Bridge* turns into *burge.*

Traditional instruction in phonics, which emphasizes blending, is usually beyond the comprehension of individuals who have auditory dyslexia. It is possible for them to achieve limited success in simple word analysis after a lot of drill and memorizing of key word patterns. This technique, *overteaching,* saturates the student with intensive, highly structured practice with regular words until an automatic response occurs. Students like Maria seldom develop true understanding of blending and word analysis, although they often can learn to read at a slow rate.

Garbled Pronunciation

Closely associated with the inability to blend is an embarrassing problem of garbled pronunciation. Persons with auditory dyslexia find themselves the object of much laughter and teasing because of scrambled speech, known as *echolalia.* Parents and teachers can identify this aspect of dyslexia by devising lists of words for the student to repeat.

Normal Pronunciation	Auditory Dyslexic Speech
aluminum	alunimum
vinegar	vigenar
animals	aminals
olive	olly
baskets	baksets
streamline	steam lion
spaghetti	pasghetti

Teachers can create pronunciation games to reveal echolalia by using sound units that are scrambled within words. These tests can be fun, as well. For example, the teacher might have the class do a Tongue Twister Race, and privately keep a record of garbled speech tendencies that appear in certain students during the game. The emphasis must be upon fun, with no one feeling shame because of a twisted tongue. The following are some good word combinations for this information observation:

- apples in cinnamon

- alum in vinegar

- baskets of olives

- she sells seashells on the seashore

- aluminum animals

- mama's spaghetti

- transcontinental train

Older students enjoy such twisters as these:

- political candidacy

- musketry maneuvers

- blueberry strudel

- a crow flew over the river with a lump of raw liver

- six long, slim, sleek, slick, slender saplings

Confusion with Dictionary Symbols

As would be expected, auditory dyslexia makes traditional dictionary usage quite difficult. To expect a student like Maria to interpret phonetic respellings, accent markings, and pronunciation guides is unrealistic. Highly motivated students with dyslexic tendencies do manage to cope with the various codes found in reference materials. However, most students with dyslexia cannot comprehend the variety of symbol systems they see in current dictionaries. This problem is further complicated by the use of *schwa* symbols showing vowel sounds in unaccented syllables. With enough careful training in word-analysis skills, these learners can benefit from studies in word origins, multiple meanings, and syllable division. However, arriving at correct word pronunciation from dictionary keys is frequently impossible.

LEARNING ACTIVITIES FOR PERSONS WITH AUDITORY DYSLEXIA

It is imperative that students with auditory dyslexia have highly structured, well-organized learning routines that do not change from day to day. Equally important is keeping materials, tools, and reference books in the same place in the classroom. Oral instructions, written instructions, and placement of materials must be consistent. Once the students learn where things are, they depend on those things being in the same places day after day. Keeping the learning environment well organized without surprise changes is essential. If the classroom arrangement must be changed, students with dyslexia must relearn the landmarks before they feel comfortable again. The following guidelines will help an educator establish a well-organized classroom environment in which students with dyslexia can learn comfortably.

Organize the Classroom

Individuals with auditory dyslexia do not respond to the usual practice of presenting a rule and practicing that rule with words that follow the rule. Instead, they must begin with a visibly structured experience. They may understand the rule at a later time, although many never fully comprehend oral or written rules. Although it is possible that they may gain a level of functional performance, it will be without being able to tell why or how they carry out the rule. Because independent literacy is the goal of education, this functional level must be considered good enough. If one has dyslexia, all of the senses must be involved in helping one to become a functional reader or speller. This, of course, poses problems for classroom management. The teacher's dilemma is to provide for the different learning styles he or she finds among the pupils. This can be accomplished if the teacher keeps a sense of humor, is not too rigid, and remembers that these pupils are human beings with exactly the same feelings others have experienced in the toughest high school or college courses they ever took. If it had not been for mercies extended by sympathetic professors, many excellent classroom teachers would never have gained professional certification.

There are thousands of ideas in professional publications for teaching reading, writing, and spelling skills to students with LD. Instructors must keep in mind the cardinal principles: *simplicity, repetition,* and *step-by-step progression* into higher-level skill areas. Almost any teaching technique can be made to fit the needs of someone like Maria if the pace is kept slow enough and the practice activities are simple and thorough.

Before students with dyslexia begin to become functional with letter–sound connections, they must have a great deal of experience with stable word patterns that follow the rules the instructor hopes to teach. The most practical source for these words is the daily vocabulary of the students. Because, unfortunately, many individuals with dyslexia will not finish school, they need to master basic literacy skills if they are to manage their own affairs when formal schooling is over.

Establish a Lifestyle Corner

Basal readers, spelling manuals, language handbooks, and arithmetic and social studies textbooks are virtually meaningless to most students with dyslexia. This is not to criticize the materials or their authors. The point is that textbooks designed for students who have reading skills are not appropriate for the extremely slow reaction time of learners with dyslexia. Because of their different styles of learning, Pete's and Maria's literacy skills must be linked to their immediate daily environment. Although they are capable of imagination, persons with dyslexia are multisensory learners. They must see it, say it, hear it, and touch it before complete mental images are achieved. The quest for independent reading, spelling, writing, and arithmetic skills for these learners thus must take a different course. The most direct route is through the experiences they encounter every day.

The most effective classroom device for enlisting the students' interest and cooperation is a lifestyle corner where functional words from these students' daily life are displayed. For example, a shelf of common grocery items might display food labels that they must know how to read and write, along with the prices to teach simple money figuring. Other shelves display other lifestyle items, such as clothing, utensils, tools, sports and recreation equipment, parts for motor bikes or cars, items for good grooming, common medical supplies, and whatever else is appropriate to the interests and lives of the students involved.

In addition to these objects, other word sources should be provided: sections of the daily newspaper, a Bible or other scriptures for students who are religious, mail-order catalogs, telephone directories, maps of the city and state, and travel guidebooks. For older students, items might include samples of checkbooks and budget-planning materials; cookbooks; income tax forms; applications for licenses; manuals outlining local hunting, fishing, and motor vehicle regulations; and reproductions of traffic signs. Another good idea is a browsing table for popular magazines the students bring to exchange, as well as comic books and paperbacks they have enjoyed. There should be a guide for television shows, reviews of movies, and current magazines on easy reading levels.

All of this is not for entertainment, and it need not occupy much space. The lifestyle corner is completely practical, as well as essential for treating dyslexia in the classroom. The packages and other materials provide immediate visual cues through colors, shapes, word forms, and unique patterns. These cues trigger quick recall of important information for students who struggle to remember details. Here the teacher finds a wealth of simple, practical language materials for teaching literacy, which is the primary educational need of students with dyslexia.

Even children in primary grades need to master basic reading, writing, and spelling vocabulary from their daily lives. Every instructor and supervisor should live for a while as these children and young people live, not knowing which door leads to the right rest room, not knowing how to find specific streets or house numbers, not being able to order a meal from a menu, not knowing how to deposit money in a bank or how to make or follow a shopping list, not being able to write the simplest kind of letter. The lifestyle corner opens up many new doors into face-saving independence, as well as providing the teacher with ready-made sources for instructional activities.

Every important phonics rule can be taught from the lifestyle corner. For example, the grocery shelf is loaded with word families: the *-am* family (*ham, jam, Pam, Spam, yam*). Different spellings of the same sound chunks are easily illustrated: *steak, cake, weight.* Homonyms are evident, particularly in traffic terminology: *right–write, wait–weight, road–rode.* Also at the teacher's fingertips are words to illustrate rules about dividing words into syllables:

1. *Dividing between consonants that are alike* (double consonants): but/ter   dol/lar   car/rot   ham/mer   pep/per   cab/bage.

2. *Dividing between consonants that are not alike:* tur/key   sil/ver   quar/ter   Hon/da   Mus/tang.

3. *Dividing after the vowel in open syllables:* ba/con   rhu/barb   pe/can   to/ma/to.

4. *Dividing between speaking vowel units:* Bu/ick   Toy/o/ta   su/et   O/hi/o   ra/di/o.

5. *Compound words:* straw/berry   pine/apple   police/man   ice cream   hot dog.

The lifestyle corner is a prime source of creative writing ideas, if the quantity of writing is kept small. The many sensory cues from pictures, packages, colors, shapes, and flavors, provide a wealth of quick stimulus material. Learners such as Pete and Maria find it much easier to write acceptably when this kind of visual library is at hand.

Maintain Accountability

Students with dyslexia should not be pampered any more than their peers. Once the teacher has provided learning sources within the skill ranges of the learners, students such as Pete and Maria can be held accountable for reasonable quotas of reading, writing, spelling, and arithmetic. If other classmates are expected to master 20 spelling words each week from a regular spelling textbook, students with dyslexia can meet a similar expectation by using a lifestyle vocabulary that fits their individual differences and needs. Each student's rate of processing should be determined, and then each can be held responsible for producing what he or she can do at his or her own pace.

The lifestyle corner is a comfortable, safe starting place. If Pete and Maria should not finish their formal education, they are prepared to shop for groceries and fill out a job application form. The hope is that by starting with this kind of lifestyle literacy base, each dyslexic learner will eventually transfer his or her literacy skills to textbook materials.

Create an Interaction Center

Overcoming auditory dyslexia in the classroom depends upon one vital element: *interaction.* If this factor is missing from the learning environment, then very little formal skill development will occur for those who have dyslexia. Several forms of interaction are needed within any effective classroom. The lifestyle corner is designed to stimulate multisensory learning for students who cannot function in silent, passive learning situations. An interaction center provides a controlled environment where physical movement, listening, and speaking are blended in active learning. Students such as Maria and Pete must blend these three aspects of interaction in order to comprehend reading, writing, and spelling. They must feel it, hold it, manipulate it, hear it, say it, and receive immediate feedback before complete mental images are achieved. This kind of interactive learning cannot occur at a passive reading circle or when students are confined to their seats.

The teacher's first challenge with interactive learning is to keep the noise level under control, but it is not difficult to create an interaction center within a mainstream classroom, if only for a few minutes at a time. Ideally, the center should be partially screened by bookshelves or portable partitions. The point is to protect different learning styles from too much conflict. Every classroom includes students who prefer a silent environment, who are too quickly distracted and irritated by nearby sound and movement. These individuals function best alone. Within the same class can be found students who function best when they are stimulated by talking things over with a study buddy because they cannot build complete mental images through silent, passive study by themselves. Still other individuals need body movement to learn best. Sitting still in a quiet place triggers too much inner distraction. If the teacher counsels students about accepting each other's needs, these different styles of learning can be accommodated within the same classroom.

The interaction center is primarily for the purpose of low-key talking and moving about while learning. At specific times each day, the teacher meets these active, multisensory students who need body involvement and oral feedback for full comprehension. The interaction center allows them to lie on the floor while talking or listening. A few large beanbags or giant pillows provide places to sprawl and squirm and let off excess energy without creating much noise. A sturdy rocking chair becomes a channel for releasing energy while the student takes part in discussion. During the day, Pete and Maria may take their books to the interaction center and spend a few minutes discharging extra energy by rocking and reading for a while. Study buddies can go to the interaction center to work on projects or help each other prepare for a quiz.

An interaction center creates positive new relationships for teachers and students. Now alternate learning styles and different energy levels can share the same, larger learning space. Multisensory learners who generate friction in traditional silent-learning environments now have an acceptable way to discharge their inner tension. Overcoming dyslexia begins by removing old silent-learning barriers that do not fit the learning styles and perceptual needs of 15% to 20% of U.S. students. As public education moves toward the full inclusion mandates of the Individuals with Disabilities Education Act of 1990 (IDEA), providing a lifestyle corner and interaction center for each classroom are ideal strategies for students who have dyslexia.

Offer Multisensory Letter–Sound Connections

Overcoming auditory dyslexia requires a multisensory approach involving all of the senses that can be brought together in the learning process. The four most important sensory learning channels are *sight, sound, speech,* and *touch.* When these sensory pathways are integrated, students with auditory dyslexia can begin to comprehend what reading, spelling, writing, and arithmetic are all about. Doing multisensory processing requires freedom to speak and hear while moving some part of the body.

Multisensory learning is like playing tennis: The player needs immediate feedback from a partner. If no partner is there to provide immediate oral and visual feedback, a student like Maria can learn to simulate the feedback process by talking to herself, listening to herself say it, and using her fingers or body motions to tie together loose ends in her mental images. Multisensory learning is not a silent event. This mode of processing generates some degree of noise and motion. It is a slow way to learn and it cannot be hurried.

Identifying Sound Chunks in Spoken Words

Adults usually think only of consonants and vowels when reference is made to sounds within spoken words. However, these building blocks of reading and spelling are not the beginning points for teaching those who have auditory dyslexia. Earlier in this chapter, it was noted that there is a neurological cause for auditory dyslexia. Figure 3.1 showed the immature cell development along the auditory pathway that makes it impossible for students like Maria to hear the hard/soft/hard/soft chunks of sounds that make up oral language. This is why teachers cannot start with traditional phonics that asks the learner to hear soft consonants and vowels. These tone deaf individuals do not know that these phonemes exist because their auditory pathways cannot hear subtle speech differences. Instead of pressing Maria to hear soft consonants and vowels, instructors must begin by teaching her how to find syllable chunks and whole words. If sight, sound, speech, and touch can be brought together in this experience, it is possible for her to bypass her tone deafness well enough to develop most of the basic phonics skills.

Hundreds of activities for teaching phonics to students with dyslexia are available in the professional literature and wherever children's books are sold. The common theme in most of these materials is the same: "Listen to the vowel inside this word _____. What sound do you hear the vowel make?" Because students with auditory dyslexia do not hear vowel sounds, a different approach must be used. First, they must be taught to *see* the softer sound chunks instead of trying to hear them; that is, a system of *visual phonics* must be provided. Second, the student must be able to link together several sensory pathways. To learn very much about phonics, Maria must see it, say it, and feel it. With enough multisensory practice, she may actually begin to hear some of the softer chunks.

Visual Phonics

Persons with dyslexia seldom have trouble learning which letters are vowels and which are consonants. In Chapter 2, the importance of mastering alphabet sequence before students like Pete and Maria move on to more advanced word analysis was reviewed. In learning the alphabet sequence, Pete has no trouble remembering that *Aa, Ee, Ii, Oo,* and *Uu* are called vowels. As they practice with alphabet sequence, Pete and Maria also may learn that *Ww* and *Yy* can be vowels, although they may not understand how or why this is so. It is simple for Pete and Maria to remember that all the other letters are called consonants. (Adults often notice that auditory dyslexic learners like Maria say "constonants" or even "consants.") This knowledge of how alphabet letters are classified lays the foundation for learning to see sound chunks when the tone deaf student cannot hear them.

The following procedures for teaching visual phonics to tone deaf learners show how this method presents phonetic information to struggling learners.

1. *Seeing vowels inside words.* The instructor begins by showing the student how to locate vowels inside words by seeing vowel letters and marking them with a pencil. The words are arranged so that the vowel letters come in alphabetical sequence. The teacher says, "Maria, let's look for vowels inside some words you have seen in reading."

cat   bed   did   stop   up

"Look for the vowel in each word. Underline each vowel you see. Now tell me the name of each vowel you underlined." Maria's task is to say the *names* (aye eee eye oh you). At this point, no other sound should be associated with these vowel letters. The teacher then says, "Now, Maria. I am going to show you some words that have two vowels."

date   meet   ride   rope   cute
_{1 2}

"Let's count the vowels in each word. What is the first vowel in date? Put a small 1 under it. What is the second vowel in date? Put a small 2 under it. What is the name of number 1 vowel? What is the name of number 2 vowel? Now let's do the rest of the words this same way."

2. *Sounding vowels inside words.* When Maria is fluent in seeing and naming each vowel letter, she is ready to take her first step in sounding the vowels she sees in short words. Her first experience with phonics will be with the *short name* of single vowels that come in short words. The teacher will say, "Maria, I am going to show you some short words that have just one vowel. Let's learn a rule: *When I see one vowel by itself in a short word, the vowel says its short name.* Now I will help you learn to say this rule." The instructor guides Maria in saying this rule until she can repeat it rather well by herself. Then the instructor says, "Now let's look at some words where the vowel says its short name."

băg   let   it   mop   up

"Now, Maria. Let's find the vowel in the first word. This time I will show you a new way to mark this vowel." Above the *a* the instructor draws the half-moon mark (∪, called breve) that stands for the sound of short *a*. "Maria, when one vowel comes in a short word, the vowel says its short name. This mark reminds you to make the vowel say its short name." This rule is practiced again and again until Maria is confident in marking the vowel letter in a short word to see that it says its short name.

When the instructor feels confident that Maria knows how to apply this short vowel rule, it is time to take the next step. The teacher then says, "Maria, let's learn a new rule: *When I see two vowels in a short word, the first vowel says its long name. The second vowel doesn't say anything.* Now I will help you learn this rule." The instructor guides Maria in saying this rule several times until she can repeat it rather well by herself. Then the instructor says, "Now, let's look at some words and make the first vowel say its long name."

dāte̸ eat hide bone rude
1 2

"Now, Maria, let's practice our new rule. How many vowels do you see in the first word? Put a small number under each vowel that you see. Now let's say our new rule: *When I see two vowels in a short word, the first vowel says its long name. The second vowel doesn't say anything.* Now I will show you a special mark that tells the vowel to say its long name." The instructor makes the long name mark (–, called macron) above the *a*. "Now we see what sound the *a* makes. Let me show you the mark that tells the second vowel not to say anything." The instructor makes a slash mark (/) through the second vowel.

As simple as these beginning rules appear, they open the door for independent reading for students such as Maria. Several dozen familiar short-vowel and long-vowel words follow these two rules in beginning reading practice. Maria and her instructor can write their own practice reading activities by choosing words that follow these beginning vowel-sounding rules. Again, the instructor and any adults assisting Maria must remember why she cannot benefit from traditional methods for teaching phonics: She cannot hear the soft sound chunks when she is asked to listen for them.

She must start with a method that teaches her how to see vowel chunks. Then she can work out vowel sounds by using the multisensory strategy demonstrated here.

3. *Finding word chunks.* Students with dyslexia often are confused by the task of locating syllables. Instructors must remember that syllable division in the dictionary does not always match the oral syllables of speech. Dividing words into dictionary syllables requires a rather high-level talent for word processing; therefore, students with limited talent for reading and spelling do not benefit from the traditional practice of dividing words into dictionary syllables. What they see in print often is different from what they say in word usage.

Both Pete and Maria need a different method for locating the breaks (chunks) as they move to higher levels in sounding out words. After they have mastered the simple phonics rules for finding short vowels and long vowels in short words, they are ready to move up to finding chunks in longer words. Again, the most effective strategy is a multisensory one.

Pete and Maria need to learn an old-fashioned word chunking technique called *chin bumping,* which was taught when children attended only a few years of formal schooling. Chin bumping is a multisensory way to feel, hear, and say the chunks of speech. In reading, Pete and Maria must learn how to translate what they see on the page into inner speech. They must literally turn printed words into a mental voice that tells them what their eyes are seeing. In chin bumping, the learner holds two or three fingers under the chin to feel what happens as the mouth says the longer word. The chin will bob (bump) downward slightly every time the mouth reaches the end of a chunk. When the chin bumps downward, the reader marks that place as a dividing point in the word. This process does not always match syllable divisions shown in the dictionary, but beginning readers are not concerned with what the dictionary says is correct word division. Beginning readers need only know how to break words into chunks to enhance the word-sounding process.

The instructor shows Pete and Maria some familiar longer words: saddle   yellow   little   Monday   summer. Together they practice chin bumping these words:

sad / dle   yel / low   lit / tle   Mon / day   sum / mer

Now would be a good time for the instructor to show Pete and Maria another piece to the puzzle of word sounding. Each of these longer words starts with a "short word" that contains one vowel. What sound does this vowel say? What mark do we make to show the sound for one vowel in a short word? A complete system for teaching visual phonics to dyslexic learners is provided in the *Jordan Prescriptive/ Tutorial Reading Program for Moderate and Severe Dyslexia* (Jordan, 1989b).

Using a Keyboard and a Tape Recorder

The value of a word processor in the classroom has only recently been recognized by educators. Because of the cost of new machines, teachers often put out of their minds the possibility of having keyboard units in the classroom. Traditional school emphasis upon penmanship for everyone has further obscured the potential that word processors hold for remediation of dyslexia.

As was discussed in Chapter 1 and will be in Chapter 4, students with dysgraphia are especially handicapped by their inability to cope with all of the handwriting expectations. Auditory dyslexia poses a similar threat for those who cannot recall word patterns correctly. When students with dyslexia are taught how to write with a keyboard, a new world of possibilities emerges.

Electronic firms that specialize in business machines predict that doing jobs by handwriting may become obsolete in the foreseeable future. With new families of electronic devices already on the market, persons with dyslexia and/or dysgraphia will be able to enter professions that now require spelling, handwriting, and composition skills. In an era of voice recorders and automatic typing machines, which offer a variety of options for encoding messages and retrieving information, the classroom should introduce all children to these alternative forms of writing.

The keyboard/tape recorder routine is quite simple. The point of this activity is to provide an integrated experience with sight, sound, speech, and touch. Practice words can be taken from any source, preferably from the student's own vocabulary. The students study a word on a card and pronounce the word into the tape recorder. Next, they spell the word aloud into the recorder. Then they type the word immediately from memory. Finally, they read into the recorder the way the word was typed. They select another word card and repeat this process. After spelling out five words, they run the tape back to the starting position and review what they typed and spoke into the recorder. They continue this routine, five words in each work segment, until all the words in the card set have been done.

This multisensory procedure produces immediate results. As the students feel their fingers tap the keys, they become aware of the sequence of letters within the words being typed and recorded. Any reversal or rotation tendencies quickly become apparent. The teacher may overhear them muttering as they work out correct letter sequence: "Where's the *b*? Uh, oh! I got it upside down again. Now, where's *o*? a-b-o-v-e. Above! OK. I got it right. Now where's *t*?" This stream of chatter is a vocal mirror of the thought patterns a student with dyslexia experiences with every school assignment. Listening to him or her work through exercises with the keyboard and tape recorder reveals much about his or her dyslexic confusion with sounds and symbols.

Recruit Teacher Aides

The Bible records a remarkable lesson in how a frustrated, overworked leader solved a major problem of group management. Moses tried to handle all the details by giving personal attention to the needs of a million people. Observing his son-in-law struggling to do everything himself, Jethro gave his famous advice: *Divide the people into groups. Then appoint aides to take care of their everyday needs.* In essence, Moses was taught how to conserve his strength for the major decisions his subordinates could not make. Because the plan worked, Moses became one of the giant figures of world history.

Like Moses, classroom teachers face a multitude of responsibilities, problems, challenges, frustrations, and even failures. When dyslexia enters the picture, a teacher must accept help. Regardless of his or her enthusiasm and personal resolve, no teacher can possibly meet all the demands posed by learning differences in the classroom. Help must be found and accepted. It is not a sign of strength for harassed teachers to reject assistance in meeting the needs of students with disabilities. In fact, it is difficult to defend a situation that pits a lone adult against the many needs of a roomful of students.

Using Older Students

A great strength of one-room rural schools was the interaction between older students and primary pupils. My own experiences as a child in a one-room country school have served as a lifelong model for behavior management. My teacher, Mrs. Keithley, could have worked herself into an early grave had she attempted to teach all her students in all eight grades in that one large room. Instead, she demonstrated the wisdom of delegating responsibility. It was a special honor to be a upper-grade student in her school. When his or her behavior proved acceptable, an older student frequently would be called upon to "listen to Johnny recite." This was a cue for the older student to take one of the little ones to the cloakroom, out to the shed, or, in good weather, down to the creek. There the upper-grade student drilled the younger one until the child was ready to recite for Mrs. Keithley. This use of older learners as tutors was extremely effective in establishing accurate perceptual awareness of phonics, arithmetic, spelling patterns, history facts, or whatever needed to be mastered.

There was a double purpose in Mrs. Keithley's classroom management, of course. She did not call upon only the better students to tutor. Quite often an adolescent boy who was struggling with elementary reading or spelling skills was assigned the task of teaching the alphabet to a child in first or second grade. Or a 15-year-old might be called upon to teach multiplication facts to a 9-year-old. This pairing of tutor and learner was intended to reinforce the older student's skills as well as to accelerate the younger pupil's achievement. In other words, Mrs. Keithley was practicing an age-old principle: *We learn much better what we teach to others.*

Many schools are revisiting these old techniques in today's struggle to solve the dilemma of dyslexia and other learning disabilities in the mainstream classroom. By using older students as tutors, teachers are finding a way to provide one-to-one attention for struggling pupils. There is tremendous motivation for a sixth-grade boy to be asked to visit a primary classroom three times a week to coach a child in learning the alphabet. Upper-grade teachers witness changed attitudes in older students, who now feel needed and involved—many for the first time in their school experience. It is impossible to say who benefits more, the tutor or the child receiving this individual attention. Both learners grow in academic skills and self-esteem.

Teachers generally have backed away from this sort of student-to-student teaching relationship on the grounds that only experienced teachers are qualified to give instruction. Although this may be true when teaching concepts, it is not always true that teachers are the best guides for skill practice. In fact, older students with dyslexia often are more effective tutors and monitors than professional adults, because they frequently can express abstract ideas in a way that is understood quickly by another who also has dyslexia. Adults frequently find themselves unable to communicate so simply or so well.

An important two-way exchange occurs when an older student monitors skill practice with a younger learner. First, an essential ego boost is gained by the older one who has struggled so hard and achieved so little. Being selected as a student aide usually does a great deal to awaken self-confidence and an interest in learning. Second, the younger child is delighted and somewhat awed to have a "big kid" alone as his or her very own tutor. This is particularly effective when the older student is good at sports or has won some sort of public recognition.

The point is that harried teachers have a ready-made tutorial staff waiting to be recruited. Care must be taken, of course, not to use immature students who are not ready to handle a tutoring situation. If a personal clash develops, if there is a lack of sufficient discipline, or if some other factor makes effective tutoring and learning impossible, then the relationship should be terminated immediately. Usually, however, enough capable older students can be enlisted to give every child with dyslexia 20 or 30 minutes of individual help two or three times each week. As Moses was relieved to discover, his new aides took much of the backbreaking labor off his shoulders, enabling him to devote himself to the larger problems affecting the entire group.

Enlisting Volunteer Help

As the 21st century approaches, it is hoped that much national attention will be focused upon service to mankind, as opposed to satisfying one's own desires exclusively. Communities will need to enlist high school students, homemakers, workers with time to spare, and senior citizens who often feel no longer needed by society. Schools near college campuses have still another prime source of energetic young talent, including future teachers. Assistance with individualized classroom teaching could be more readily available than at any previous time in our history. Teachers and administrators who have taken the initiative to enlist volunteer tutors have seldom been disappointed.

The main difficulties in enlisting volunteers are finding adequate space for one-to-one tutoring and having time to give the aides sufficient guidance about specific details of their work. Once these volunteers have settled into a regular tutoring experience, they need surprisingly little direct attention from the classroom teacher because they are monitoring basic skill drills, not teaching new concepts.

Parents of children with dyslexia are among the most helpful volunteer aides, but it is almost never wise for parents to work with their own children. Rarely can a parent remain calm as his or her own flesh and blood struggles with symbol mastery. Emotions are too near the surface between these children and their nearest kin. For children of other families, parents and grandparents make good tutors and teacher aides.

PRINCIPLES FOR OVERCOMING AUDITORY DYSLEXIA

Massive attention has been directed to the teaching of auditory skills, those skills that enable a person to identify specific elements of speech. It often has been assumed that once the student can identify the component sounds of oral language, there should be little difficulty connecting written letters with spoken sounds. In other words, if a student hears speech sounds accurately, he or she should have no trouble making letter–sound connections. Students are expected to learn to write the language they speak and hear. The reverse process, of course, is turning printed symbols into the spoken language.

On the surface, this process of matching oral and written codes seems simple enough. After all, if students will only listen and pay attention, they can grasp the encoding and decoding processes that will lead into higher-level reading ability. Armed with this assumption, authors, publishers, and classroom teachers have created mountains of materials and techniques for teaching "auditory acuity," "auditory discrimination," "phonetic analysis," or just plain "phonics." To our great dismay, almost half of today's workforce cannot do this successfully. Most students who do not develop auditory discrimination have dyslexia. Earlier in this chapter, auditory dyslexia was compared to tone deafness in music, meaning that the student does not hear differences between similar sounds in speech. This condition ranges from the inability to distinguish only two or three basic sounds to the inability to distinguish whole words. Some students confuse only a few short vowel sounds. Others recognize no vowel distinctions at all. The problem is not poor hearing; it is the inability to interpret what is heard.

As has been shown, traditional phonics drill largely is wasted on students with auditory dyslexia, like Maria. If the tone deaf learner is to become a proficient reader and speller, different techniques must be used. Simply giving this student a stringent diet of phonics does not solve the problem. A major factor in auditory confusion is the way phonics is presented in most reading programs. Only a few commercial reading programs begin reading instruction with carefully sequenced spelling patterns that follow the rules until the learner is confident enough to handle variations from those rules. Beginning students usually are faced with a conglomeration of whole words in which the letter–sound relationships are randomly variable and inconsistent. It is not unusual for a beginning reader to see several spellings of certain vowel or consonant sounds in the same story.

For example, a learner with auditory dyslexia would be frustrated by the following reading experience:

> "Run, Sue!" called Mother. "Here are four cookies for you."
>
> "Good-bye, Bootsy," Sue said to her doll. "I will eat a cookie for you."

In spite of weeks of drill on individual sound units, Maria cannot cope with all these different spellings of the same sounds: *run/Mother, Sue/to/you/Bootsy, for/four, I/good-bye.* She is equally confused by different sounds for the same letters: *run–Sue, Here–her, cookies–Bootsy, for–four, I–good-bye.*

It is virtually meaningless to a student with dyslexia to be told, "Listen for the long vowel sound in Sue. Do you hear *u* say its name?" The student seldom hears the vowel at all. When the mysteries of decoding are presented in random order, this individual is lost from the start. Thus, in seeking to remediate auditory dyslexia, parents and teachers must keep certain principles in mind.

Principle 1: Immediately Apply Abstract Rules in Tangible Ways

Rules about phonics almost always are taught in the abstract, even when parents and teachers think they are providing simple, concrete illustrations. For example, a teacher would be dealing in abstractions when he or she shows the word *road* while emphasizing the "long sound of *o*." When shown the word *road* and told, "Listen to *o* say its name," Maria is confronted simultaneously by three abstractions:

1. The intellective act of attending to what the teacher says (tuning out distractions);

2. The printed word that represents the concept; and

3. The abstract concept of "sound of *o* saying its name."

Because she cannot filter out a single point from all the stimuli bombarding her, Maria cannot cope with even this simple cluster of listening, speaking, and seeing relationships. As a result, she does not comprehend what the teacher means. What appears to an instructor to be a simple learning exercise to Maria is a confusing jumble—a "roar"—from which she gleans no meaning. Consequently, she fails to please the teacher.

It is difficult for instructors to believe that older students, even at the high school level or adults, may still need to work with concrete objects in order to nail down such foundation concepts as "Listen to *o* say its long name." Even tone deaf adults must experience beginning-level activities, such as handling movable cutout letters, if they are to comprehend separate sounds in words. If students with auditory dyslexia are to master the foundation concepts of letter–sound relationships, they must experience immediate, tangible reinforcement. Teachers must realize that traditional reading instruction has not worked for these individuals precisely because there is not enough concrete reinforcement of abstractions.

Principle 2: Provide Multisensory Experience

Most teachers, and many parents, recall a concept from introductory psychology: *The more senses that are involved in a learning experience, the more fully the experience is learned.* This oversimplification of learning is a key to successful remediation of auditory dyslexia. If a student sees it, hears it, says it, feels it, moves it, even smells or tastes it, he or she can begin to comprehend it. In other words, the more sensory channels that are used while learning, the more comprehension will be attained.

There is some risk of overanalyzing if emphasis is placed on sounding out words, especially when dealing with isolated sounds and symbols. Some students misperceive sound–letter patterns, resulting in grossly exaggerated sounding out of words that makes reading impossible. For example, some learners have the mistaken idea that each letter of the alphabet is a "word." *A* is "aye" or "aaaaa." *B* is "bee" or "buh." *C* is "see" or "kuh" and so forth. It is perfectly natural, therefore, for students such as Pete and Maria to perceive the word *cat* as three words, not three letters. Thus they would drawl, "cuh-aaaaaa-tuh." Because this is like nothing heard in their daily language, Pete and Maria completely miss the word.

Students with auditory dyslexia usually must begin with cutout letters—matching them, arranging them in sequence, and spelling out simple words the instructor provides as models. Gradually, by using movable letters that they can feel, they begin to connect names and sounds to the letters they touch, feel, and manipulate. Many teachers have clinched such learning by adding taste and smell with cookies shaped like alphabet letters. The point is that whatever sensory stimuli are necessary to imprint the concepts within the learner's memory should be used.

For example, the only way Maria can master phonics is to see the patterns rather than try to hear them. Her instructors follow a drill procedure that teaches Maria how to combine several sensory pathways at the same time. She must see, say, hear, and touch all together, which is accomplished easily by following a simple 5-step procedure in drilling with visual phonics. Maria's instructor makes a set of flash cards showing several words of the same spelling family: *cat, bat, rat, sat, hat, fat,* and *mat.* Maria then performs the following steps for each card:

1. *See the word.* Look at it. Touch it. Trace the letters with a finger.

2. *Say the word.* Say it from sight-memory or sound it out, if possible. If Maria cannot say the word, then her instructor pronounces it and listens as Maria repeats.

3. *Spell the word orally.* Maria carefully says each letter in correct sequence while touching each letter to guide her eyes in refocusing correctly. If she says any letters out of sequence, or if she calls a letter by a different name, the instructor helps Maria work out the correct spelling sequence. She practices this oral spelling until she has memorized the word.

4. *Type or write the word from memory.* Without looking at the card, Maria tries to encode it on the keyboard or with a pencil. She whispers each letter as this writing is done.

5. *Check for accuracy.* After the word is typed or written, Maria compares her writing with the flash card. If any mistakes have been made, the procedure is repeated until she can encode the word correctly.

This 5-step visual phonics procedure moves slowly, and students may become bored doing this kind of practice. However, it is the most effective technique for helping individuals with auditory dyslexia overcome the tone deaf block in spelling. Over a period of time, this kind of drill with word-family patterns implants basic phonetic patterns within the student's memory better than any other technique.

Principle 3: Provide for Kinesthetic Reactions

Many teachers control their classes by the dictum, "I want silence and plenty of it!" This mode of instruction sometimes is supported by administrators who judge the quality of teaching by the degree of silence in the classroom. Unfortunately, a habitually quiet classroom is a poor learning environment for many students with auditory dyslexia. When body movement and vocal response are sharply curtailed, Pete and Maria are immobilized because essential learning channels are shut off.

During the 38 years I have worked with the dyslexic population, I have seen three basic behavior patterns in virtually every classroom.

Number 1: The Silent Learner

This person absorbs information in a mostly passive, quiet, and private manner that would delight librarians. The silent learners gain knowledge by concentrating through one sensory channel at a time. If they are reading, they use only the vision pathway. They rarely mix sensory channels. These single-channel processors want to be left alone during study time, and they are intensely aware of personal space. They resent having their privacy interrupted or their territory invaded during their times of concentration. These students seldom have dyslexia, although occasionally an individual with LD will fit this quiet, passive learning style.

Number 2: The Noisy Learner

Noisy students must combine three learning channels simultaneously in order to acquire new information. They must see it, say it, and hear it all at once. If these students are denied speech and hearing during study time, they do not completely internalize what they read or hear. They can be forced into submission by overbearing instructors, but they always want to whisper or mentally say each word while reading or working math problems. Noisy "Number 2" students eventually drive the quiet "Number 1" workers up the wall unless instructors take steps to separate them during study time. Noisy students must have the feedback of conversation and voice response, and they do not notice the privacy signals set up by the silent learners. In other words, they are natural classroom enemies. If these opposite learning styles must exist in the same space, there will be friction and dissatisfaction before the class is over.

Number 3: The Body Learner

These individuals cannot cope with learning unless body motion and muscle reactions are involved. They must see it, say it, hear it, and manipulate or touch it before mental images come together. When forced to sit still and be quiet, they cannot learn successfully, and they become discipline problems in traditional classrooms where silent, passive learning is required. Body learners usually are considered to be hyperactive.

Students with auditory dyslexia are especially frustrated when talking, moving, and touching are denied in learning situations. If they are forbidden to use their overall body as a global learning channel, being forced to sit passively and think silently, they cannot interact successfully with the teacher's instructions. Rather than being a hallmark of good teaching, forcing them to work quietly virtually guarantees illiteracy in many cases. Effective teaching means encouraging each individual to exercise his or her own learning style, even if this requires separating students into groups for studying.

Principle 4: Build a Stock of Memory Cues

Even when they master the fundamental letter–sound connections for reading, persons with auditory dyslexia seldom become fluent spellers. The missing links between the middle ear and the auditory cortex block their ability to build memory images of word patterns. Because Maria does not "see" word forms in her mind while working from memory alone, she has no reliable cue system for accurate recall of word patterns. When there is no visual model, she is helpless to reconstruct accurate words on paper.

Adults with dyslexia who have achieved academic success have done so by devising their own systems for recalling spelling patterns. Few persons with dyslexia ever describe their private memory tricks, for fear of being thought silly. It does sound strange to listen to Pete or Maria whisper as they work out spelling patterns: "Let's see . . . 'mother' is *t-h-e* with *mo* in front and *r* on the end. Warm is *a-r-m* with *w* in front." Because they cannot build mental images of sound patterns, persons with auditory dyslexia remember bits and pieces of spelling patterns, tacking on letters to flesh out the skeletal word structures as they are recalled.

When parents and teachers are aware of this perceptual need, they can help Maria a great deal. After assigning the week's spelling words, the teacher helps Maria figure out memory cues that trigger recall of word patterns. It is completely irrelevant whether Maria's memory tricks make sense to anyone else. The important thing is whether they help her recall spelling patterns.

Principle 5: Concentrate on Consistent Spelling Patterns

An old-fashioned technique that drills with word families was reviewed previously. This technique introduces students with dyslexia to stable, similar patterns that stay with the rules, and has been used by many teachers under the label of *consonant substitution.* The basic idea is to present a root spelling, such as the *–at* family. Pete and Maria practice building familiar words by placing different consonants in front of *–at:* b*at* c*at* r*at* f*at.*

Many teachers shy away from nonsense words (e.g., *lat, wat, dat*). However, students with dyslexia often enjoy creating nonsense words that fit the word family. In fact, most youngsters with LD spend a great deal of their private fantasy time devising word games. In a form of solitaire, they mimic words they hear, creating nonsense vocabularies just for the fun of it. Successful teachers know that making nonsense words is a highly motivating activity for many reluctant readers and spellers.

Adolescents and adults respond well to this activity, so long as the instructor turns a deaf ear to the double entendre items that inevitably occur. If things become too earthy when streetwise adolescents are involved, the teacher should stop the double talk at once by informing the culprits, "I know exactly what that means, and I don't want to hear it again." Before calling a student's bluff, however, the teacher must be sure the learner is consciously trying to be cute. Some naive youngsters (as well as adults) have no idea that their words or phrases carry a double meaning.

The important point is not to confront these students with variable spellings that violate the rule they are trying to comprehend. For example, if Maria is coming to grips with the fact that when *o* comes by itself inside a short word, it has the sound of *o* in *hot,* she should not suddenly be exposed to the word *cold.* At this point, it is irrelevant for Maria that "*o* before *ld* has its long name." This kind of generalization has no meaning to her. Her mastery of letter–sound connections is built upon visual cues, not upon abstractions. In fact, even intelligent adults with dyslexia seldom become skilled with phonics rules. Teachers must realize that these unique students seldom respond to abstractions, but rather to structured systems of memory tricks and visual cues.

Principle 6: Provide Visual Cues

A firmly entrenched attitude among many instructors is that tests must be taken strictly from memory in order to determine what the student has learned. Consequently, all visual cues to answers are removed during test time, forcing students to retrieve information or organize responses only from memory. This rather curious custom is unfair to those with learning differences. Taking tests from memory arbitrarily labels talented test takers as "good students," whereas those who perform awkwardly are called "poor students." Persons who are gifted with quick, accurate memory (retrieval) are the star performers, regardless of whether they can make a practical application of their knowledge. In fact, the term "test wise" is often heard, denoting those who know how to pass tests even when they do not understand the content. Also in current use is the cynical student phrase "multiple guess," referring to the so-called objective tests that force students to select one of several arbitrary choices.

Forcing students with dyslexia to work from memory alone when their retrieval is erratic is a questionable educational practice. When a specific learning disability has been diagnosed, this educational practice becomes illegal. If Pete and Maria can function well if given visual models for points of reference, then teachers should provide this kind of reinforcement.

For example, it is not cheating on a spelling test when Pete glances at the cursive writing chart to remind him of how to write a certain letter. This is survival. Nor is it showing favoritism for the teacher to display model spelling patterns while the class is doing written test items. If navigators need trustworthy directional instruments to point the way to specific destinations, students with dyslexia must have visual cues. The purpose of education is to produce independently literate individuals who know how to read the signs and do what they say. Those who have dyslexia are placed in hopeless situations when instructors hide all the visual indicators, forcing them to work from memory. The same teachers would be horrified to see a track coach confiscate the crutches of a boy with a physical disability, then force him to hobble after his able-bodied peers just to "test" his track skills.

Visual cues can be in the form of pictures, graphs, charts, colors, or textures—whatever is appropriate to the particular classroom situation. Regardless of the visible code, Pete and Maria prove remarkably knowledgeable when allowed to work where they can see visual reminders. Without such reinforcement, they become understandably restless, uncooperative, and eventually hostile toward school.

Principle 7: Allow Oral Answers on Tests

Parents and teachers both can recall personal experiences of frustration in taking an examination. Adult educators are aware of the near panic felt by many adult students, including teachers taking graduate courses, when they are forced to work strictly from memory in answering comprehensive test items. Physicians who practice near universities know when qualifying exams are scheduled for doctoral candidates because their medical clinics are besieged by graduate students seeking relief from hypertension, ulcers, and near collapse under the strain of taking tests without benefit of visual cues. It is unfortunate that adults who experience such trauma seem to have so little understanding of the feelings and needs of children with disabilities.

Students of all ages who have dyslexia show the same behaviors as worried adults at test time. When required to write what they should have learned, working entirely from memory, they face a difficult choice: They can either endure the pain and embarrassment of flunking another test, or they can avoid the test, if possible. This intense frustration causes much of the ugly classroom behavior seen in students who decide to fight the system, a form of confrontation that is unnecessary.

When alternative ways to respond to tests are provided, students such as Pete and Maria usually exhibit satisfactory knowledge. Through listening and some reading, they gain a great deal of accurate information. Classroom teachers who understand the dyslexic dilemma have discovered that these students can be held responsible for specific information if allowances are made for their handicaps in reporting or writing. Oral tests have proved to be the answer for many such students. When they are tested orally, they experience success, which is, of course, what education should be all about.

Chapter 4

Overcoming Dysgraphia

The first explanation of chronic poor handwriting appeared in 1869 when English neurologist Henry Charlton Bastian published his studies of written language deficits in adults who had suffered aphasia (Bastian, 1869). A full century later, the cause of lifelong handwriting dysfunction was discovered (Jordan, 1995). Toward the lower region of the transcortical motor area (TCM) of the left brain is a cluster of specialized nerves that control fine-motor coordination for penmanship. A form of dyslexia called *dysgraphia* occurs when this specialized portion of the brain is underdeveloped or develops in a different way. In Chapter 1, two types of brain cell differences that cause dyslexic tendencies were described (see Figures 1.1 and 1.2). When clusters of cells within the TCM region of the left brain skip developmental steps or fail to prune away unneeded dendrites, otherwise educated persons cannot master fine-motor skills for legible penmanship. Figure 4.1 shows the regions of the left brain that control finger motions in handwriting.

Bastian's observations toward the end of the U.S. Civil War have been authenticated through recent brain imaging science and anatomical studies of dyslexic brains. Many persons with dyslexia in reading and spelling also have handwriting problems. No matter how hard they try, it is neurologically impossible for them to develop fine-motor coordination skills in this area.

Handwriting is a sensitive, personal matter. Partly because of this personal nature, penmanship practice has

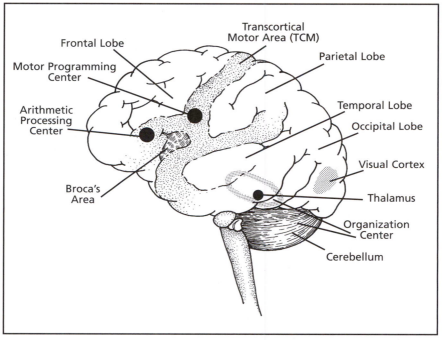

FIGURE 4.1. These regions of the left brain are involved in the act of handwriting. Incomplete cell development makes it impossible for individuals to master legible penmanship skills.

been one of the least popular school activities, especially for boys. In recent years, educators have removed pressure from children to make their handwriting perfect. Students no longer have to fill pages with push–pulls and curlicues that are well remembered by older persons. Today's teachers tend to accept uniqueness in children's writing, so long as the writing is legible.

There is a technical difference between dysgraphia (the inability to write legibly with a pencil or pen) and *dysorthographia* (the inability to spell correctly from memory). Many poor spellers develop good enough penmanship to win praise for their handwriting, but they never master basic spelling rules. This poor spelling pattern has been described in previous chapters. On the other hand, it is not uncommon to find good spellers who cannot write legibly. The struggle to write clearly often masks adequate spelling ability, which emerges when the poor writer uses a word processor. Dysorthographia is not always related to poor penmanship.

Ironically, old-fashioned penmanship drills previously may have corrected a form of dyslexia that is a serious educational problem in modern classrooms. Since the introduction of manuscript printing to primary grades during the 1930s, many intelligent youngsters have not learned to write acceptably. Fifty years ago, penmanship drills saturated children with perceptual awareness of letter formation. Today, thousands of students fail at handwriting. The penmanship drills that filled many classroom hours for our parents and grandparents provided inadvertent remedial treatment of borderline and moderate levels of dysgraphia. Even those with severe dysgraphia developed legible writing through seemingly pointless graphic training.

Dysgraphia involves faulty control of the muscle systems needed to write letters and words accurately. Learners who have dysgraphia usually have a clear mental image of what the left brain intends to encode, but the student keeps "forgetting" how to write specific symbols. Certain letters and numerals are made with backward or upside-down motions. Handwriting is generally so awkward and unsatisfactory that dysgraphic writers try to avoid situations that require them to practice penmanship.

Most persons with dysgraphia learn to read, although dysgraphia usually is associated with both visual and auditory dyslexia. Teachers and parents seldom see one form of dyslexia that is not complicated to some degree by other signs of symbol processing struggle. When individuals who have severe dysgraphia are taught to use alternate means of writing, such as word processors or dictation technology, the handwriting disability largely can be removed as an educational problem. So long as educators insist that all students master manuscript and cursive penmanship skills, dysgraphia will continue to be a frustrating educational handicap.

DYSGRAPHIA SYNDROME

Because educators tend to judge student competence by the neatness of written work, students with dysgraphia are at a serious disadvantage. Teachers must distinguish between careless handwriting habits and the neurological inability to develop penmanship skills. For example, boys often reject the self-discipline required for an attractive writing style. A cluster of unique characteristics differentiates dysgraphia from carelessness, and the syndrome is not difficult to identify if the teacher studies a variety of handwriting samples from each student's daily written work. The following sections describe the characteristics of dysgraphia. (Appendix D contains a checklist of dysgraphic symptoms.)

Difficulty Learning Alphabet Forms

The primary characteristic of dysgraphia is difficulty remembering how to write certain letters and numerals. Instructors might not identify this flaw unless they watch the student write. The cursive writing style is intended to flow from left to right, whereas dysgraphia involves the tendency to make backward strokes (from right to left). So long as younger pupils print isolated letters in manuscript style, this backward tendency may not be a major problem because the letters are not connected in a series. Dysgraphia therefore may not be noticed until children are expected to develop skills in left-to-right cursive writing style, which usually occurs at the third grade.

Few adults are aware of the staggering perceptual burden modern education has placed upon beginning pupils when it comes to writing the symbols of the English language. Adults who have good literacy and handwriting skills assume that children must master only 26 alphabet letters. Unfortunately, this is not true. Since the early 1930s, U.S. educators have taught manuscript print in kindergarten and first grade, but the alphabet seldom is taught in the sequence of A through Z. Instead of learning only 26 letters, primary pupils are expected to master two sets of alphabet symbols: the 52 capital and lowercase manuscript symbols and the 52 capital and lowercase cursive symbols—a total of 104 alphabet letters.

Manuscript print usually is taught throughout the second grade. At the same time young pupils are mastering the first 52 alphabet symbols, they are exposed to a wide variety of type styles in all kinds of media. In fact, the Library of

Congress lists more than 100 typefaces commonly found in U.S. reading materials. Near the end of second grade or by the middle of third grade, children are told that manuscript style no longer will be satisfactory—they now must master a new style of letter writing. The 52 isolated, unconnected manuscript letters mastered through 2 or 3 years of drill are gradually discarded, while a new handwriting style, called cursive, is introduced. By the beginning of fourth grade, young students are expected to have memorized the entire set of 104 alphabet forms.

Along with learning to cope with 52 manuscript symbols, primary pupils are simultaneously confronted by more than 30 printer's cues commonly used in basal readers, library books, textbooks, and other sources of reading at home and in the classroom. At the same time, they are expected to distinguish among several marks of punctuation, color cues, boldface type, italic, indentation, chapter and story headings, unusual page format, and other markers. These symbol systems take on meaning only when the students understand how all these visual signals match what they say and hear in oral communication. Few adults would willingly attempt such a staggering burden of language symbol mastery within a 3-year span. The wonder is not that many children fail, but that so many succeed. To start a child's quest for literacy with manuscript printing is a serious barrier for children with LD, who are more confused than edified by so many alphabet symbols.

Dysgraphia becomes a crippling factor when it brings the student into conflict with tradition, especially the left-to-right orientations of reading and writing. Cursive letter forms involving closed, circular strokes are difficult for students with dysgraphia. Equally difficult are letters that require a change in direction of hand movement. Writers who have dysgraphia frequently have problems remembering where to stop a sweeping or circular movement, how to swing back, and how to connect the lines within complicated letter formations. They have great difficulty remembering where and how to stop circular motions in order to swing accurately into the next letter. These difficulties are dramatically reduced when they are taught the continuous-stroke cursive style first instead of starting with the isolated letters of manuscript printing.

Mirror Writing

A rather puzzling form of dysgraphia is commonly called mirror writing because it actually can be read when held up to a mirror. A complete mirror image is rarely seen by parents or teachers, but varying degrees of this tendency commonly are found in dysgraphic work. As a rule, only certain words or portions of words will be written backwards.

The counterpart of mirror writing is mirror reading, in which whole words are read from right to left (*was* for *saw*, *tub* for *but*, *no* for *on*). Figure 4.2 is an example of mirror writing done by Vanessa, a bright second grader who did not exhibit mirror reading tendencies. Because she had partially adjusted to the left-to-right sequence, she was able to overcome her tendency to mirror write rather quickly when the teacher understood the nature of the problem. A study buddy helped Vanessa work through a series of tracing and copying activities that taught her to think left to right, and within a few weeks, her mirror writing habits had largely disappeared. Occasionally, there will be a person who has such severe dysgraphia that he or she cannot make the transition from mirror image to left-to-right orientation.

Scrambled Sentence Structure

A significant clue to the language potential of a student with dysgraphia is sentence structure, or syntax, which is largely camouflaged by poor handwriting. Two examples of frustrated creativity are presented in Figures 4.3 and 4.4. The passages have been translated to illustrate the language maturity of each struggling writer. In each case, an interested teacher took time to decipher the messy, crudely done handwriting that at first glance seemed not worth wading through. When the dysgraphia patterns had been recognized, these students no longer were regarded as lazy and careless. They

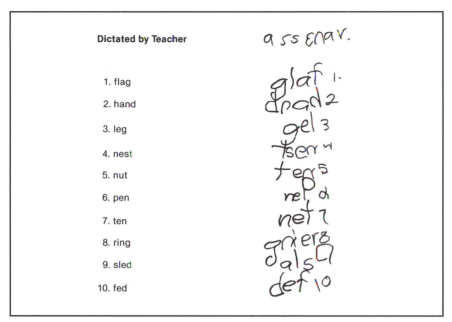

FIGURE 4.2.   An example of mirror writing produced by a student in second grade.

made rapid progress by mastering the D'Nealian writing style.

Figure 4.3 is Donna's response to an unfinished story in her reading class. After reading a brief story about children picking blueberries and being startled by "a loud, astonishing noise" from the woods, she was asked to imagine what happened next and then write an ending in her own words.

Figure 4.4 is Andrew's Christmas story. In second grade Andrew was severely dysgraphic. A poorly interpreted psychoeducational assessment wrongly labeled him as being emotionally disturbed. The *Wechsler Intelligence Scale for Children–Revised* (WISC–R) (Wechsler, 1974) yielded a Verbal IQ of 103, a Performance IQ of 110, and a Full Scale IQ of 107. Because the examiner did not ask Andrew to write, his severely dysgraphic tendencies were not observed. To explain why he was not keeping up in classroom learning, the psychological examiner concluded that Andrew must be suffering from some type of emotional trauma that was keeping him from learning on schedule. It was further reasoned that

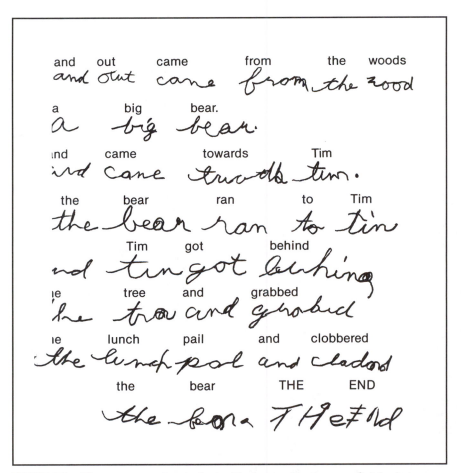

FIGURE 4.3. The response of a student with dysgraphia to an unfinished story. The sample shows language maturity that is masked by poor handwriting.

Andrew could not have a learning disability because there was not enough discrepancy between his IQ and his scores on a standardized achievement test.

This reliance upon standardized test scores was challenged by Andrew's classroom teacher, who had noted a sophisticated language structure in the boy's work. A reading diagnostician identified the problem as dysgraphia, which does not always show up on clinical tests for motor development. Older students helped the classroom teacher guide Andrew through daily training in D'Nealian handwriting skills. Within 6 weeks, his dysgraphic symptoms had begun to disappear. This incident illustrates the danger of

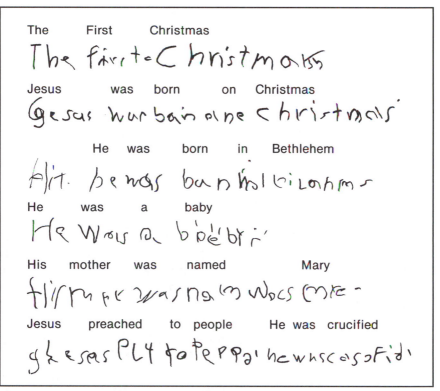

FIGURE 4.4.   A sample of poor handwriting by a student with dysgraphia. Based on test scores that showed no impairment in coordination, this student was originally misdiagnosed as severely emotionally disturbed.

professionals looking only at scores instead of at actual classroom performance.

The major flaw in Andrew's manuscript print is broken letter patterns. Lowercase *a, h,* and *m* are usually fragmented, with the strokes scattered apart. This gives his writing the appearance of "bird scratches." Several letters are rotated toward the left, adding to the disoriented appearance of his work. These faults were quickly remedied as Andrew mastered the D'Nealian writing style.

Poor Directionality

A crippling aspect of dyslexia is the inability to see how parts of a whole pattern relate to each other and to the whole. For example, students are expected to read horizontally from left to right. In writing, the right-handed student is supposed to progress horizontally left to right with the page tilted slightly toward the left. If a page is divided into columns, the student is expected to progress downward until the eyes or hand reach the bottom line, then move directly upward and to the right for the next column. Because the U.S. literacy system is based upon this left-to-right, top-to-bottom orientation, anyone who perceives reading or writing differently is "wrong." Persons with a poor sense of directionality do not automatically interpret book pages or work pages in this standard way. They continually lose their place and need guidance to follow the "normal" format.

Left-handed writers frequently develop a legible writing style, although they often appear to write upside down or backwards. This unorthodox compensation of "lefties" has frustrated many instructors who do not understand what is involved for left-handed accommodation to a largely right-handed world.

A subtle but not uncommon problem associated with dysgraphia is confusion with horizontal and vertical directionality. Occasionally, clinicians will see someone who demonstrates totally inverted perception. Such individuals read exactly upside down, perceiving symbols at 180 degrees rotation from normal. Because these students usually are capable readers, their upside-down orientation often is not discovered until they have to write. Teachers sometimes will notice a student turning the reading page halfway around, indicating that the individual perceives at 90 degrees rotation. For these readers, the print becomes legible only when the rows of words are vertical. This rotated orientation usually disappears as the students are indoctrinated to correct orientation. The need to rotate lines or turn them upside down bothers instructors much more than it does the individuals who are working in these ways.

Directional confusion does create a problem in handwriting. This form of dysgraphia frequently is camouflaged by extremely poor letter formation and by the messy appearance of the student's papers (see Figure 4.4). As the student with dysgraphia attempts to write, particularly with no visual model to copy, directional confusion creates jerky production, with much erasing and writing over. The writing usually cuts through the line or wobbles up and down about the line. When moving from the bottom of one column to the top of the next, the writer sometimes switches to mirror image, writing on the left-hand side of the midline instead of on the right.

Difficulty Copying Simple Shapes

A hallmark of dysgraphia is the inability to copy simple shapes without distortion, as mentioned in Chapter 2. Teachers assume that students can hold mental images of what they see while those images are translated through fine-muscle coordination onto paper. Dysgraphia greatly inter-feres with this complex perceptual task. Instructors can use any activity that involves copying circles, squares, dia-monds, triangles, or rectangles to see how well a struggling pupil can do this simple work. (It is important to allow for immaturity in younger children in the primary grades.) Dysgraphia is indicated only when other symptoms also are present in the learner's handwriting. The *Jordan Written Screening Test* (Jordan, 1989b) quickly identifies this dys-graphic tendency. Figure 4.5 demonstrates how a simple copying activity reveals dysgraphic tendencies. This work was done by a sixth-grade boy (age 12 years 9 months) who had a mental ability within the average range.

A frequently observed flaw in copying shapes is the ten-dency to draw "ears" on the corners of simple figures. Teachers can see this tendency on math pages and art activ-ities that ask students to sketch or copy shapes and figures. Figure 4.6 shows examples of "ears" that indicate left-brain inability to handle right-brain images.

Telescoping

When students with dysgraphia are laboring to write longer words, they commonly leave out portions of the letters or syl-lables without being aware of this error. The effort of putting word units onto paper is a labored process for them. After

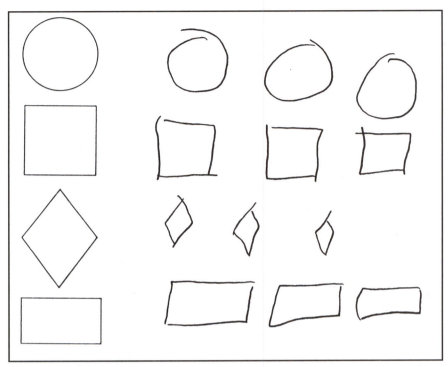

FIGURE 4.5. A copying activity revealing dysgraphia in a sixth-grade boy.

writing for a brief time, they start to lose track of how much of a word has been encoded. This habit, called *telescoping,* was illustrated in Chapter 3 in the spelling errors under "Sound Chunks Omitted" (see p. 123). Learners who tend to telescope usually have auditory dyslexia as well as dysgraphia.

Perseveration

The opposite of telescoping is *perseveration,* mentioned in the spelling error examples in Chapter 2 (see the "Oral Reading" section). Once the brain starts a signal pattern commanding the fingers to write, the student with dysgraphia cannot stop. The fingers keep making the same pencil strokes again and again. Perseveration is often heard in oral reading or in conversation as persons with dyslexia inadvertently repeat vocal patterns. It also often occurs during rhyming drills, as when a student responds to *cat* by

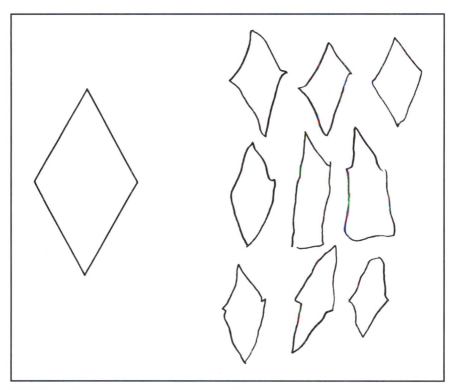

FIGURE 4.6. Copying activity showing "ears" on corners, revealing dysgraphia.

saying "vat, dat, lat, nat, wat." This run-away verbalizing is not an effort to be amusing, but an involuntary reaction. At that moment, the person cannot stop the repeating reflex. In the same way, writers with dysgraphia cannot halt the reproduction of certain letter or syllable patterns without completely stopping their writing, then starting again. Perseveration also results when the writer habitually lifts the pencil from the paper midway through writing a word. This break in continuity leaves the person unable to remember where he or she stopped in the word pattern.

OBSERVATION SKILLS FOR TEACHERS

Instructors must develop two skills of observation if they are to detect dysgraphia quickly. First, they must actually observe the student at work. Individuals with dysgraphia often mask their difficulties so that the problem may not be apparent on sample papers collected for evaluation. Second, teachers must learn to re-create the student's writing style by slowly tracing over the handwriting. This hands-on experience of feeling and observing the flaws in directionality lets the instructor discover where the writing breaks down.

Figure 4.7 is a sample of writing by an intelligent fourth-grade girl. This was Glenda's attempt to write the alphabet from memory. Her confusion in transferring from manuscript to cursive style is apparent because she mixes the two writing styles. Dysgraphia is noted in Glenda's difficulty forming the loops on *d, b,* and *p.* She also confuses *d* and *b* because of her initial experiences with these letters in isolated, unconnected manuscript style. Capital *Z* causes Glenda considerable confusion, as indicated by her erasures and awkward overprinting. By tracing over her writing, the reader can feel the confusion Glenda experiences.

Figure 4.8 displays the spelling test of a fourth-grade student with dysgraphia, which illustrates that any example of writing can be used to look for dysgraphia. The instructor should slowly trace over the student's writing while saying

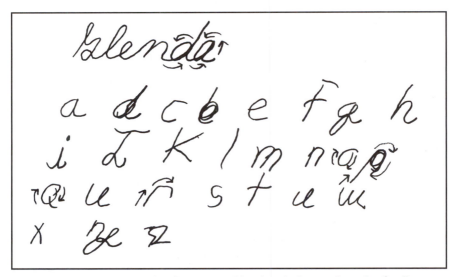

FIGURE 4.7. A writing sample of a 9-year-old girl with dysgraphia who finally mastered good cursive writing skills by learning the D'Nealian technique of continuous stroke writing. The small arrows show direction of stroke.

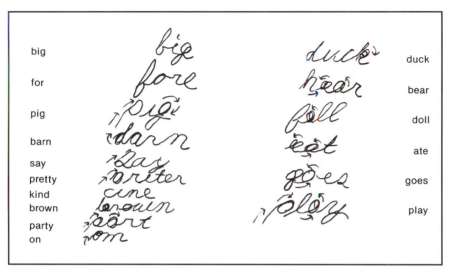

FIGURE 4.8. A spelling test of a fourth-grade student with dysgraphia. The small arrows indicate backward strokes.

the words over and over as this student did while he wrote. The small arrows in Figures 4.7 and 4.8 indicate the backward strokes these students used in their writing, which is the reason why such students are extremely slow, insecure writers.

A careful observer will note the many broken letters in Figure 4.8. This boy's writing is actually a series of pieces strung together. In words such as *pig* that begin with *p*, the child started at the bottom and marked upward, ending in a backward loop to form the top of the letter. Because this caused him to finish the pencil stroke inside the letter, he was forced to break writing continuity by starting the next letter somewhere near the bottom loop on *p*. Initial *f* was often patched together because the writer could not recall how and when to change the direction of the pencil motion. This lack of continuity caused him to circle again and again when writing *d, b, a, o,* and *e,* as illustrated in the words *barn, brown, party, duck, bear, doll, ate, goes,* and *play*. The reader can easily imagine the panic this boy experiences during pressured writing activities in school.

A more serious form of dysgraphia is illustrated in Figure 4.9 in the writing of a highly intelligent boy in the third

Dictated by Teacher	Student's Dyslexic Responses	
big		*d* reversed for *b*
for		*r* consistently resembles *i*
pig		began to reverse *g*, then overprinted *P*
barn		*b* reversed for *d* *o* intended for *a*
say		phonetic spelling *sae*
pretty		began with *Pertr*, then overprinted reversed *P*, then overprinted final *t*
kind		
brown		reversed *b* for *d*, mutilated *o*, repeated *o* but changed to *n*
party		phonetic spelling *parte* with final *e* rotated forward
on		
duck		reversed *d* for *b*, then had difficulty forming *c*
bear		began *b*, then changed to *d* *r* looks like *i*
doll		reversed *d* for *b*, then made *o* backward with both *l* letters written bottom to top

FIGURE 4.9. A writing sample of a third-grade boy with combination visual dyslexia and dysgraphia.

grade. This student's work was troubled by a combination of visual dyslexia and dysgraphia, as revealed by backward letters and reversed word elements. These dyslexic tendencies were almost entirely corrected during a 14-week cycle of intensive training that supplemented his regular classroom activities. The key to success was his mastery of D'Nealian cursive writing, an excellent writing program (Thurber, 1993). The student practiced an hour each day until he had mastered the cursive lowercase alphabet in D'Nealian style. As alphabetical order and sequence became automatic, the dysgraphic problems shown in Figure 4.9 began to disappear. By the end of third grade, this boy was meeting grade-level expectations in writing and spelling from dictation.

ACTIVITIES FOR OVERCOMING DYSGRAPHIA

The following sections describe activities that can be used in the classroom to overcome dysgraphia, including activities dealing with directionality, handwriting, poor eyesight, dictation, checking for errors, and increasing work output.

Establishing Directionality

The primary disability underlying dysgraphia is the inability to deal with directionality, which means that when the learner attempts to write symbols on the page, he or she does not have a clear, automatic habit of proceeding left to right or top to bottom. Instead, the writer tends to mark circular strokes clockwise, which is backward from what educators call correct. The writer with dysgraphia also tends to start at the bottom of the letter or numeral and mark upward, which also is backward from the standard orientation. There is nothing wrong with backward orientation as such. If left alone to adapt to reading, writing, spelling, and arithmetic in their own way, most students who have dysgraphia would devise ways to cope with literacy requirements. The major obstacles around which they cannot move are stereotyped expectations regarding handwriting. When these artificial penmanship restrictions are laid aside, these learners are as able as most others to do the work of educated persons.

Instructors who work with learners who are dysgraphic must follow certain procedures to help these struggling writers think of directionality. First, individuals who are dysgraphic should write with hard lead pencils that do not become dull quickly. Using a 4-F pencil instead of a Number 2 pencil prevents smudged, messy writing. Second, all writing must be doublespaced. It also may be necessary to teach the student who is dysgraphic to lay a finger between words to make sure that the student does not inadvertently write the words too close together. Third, learners who are dysgraphic must be reminded where to start on the page. A starting mark, such as a brightly colored dot or a star, should be placed where writing should begin on each page. The struggling learner is taught always to touch the starting place before he or she starts to write. Fourth, learners who are dysgraphic must be coached repeatedly in left-to-right, top-to-bottom orientation. As these students write, they must be reminded to move the pencil systematically from left to right, and they must be reminded to check their work for anything they may have written backwards or upside down. Fifth, margins must be clearly marked. Instructors should use a felt-tip pen to draw margin lines down the left and right sides of the paper. Then learners who are dysgraphic must be coached in "bumping the margin" as they write. Finally, each student who is dysgraphic must have a study buddy who patiently guides the LD writer in reviewing each written activity. Together they should find any reversed or upside-down letters or numerals, and they should talk about pencil strokes that cut through the line or float above the line. As a team they can practice bumping the left margin and keeping the pencil inside the correct spaces. Over time, these coaching strategies teach learners who are dysgraphic how to monitor their own work and correct most of their errors in directionality.

Educational hostility toward those who deviate from the norm inflicts permanent damage in students who have dyslexia. By the time they reach fourth and fifth grades, their interest in developing writing skills has been extinguished, or they have become too defensive to respond to usual classroom procedures. The fight to preserve individuality has absorbed all of the person's time and energy. Older students with dysgraphia often have little inclination to develop the niceties of correct writing because for too long it has been perceived as the enemy responsible for their rejection by instructors and classmates. Youngsters with dysgraphia are among the most seriously damaged casualties of our educational system. Overcoming their writing disabilities is a long-range undertaking, but the good news is that, in most cases, it can be accomplished.

If parents or teachers wonder whether this description of the child's plight is overly dramatic, they should listen as these struggling students verbalize their feelings to counselors and tutors. Whereas students with visual and auditory dyslexia appear to enjoy school, most students with dysgraphia do not. The difference seems to lie in the attitudes of parents and teachers. Most students at least can trace adequately or draw acceptable pictures, thus earning praise and a degree of status; however, the person with dysgraphia lacks even these means of gaining acceptance. Their struggle is compounded further by the messy appearance of their work. Correcting dysgraphia calls for a great deal of patience on the part of teachers and parents. Not only must they teach writing skills, but they also must convince children that it is safe to try.

Mastering Handwriting Skills

Regardless of the student's age or grade placement, the essential starting place for correcting faulty concepts of directionality in writing is cursive writing. This proposition contradicts the philosophy of most educators, who, for half a century, have insisted that manuscript printing must come first. The reader should keep in mind that this book concerns exceptional children, not those who fit the mold of the majority. Although most children do prosper when they learn manuscript printing first, a different approach must be used in teaching handwriting to children with dysgraphia.

Most U.S. elementary schools now use one of the most effective handwriting programs created during the 20th century. In the 1950s, a creative elementary school teacher and principal, Donald Thurber, realized that children with dyslexia/dysgraphia could not become fluent with the traditional ball-and-stick manuscript writing style. Those who developed legible printing faced great difficulty transferring to cursive writing later on. Thurber developed a unique handwriting system based upon single-stroke pencil movements instead of the isolated ball-and-stick ones. This different approach to handwriting, the D'Nealian Writing Program (Thurber, 1993), has been mentioned previously in this book. The title is an acronym devised from Thurber's own name: Donald Neal Thurber. Many children, adolescents, and adults now are writing legibly with great pride, thanks to the creative work of Thurber. The D'Nealian system of writing gives the student a simple, dependable way to write in cursive style with only a few instances where the pencil must be lifted to make certain letters. Single-stroke writing solves penmanship problems for students who cannot master handwriting skills in the traditional manner.

Coping with Poor Eyesight

Students with dysgraphia often have major problems with vision control. Certain characteristics of letter formation, irregular spacing, ragged left margins, telescoping, loss of place, and poor placement of writing on the page often signal problems with eyesight. Teachers frequently see dramatic disappearance of dysgraphic symptoms when faulty vision is corrected. Students who cannot team the eyes together (maintain saccadic movements) or who cannot maintain clear focus in sustained work are handicapped in copying, doing workbook assignments, and coping with penmanship activities. Instructors must make sure that students can see well enough to do written work before assuming that dysgraphia is the cause of poor penmanship.

Practicing Dictation

The goal of most educators is to teach students with dysgraphia to write legibly and with reasonable accuracy when taking dictation or writing from memory. Weekly spelling quizzes provide an ideal channel for emphasizing dictation writing skills. When working with learners who are dysgraphic, the instructor must let them know ahead of time what they will be expected to write from dictation. The teacher should start with one or two brief sentences that will be dictated at a specified time. This practice dictation must not be graded—it is a training procedure whose purpose is to teach these students to cope with increasingly complex dictation, as time goes by. Gradually during the school year, the teacher should expand the quantity of dictated material until the students can write successfully five or six sentences at one sitting. This kind of structured drill increases these children's confidence in writing from memory without having models to copy.

Checking for Mistakes

An essential survival skill for individuals with dysgraphia is knowing how to edit their own written work for errors. This is an especially sensitive area because these students often react strongly to criticism. The teacher can provide ample opportunities to let students check their own work against whatever model is being used. Spelling tests, arithmetic assignments, social studies exercises, or science quizzes all are suitable for this purpose. If these students are taught how to use answer keys and other scoring devices, they can protect personal territory and pride by being the first to see their failures.

Once errors have been checked, the students do not mind so much if the teacher or classmates see their work. Damage to self-confidence and self-esteem occurs when apprehensive writers turn in work that they suspect has many errors. Suspense builds to painful peaks before the paper is returned. If indeed it has not been good work, the student's ego once again is deflated by the sight of red ink all over the paper. Checking one's own work first, a face-saving device, is very important to insecure learners.

It should be noted that the risk of cheating occurring is no greater among students with dyslexia than it would be among honor students. In fact, cheating almost always is a direct measure of the pressure a student feels to be accepted by the system. If instructors discover dishonesty as students do self-checking, they should reexamine their educational values regarding the importance of grades. The presence of cheating often is a reliable cue that too much emphasis has been placed upon achieving good grades. Insecure students will resort to cheating to find acceptance within a learning situation. If the pressure to make good grades is coming from home, the teacher's options are limited. Aside from counseling such a frustrated student, there may be little the teacher can do to relieve anxieties about grades. If the pressure is from within the school, grade standards should be adjusted.

Increasing the Quantity of Finished Work

Regardless of good intentions by parents and instructors, no struggling learner can be fully protected from dealing with failure or criticism. Sooner or later, writers with dysgraphia must cope with arbitrary demands for finished work where little or no consideration will be given to their problems. Eventually these students must either cope with written assignments or drop out of the system.

Raising Production Quotas

It is not difficult for instructors to map out production schedules for students with dysgraphia. One example is the use of "thermometer" charts. Movable colored strips are raised by degrees to indicate new writing quotas the student is expected to reach. By using color codes along with other symbols, each student's production goals constantly are shown. Each week, the teacher reevaluates each student's work. If he or she is making sufficient growth, his or her quota for the coming week is increased by a small amount.

If, however, the student has not yet conquered a specific dysgraphic problem, the quota remains unchanged. Occasionally the expectation must be dropped lower for someone who has become discouraged. The point is to cause the student to stretch in small increments to make sure that steady growth is maintained.

The key to growth lies with the instructor, who must sense when quotas are reasonable or when too much is expected. If the student accepts the new goals in stride, all is well. He or she is ready to meet the higher output schedule. If frustration and signs of insecurity emerge, the new goals are too high. The learner's reaction to the thermometer chart usually is a trustworthy indicator of how ready he or she is for greater productivity.

Maintaining the production charts need not require a lot of bookkeeping. If the student is working in three areas—reading, writing, and arithmetic—the production chart has three thermometer columns, each equipped with a color strip that moves up or down to indicate changes in the teacher's expectations. Each column is labeled at the top, and up the side of the chart are numerals, with lines running across the face of the chart.

For example, if Wayne is expected to finish three written language papers this week, the colored strip under Language is raised to Line 3. If he is also expected to finish five papers for Math, that strip is positioned at Line 5. If Wayne must turn in four written assignments for reading, that thermometer strip would rest on Line 4. A clear, visual monitor has been provided for Wayne as well as the teacher. On Wednesday the teacher can ask how Wayne is coming on his weekly work schedule. By comparing the number of finished papers in his folder with the color code on the chart, both Wayne and his teacher have an instant check of how much more work must be done before Friday afternoon.

Wayne can be held accountable for meeting his quotas because this kind of visual cue system is fair. Wayne knows on Monday exactly what the teacher expects for that week. The teacher is relieved of trying to remember these details because Wayne's assignments are reflected on the chart. This visible right-brain contract with Wayne permits the teacher to respect his self-esteem by not nagging him to do his work. By reminding him each day to check his own progress, the teacher avoids the likelihood of conflict that is triggered when instructors trespass on a student's private space. On the other hand, Wayne has no excuse for failing to meet his production schedule. This is a fair way to teach him how to accept increasing amounts of responsibility. If Wayne "goofs off" during work time with his responsibility fully in view, he must suffer the consequences. As part of the working agreement, Wayne already knows what the consequences will be because the teacher informed him of the penalty for failing to carry out the contract.

This sort of visual contract is as effective in kindergarten as it is in high school. For many years, the workplace has used similar systems for adult workers. Employees who receive incentive pay according to their output are far more productive than those who receive only a base wage. Parents and teachers who work on a contract basis, giving worthwhile rewards for acceptable work as well as significant penalties for work failure, have been amazed at the differences they see in student attitudes.

It is hard to nag students into doing their tasks. Wise parents and teachers use incentive programs that do the nagging. The production chart is harder for Wayne to ignore than the nagging voice of a parent or instructor. There is something about the silent, persistent presence of a quota chart that spurs on most students to fulfill their obligation. This sort of self-discipline is critical for those who have dyslexia. Lifelong lessons in timing and self-programming are instilled when they are held accountable by a production chart. When Friday afternoon comes, there is no way Wayne can escape the truth. If his week has been wasted, then he faces judgment. If the week has been spent productively, then he receives the reward.

The quota chart also allows parents and teachers to present alternatives. Students with dysgraphia need to be allowed to choose which written assignments they will submit for evaluation. If Wayne has done several more papers than the chart requires, he chooses to hand in the papers he considers best for the week. Thus both student and teacher are allowed to save face. When given this opportunity to decide his own fate, Wayne cannot blame the teacher for low marks on his work. In turn, the teacher is free to make whatever candid suggestions are necessary. When the full decision has been the teacher's, both instructor and student are placed on the defensive.

Self-Discipline

Probably the most important learning derived from a quota system is self-discipline. Of all students in our schools, those with LD usually are the least self-controlled. Their perception of life is a scrambled blur of events, pressures, obligations, and information, much of which appears disorganized and incoherent. Without a highly structured system that keeps their lives ordered, they seldom achieve a sense of well-being. Adults with dyslexia who have succeeded in spite of their handicaps have learned how to order their circumstances. The primary social need of students with LD is self-control, which, of course, includes literacy. Production schedules also are essential for persons who cannot comprehend chronological time lapse. If these young people are to manage family budgets, job responsibilities, and leisure activities well, they must be taught the ingredients of self-discipline over a period of several years.

Keyboard Writing

A wide array of new technology has opened the door to good writing for students who struggle with penmanship and paper-and-pencil tasks. Federal guidelines such as the previously mentioned Education for All Handicapped Children Act of 1975 and the newer Individuals with Disabilities Education Act of 1990 permit students with dysgraphia to bring laptop computers into the classroom instead of struggling to keep up with paper and pencil. These guidelines and other regulations permit students like Wayne to do his written assignments on word processors instead of by penmanship. If using a keyboard system is not feasible or possible, students like Pete, Maria, and Wayne may dictate orally to someone else, or they may carry tape recorders to class, then listen again to necessary oral information. Future generations of students will have the technology to compensate for their lack of talent in handwriting. Keyboard writing opens the door for intelligent expression of knowledge, as Steeves (1987) demonstrated in her computer projects with boys with severe dyslexia at Johns Hopkins School of Education.

PRINCIPLES FOR OVERCOMING DYSGRAPHIA

In spite of recent prophecies that a new day is coming when handwriting will be obsolete, classroom teachers still are very much concerned with each student's ability to communicate in written form. It is essential that all students develop enough handwriting skills to cope with the workplace. The ability to put one's thoughts into legible written form will remain a vital issue into the next century.

Earlier in this chapter it was mentioned that students with dysgraphia usually know what they want to write. They may even have a model from which to copy. The dilemma is how to transfer those ideas and information into a legible written code.

Correcting dysgraphia in the classroom is possible if certain principles of instruction are observed. Teachers must keep in mind at all times that students who have dysgraphia are not just being messy or careless. Unless they become bitter and hostile through repeated failure, they will do their best each time they write an assignment. The teacher holds the key to these individuals' attitudes and self-concept. If they do their best, but it is never good enough, serious damage will occur to vulnerable self-esteem and self-confidence. If, on the other hand, the teacher can practice patience and exhibit long-range optimism, these students often can enjoy success over a period of time.

Principle 1: The Learner Is Doing His or Her Best

I learned a painful lesson about dysgraphia the second year I taught school. My sixth-grade students were asked to write stories built around "trigger words" written on the chalkboard. Wayne seemed especially interested in the project because the trigger words suggested a science fiction theme, his favorite fiction form. I graded the stories with my usual thoroughness, marking every spelling, grammar, punctuation, and penmanship error with a blood-red pencil. Wayne's story content was unusually good, but the writing mechanics were awful. At that time, I had no knowledge of dysgraphia. My attitude was that every student could do good work if he or she tried hard enough. I handed back the papers at the end of the school day, then dismissed the class. As Wayne passed me, I saw tears in his eyes. "I liked your story," I said. "Then why did you bleed to death all over it?" he sobbed, running from the room.

As a teacher I had failed to understand a vital fact: *Wayne had done his best.* The messy, smudged paper I had rejected was the best he could do at that time. In "bleeding" all over his mistakes, I had failed to perceive that he had done his best for me, and I had rejected him. Like most proficient grown-ups, parents and teachers tend to think of children as miniature adults, which blinds us to many vital elements in educational growth. Because we assume that what we see is what really exists, children are judged by the surface characteristics of neatness, punctuality, quietness, dignity, poise, and how well their work fits the mold. The stereotypes by which we judge student achievement can be cruel, if we mistakenly assume that imperfect papers are evidence that the child has not tried. Such rigid expectations may have some validity for nondisabled students. However, sensitive children like Wayne are hurt day after day, year after year, because their inability to fit the mold brings false judgment upon them. The truth is they usually try harder than their peers who always make good grades.

How does an instructor or parent determine whether a struggling learner is doing his or her best? The only feasible way to make such a judgment is to note indicators of improvement. For example, if Wayne has always disregarded (failed to perceive) small details in copying from the board or from a book, his work would have poor punctuation, failure to indent for paragraphs, disregard of capital letters, and word chunks left out. The instructor will know that Wayne is doing his best when he begins to perceive minor details that affect the quality of his work. In other words, improvement must be judged by the small self-corrections students begin to make on their own, after these deficiencies have been pointed out by the teacher or study partner. If over a period of time Wayne's finished papers show fewer and fewer mistakes, this is proof that he is doing his best.

An essential factor in correcting dysgraphia is mercy. Although mercy, patience, understanding, and forgiveness are not directly related to phonics or word analysis, these attitudes are of critical importance in the classroom treatment of dyslexia. The merciful teacher is one who begins to look for bits and pieces of improvement, instead of continuing to "bleed to death" over the multitude of errors. If Wayne and students like him begin to observe capital and lowercase letters, this represents a tremendous stride in achievement for them. What might be 1 inch forward for the teacher may represent 100 feet of progress for the student with dysgraphia. It is cruel and harmful to judge progress always by large increments. If these students must leap all the way from C to B to demonstrate that they are doing their best, there is no hope for them in the classroom or the workplace. When instructors can accept small tokens of progress as being giant steps, then mercy will begin to heal bitter attitudes, allowing additional progress to be made.

The first step toward correcting dysgraphia is not more handwriting practice—it is for the instructor to believe that even the messiest, grubbiest papers may represent the best the student can do under the circumstances. Far too many educators are biased against students with dysgraphia solely because the written work is messy.

The secret is to scan Wayne's work for molecules of improvement: certain letters no longer reversed, punctuation marks now being used, and/or capital letters where they are supposed to be. Many teachers have reversed their marking systems, using the student's favorite color to mark only the points of progress. A paper with no marks would signify no improvement. From this point of view, Wayne cherishes the days when marks cover his work, heralding the fact that his instructor sees improvement.

Principle 2: Handwriting Is Intensely Personal

It would be profitable if every parent and classroom teacher could relive his or her most sensitive experience in which personal writing or another academic attempt was criticized. Most adults, especially those enrolled in graduate courses, are extremely sensitive when their written work is judged. Any professor who returns research papers, essay test responses, or written reports can testify to the acute pain experienced by adults who find critical notes on the margins of their work. It is not unusual for grown-ups to burst into tears over criticisms professors have made. None of us is immune to feeling sensitive about what we have written. Editors are especially aware of the problems new writers face in learning how to accept editorial suggestions. Of all the sources of dread that professionals feel, having one's writing criticized, misunderstood, or belittled is among the most acute.

This universal sensitivity toward one's written work is reflected in the way adults carefully guard personal diaries and intimate letters. Although schoolwork by no means is as personal as one's private notes, there is a common feeling of caution when individuals are required to commit themselves to written form. Oral communication is not remembered verbatim. A speaker's clever use of intonation and mannerisms can distract listeners from any personal revelations that might be uttered. But thoughts put into writing become permanent. An intimate part of the writer's self becomes vulnerable once it is on the page for all the world to see.

Sensitive instructors are aware of how this timidity in writing affects classroom behavior. From the earliest grades through graduate school, insecure students slip up to the teacher to ask, "Do you want to see what I wrote?" Instructors do great damage when they impatiently send these students back to their seats without glancing over the written material. Professors who do not take time to scan a nervous graduate student's first draft inflict similar pain. When students reach out this way, they are actually pleading, "Please don't be too critical. This is the best I can do. Is it good enough yet?"

As students achieve success, they need less reassurance from instructors and others. Repeated success with writing, especially if one is talented in language usage, brings enormous satisfaction. Teachers always look forward to having students who write well and have an interesting style. This kind of success seldom is available to the person with dysgraphia. By nature, most persons who have dyslexia are overly sensitive. The struggling students introduced in earlier chapters often compensate by appearing indifferent to praise. In reality, they are hungry for the acceptance experienced by more talented individuals. When forced to commit themselves to written form, those who have dysgraphia are left defenseless. For them, writing becomes a threatening experience in which their weaknesses are fully exposed. Their choices are to muddle through or become defiant and refuse to try. If they hand in messy papers, the teacher "bleeds all over them." If they choose not to write, then they are publicly branded as lazy, careless, uncooperative, or even "dumb." No matter which way they turn, they cannot win, from their point of view.

I began this book by reviewing the vast knowledge now available about brain-based LD. In Chapter 1, the evidence that forms of specific learning disability are beyond the choice or control of the struggling learner was presented. From this point of view, there can be no such thing as the "correct" way to hold one's pencil, or slant the paper, or sit in one's chair while writing. Neither can educators logically dictate the angle at which handwritten letters must slant, nor the balance a writer should maintain between ascenders and descenders or circles and loops. The penmanship standards demanded by earlier educators were based more upon bias than upon perceptual reality.

In recent years, handwriting has come to be recognized as a unique signature of the writer's personality. Wayne slants his letters toward the left, not because he is "incorrect," but because of unique tendencies of his individuality. The size of the writer's script can have a definite correlation with his intelligence, just as the way Donna dots the letter *i* and crosses *t* indicates specific character traits or dispositions or mood. It is terribly presumptuous for a teacher to declare that a student is wrong just because the person's script does not flow like the instructor's. A great deal of ignorance has been involved in handwriting methodology, especially where children with dysgraphia have been concerned. Fortunately, the term *correct* is being supplanted by the more realistic term of *acceptable.* Having one's best efforts accepted does not imply that further progress is not needed, but being labeled acceptable allows room for growth, a step at a time.

If writing is indeed a sensitive, personal affair, then parents and teachers should handle the subject accordingly. The rule of thumb should be a practical one: *So long as the student's writing is legible, and so long as it is the best he or she can do, I will accept it without making the writer feel inferior.* Gradually, the student will learn to write more acceptably in order to avoid embarrassment as he or she matures.

Principle 3: Respect the Learner's Territory

During my final year as a classroom teacher, I learned a lesson that has shaped my professional life for the past 30 years. A dramatist turned popular science writer, Robert Ardrey, wrote two fascinating books, *African Genesis* (1961) and *The Territorial Imperative* (Ardrey, 1972). Ardrey drew hundreds of examples from the animal world to support his thesis that human beings, like lower animals, possess a strong territorial imperative that we will defend at all costs. Ardrey contended that this instinct to stake out one's territory, then defend it against threatening intruders, explains human behavior. According to his idea, every aspect of human civilization—religion, education, politics, family life, recreation, technology, war—is governed by the driving need for territory. From his observations, Ardrey inferred that, to be a wholesome individual, every person must have a certain degree of privacy (territory) in which he or she is safe from intrusion by outsiders. The theory holds that, when human beings are deprived of private territory, they become neurotic and cease to be emotionally well balanced.

Ardrey's concepts have suggested some useful applications in education. Numerous studies have documented excellent learning results when territorial needs have been provided for in teaching situations. There are critically important lessons for educators, parents, and workplace supervisors within the concept of territoriality.

If we are to help students who are struggling to overcome learning problems, close attention must be given to the interactions between these frightened, insecure individuals and confident, sometimes overbearing instructors and supervisors. Few educators realize that one talented, self-confident instructor alone with one apprehensive low-talented learner is not a one-to-one relationship. If the instructor is overbearing and the student is insecure, the relationship often is overwhelming for that student. This explains why some individuals often do not respond when tutored by well-educated persons. When viewed through the perspective of territorial imperative, dyslexic behavior does indeed appear defensive because the person feels that his or her territory (inner privacy) is threatened. This accounts for much of the disruptive behavior encountered by teachers of students who have learning disabilities. Most adults do not hesitate to defend their rights (territories) against outside threats. Walkouts, strikes, professional holidays, and other forms of protest have become common among educators. If professional adults react this way when their workplace territories are violated, then certainly one would expect overly sensitive students with LD to do the same.

My classroom experience with Wayne illustrates this principle. As his teacher, I had carefully "motivated" him to respond to the creative story assignment. I wish I could say that I coaxed him out of his shell. What actually happened was that he let me enter his private world of make-believe. I was proud of the expertise with which I manipulated the class into writing stories from the trigger words. After all, did they not decide to use my words instead of theirs? Until I saw Wayne's angry tears, it did not occur to me that I had made an unspoken contract with my students:

> If you will write a story as I have suggested, I will read it carefully. I know it's hard for you to spell and punctuate accurately. But don't worry about that. The main thing is for you to express yourself. Be creative! You can trust me to appreciate the part of yourself you put down on paper. I won't betray your trust!

Then I "bled to death all over it," as Wayne so accurately stated.

The fact that I was a young teacher was no excuse for my violation of that boy's trust. As a sensitive adult, I certainly knew the pain and embarrassment of having my own writing (territory) violated by stern graduate professors. Not 6 months prior to that day with Wayne, I had driven home in tears of rage because a professor had belittled a paper I had written for his graduate course. The mistake I made with Wayne was not to respect his territory. I betrayed his trust by "bleeding" on his mistakes, and then I compounded the injury by saying, "I liked your story." He reacted as any healthy person should react by thrusting me out of his inner territory. It was several weeks before he let me back in. There are times when teachers never regain a comfortable relationship with students whose territories they have failed to respect.

Develop a Contract

If educators are to gain entry into the inner space of students with dysgraphia, they must establish ground rules that will govern the behavior of both parties, which sometimes is called a contract. The teacher has a frank, private conversation with the student, explaining the skills that must be developed. The teacher presents a checklist of the trouble spots in the student's work, along with samples of work to illustrate these deficiencies. Then the teacher proposes alternatives, naming the kinds of activities available for correcting the problem, specifying the amount of individual attention he or she can give, explaining the grading system, and telling who the aides or tutors will be, if such help is available.

Approach with Patience

At first, not all students who are struggling are mature enough or interested enough to receive this much information. The instructor must use good judgment to determine when enough has been discussed at one conference. The point is to present a simple outline of the student's needs, explain what can be done about it, and specify his or her responsibilities in overcoming the problems.

There are many reasons why a student like Wayne might be reluctant to admit the teacher into his confidence (territory). In the first place, Wayne probably will not trust the outsider to keep the bargain. A wise teacher does not push to get in. There is nothing more devastating to someone who has trouble expressing ideas than for an articulate, outgoing educator to bombard them with personal questions. The teacher must not try to pry answers from the student. If no interaction is forthcoming, the instructor takes the initiative by making direct statements about how, when, and where the corrective work will begin. As Wayne digests this offer of help, he will realize that the instructor is genuinely ready to accept his efforts, weaknesses and all. At this point, Wayne and his teacher begin to have a more open dialogue. In fact, one of the dilemmas of tutoring students with dyslexia is how to persuade them to stop talking in order to accomplish drill work.

The gist of this principle is simple and direct. The teacher does not overwhelm the apprehensive learner by entering private, personal territory before the student is ready to allow the outsider in. Until Wayne offers cues that he is ready for a more personal relationship, the teacher should confine the relationship to simple drill routines, explaining whatever Wayne seems interested in knowing. Above all, written work must not be condemned, even when it is illegible. Tactful ways to require that unacceptable work be done again can be devised. One of the best methods is to let Wayne evaluate his own work against a model. Above all, the teacher must not write all over Wayne's paper to the point where he becomes hurt or overly discouraged.

When the instructor genuinely respects Wayne's territorial boundaries and is careful not to betray the subtle trusts he begins to show, great strides toward improvement will be seen. Abrupt, impatient, and domineering educators see virtually no growth among the students with dyslexia in their charge. Persons with strong, forceful personalities seldom realize the effect they have on sensitive individuals. Most domineering teachers perceive themselves as excellent instructors because their rooms are quiet and their students busy, but such teachers rarely should be in charge of individuals with dyslexia. Territorial boundaries are so fragile in these students that a heavy-footed instructor tramples down the fences many times each day without realizing the emotional devastation this aggressive behavior is causing. Teachers should be chosen for corrective work because of their skills in sensing these territorial boundaries. Strong-willed adults work best with outgoing, competitive students who thrive upon competition for territorial dominance in the classroom.

Chapter 5

Overcoming Failure and Developing Self-Confidence

The most critical problem with which a person with dyslexia must deal is stress. From the first experiences with language until the end of their lives, persons with language-processing disabilities wrestle with the ever-present factor of stress. The left-brain language dysfunctions described in Chapters 1 through 4 are operative from early childhood as the youngster tries to comprehend oral language, remember things accurately, and interpret the hundreds of signals that must be understood if one is to be a functional member of society.

As Chapter 3 described, children with dyslexia continually mishear, misperceive, misinterpret, and misunderstand the complex world in which they live. Having dyslexia means experiencing the never-ending stress of trying to do one's best, but continually disappointing key people in one's life. The chronic social and academic stress experienced by such individuals is similar to living with chronic pain. On better days the pain can be ignored, but it is still there whenever the body moves a certain way. In the same way, on better days, persons with dyslexia almost can forget their language dysfunction, but it is always there, ready to trip them up without warning. For those who have dyslexia, this continually haunting background of language disability colors all relationships with a depressing shade of gray. As the child with LD matures into adolescence, and as the adolescent becomes an adult, this chronic pressure from stress takes its toll. Self-image, self-esteem, and self-confidence must grow in a rocky soil that never is free from the arid influence of stress.

In earlier chapters, it has been shown that the hallmarks of dyslexia range widely from mild (merely an occasional nuisance) to severe (a serious disability). To understand how stress influences individuals with dyslexia to such a great degree, it is necessary to review the severity scale:

0		1	2	3		4	5	6	7		8	9		10
none		mild				moderate					severe			total

Stress follows this continuum closely. A person who occasionally reverses certain symbols, tangles the tongue in saying longer words, misunderstands several words that sound alike, and must consult a dictionary to make sure certain words are spelled correctly will feel stress from time to time. These episodes come more through frustration with one's self than from outside pressure. This mild dyslexic level triggers frequent flashes of irritation. Occasionally, it brings criticism from a teacher, parent, or boss, who complains about the dyslexic "blips" that cause errors. This kind of stress comes and goes. It is embarrassing and frustrating, but it is not chronic or severe. Persons who have only mild or occasional dyslexic patterns can handle this degree of stress, although sometimes an overly sensitive person will blow this kind of periodic stress out of proportion. With affectionate support from family and friends, most persons who have mild dyslexia handle their stress with no significant ego damage.

Stress does become a problem, however, when dyslexia is within the moderate range of severity. As discussed in earlier chapters, persons who are at Levels 5, 6, and 7 make continual mistakes: Spelling is never fully accurate, details continually scramble out of sequence or become cluttered, listening comprehension is faulty and creates a lot of misunderstanding, and reading is slow and labored. These individuals with moderate dyslexia have difficulty taking accurate notes rapidly enough to keep up with the flow of new information. They confuse or reverse body-in-space directions (east/west, north/south, up/down, top/bottom, left/right). They continually forget important things unless they keep written lists and daily schedules, and they are late for meetings and appointments. They are usually slow doing certain kinds of activities that require recall of specific information. They lose their words as they speak, or as they tell or describe. They forget the names of people and cannot always remember what to call familiar objects. These persons are socially awkward, hesitant, slow, and prone to make many more careless mistakes than same-age peers. These persons live under a constant weight of stress because they do not meet society's expectations. They almost never find safe places or circumstances where they are completely accepted without some kind of judgment or criticism coloring the relationship.

Individuals who have dyslexia at the severe level live in a constant state of heavy stress. Few persons at Levels 8 and 9 know what it is to be free from social, educational, economic, or family stress. Those individuals at Level 10 often do not survive without serious mental health problems because their developmental years are so heavily saturated by stress that ego structures are crushed beyond recovery. These individuals grow up under a dark cloud of constant criticism. They constantly hear, "You messed up again!" or "Why don't you ever try to do it right?" or "Don't you ever listen to what I tell you?" If they are lucky enough to have parents who are compassionate and supportive, this often is offset by teachers who are not. If a brother or sister seems to understand, grandparents or other relatives may not. If a boss is tolerant and forgiving, other supervisors are critical and demanding. If adolescents or adults with severe dyslexia allow themselves to seek romance by dating, they run the high risk of being rejected once that special friend finds out.

Individuals with severe dyslexia also face overwhelming emotional trauma trying to find work. If they reveal their condition, few employers will hire them and they will not be admitted into military service. If they say much at all about having dyslexia, they are told, "Well, we all have our problems," or "You use your dyslexia as an excuse." They frequently meet adults who believe that dyslexia is linked to mental retardation, or that there is no such thing as dyslexia. Everywhere these persons turn, they face the stress of either dealing with the problem alone or being rejected and criticized because of it. From the earliest years when toddlers begin to interact with their larger world, youngsters who struggle with language development feel the stress of being different and not being correctly understood.

No human being can develop normally and wholesomely if he or she cannot find respite from stress. Even in persons who do not have dyslexia, stress takes a heavy toll in heart disease, digestive problems, anxiety, mental health breakdown, ruptures in personal relationships, and so forth. It is impossible for anyone to be a whole person if stress exists day after day, year after year. The irony of dyslexia is that the language-processing deficits that trigger stress cannot be removed through counseling or therapy. This chronic life pattern either is built in from the stages of fetal development or, occasionally, is caused by injury to the brain. It thus will always be there to some degree. Persons who have dyslexia must develop ways to cope with their chronic patterns so that stress can be reduced as much as possible. It is critically important that the significant people in the life of the individual with dyslexia understand what causes stress for him or her. The following factors are keys to helping such individuals overcome failure and develop adequate self-confidence. If the important people understand these critical issues, the effects of stress can be reduced to the level of being a tolerable nuisance instead of an intolerable, crippling condition.

STRUCTURE

The most critical skill persons with dyslexia must develop is knowing how to maintain structure in their lives. It is the nature of dyslexia that details are out of order or sequence. Having dyslexia means not holding on to clear mental images of how parts go together in a specific order to produce a functional whole. Every moment of every day, the person must cope with mixed images; partial memory of details; confused sense of passing time; incomplete awareness of direction; and an inability to recall where things are located, when it is time for the next important activity, how much money has been spent already, how much money is left to meet the budget before the next payday, how many steps are yet to be done before the job is completed, and so forth.

Persons at Level 3 or lower on the severity scale have little difficulty learning how to stay organized because they learn early in life to use cues and reminders. They learn to cover their scrambled thinking well enough so that few outsiders ever suspect that these invisible stumbling blocks exist. Persons at Levels 4 and 5 cannot fully hide their trouble with structure. However, they manage to get by, although they face continual criticism and complaints about being "forgetful" and "scatterbrained." Persons at Levels 6 and 7 face a lifelong struggle keeping their lives structured. Those who stay at Levels 8 and 9 all their lives suffer tremendously because their lives are so poorly ordered.

Until puberty has fully begun during the early teens, youngsters with dyslexia need help structuring and organizing their lives. Preschool youngsters are much more clumsy, are poorly plugged into their world, and are less able to manage themselves than are peers who are developing normally. Delayed language development (DLD syndrome), which in early childhood creates problems with specific memory, places great stress upon the child as adults urge him or her to tell, describe, remember, and perform. "Jay, tell Grandma what we saw in the park yesterday," Mom says. Jay is stuck. He is partly blank. He remembers going to the park, but he does not have a full image of what went on there. "You know, Jay," mother says as she tries to show him off to his grandmother. "We saw that great big brown animal with the big teeth!" Still Jay is partly blank and confused. "Dog?" he finally blurts out. "No, Jay, you know it wasn't a dog. Think hard now. Tell Grandma what animal we saw." If Jay is a sensitive child, he already is close to panic. If Grandma joins in urging him to remember and tell her, he suddenly is under stress from two key people in his life. If Grandma also should add a bribe by saying, "I've got something nice in my purse for a little boy who can tell me what he saw in the park," the stress may become unbearable. Before anyone has discovered that Jay has dyslexia, he is living with stress.

Many children like Jay are too sensitive to cope with this kind of early failure. They burst into tears as others press for specific language structure that these children cannot give. Jay's oral language processing is too loose to let him remember specific details in a given order. He needs help, but, instead, he often receives criticism, even though it may come under the camouflage of loving adults pressing him too hard to remember. Time after time during delicate years of ego formation, stress takes its toll on self-confidence and self-image. Delayed language development in early childhood imprints lasting scars upon self-image and self-worth, especially if Jay has a sibling who blurts out answers for him or "shows him up" by being more successful.

In Chapter 1, Wilson's landmark studies of the impact of DLD syndrome on young children were reviewed. This and other studies have documented the effects of stress related to early language struggle in children. Enormous frustration and damaged ego development are integral components of delayed language development.

Earlier, it was pointed out that labels such as dyslexia never should be applied until a body of evidence has been accumulated. It seldom is possible to make a definite diagnosis of dyslexia until the child reaches the age 7½ or 8 years. Many youngsters who stumble over poor structure are late bloomers. However, whether the child is poorly organized because of a brain-based dysfunction or due to late maturity, the helping process must be the same. Poorly organized learners must have help with any task or situation that requires them to deal with structure.

SUPERVISORS AND SUPERVISORY STRATEGIES

Perhaps the greatest problem adults face in working with children who have dyslexia is the youngsters' resistance toward being supervised. Yet, these vulnerable young persons cannot learn to cope with stress without supervision.

This universal stubbornness is due partly to their different views of the world. They do not perceive the same panorama of events, scan their world with the same degree of insight, come away from experiences with the same quality of impressions, or look back with the same perspective. They do not judge time, dimension, distance, space, or reality the same way others do. They do not react to stimuli with a whole, fully integrated response. They continually leave out important ingredients that alter how they should have reacted, and they tend to respond more slowly than others, which causes their understanding to be delayed. They have the tendency to "freeze" in unexpected situations, which looks very much like balking or stubbornly refusing to cooperate. They often do not know what to do in situations where others know automatically or quickly figure out the right response. Having dyslexia in today's heavily loaded culture is like standing in the middle of a busy freeway. If these individuals are left alone to decide for themselves, they are out of step, in conflict, at cross-purposes, and in emotional danger as the fast-moving traffic of their society whizzes by on all sides. Because of slow reaction time, faulty interpretation, incomplete recall, misunderstanding of signals, scrambled impressions, cluttered mental images, and uncertain body-in-space orientation, persons with dyslexia must have outside help to handle all the traffic on society's freeway.

Reducing Fear Levels

Parents of children with dyslexia face the never-ending task of keeping the child's life structured so that as few loose ends as possible are faced each day. It is impossible for these youngsters to be on time for meals, gather up necessary things for school, get dressed on schedule, remember a string of oral instructions, do a series of jobs that were listed verbally that morning, keep everything picked up in their rooms, bring all outside things into the garage at night, take care of pets, and so forth.

Because their memory cannot cope with the hundreds of facts and sequences that are part of normal living, these children must have supervision—kind, nonaggressive, helpful, not overly critical supervision. The "supervisor" must be patient, must stay calm, must not yell or lash out at the confused child. He or she must walk by the child's side as a guide, not push from the back as a prodder. Such children need supervision because they cannot see the next few steps clearly, much like someone peering into a dark corridor, wondering what is just ahead. Anyone would naturally pause before starting down a dark, unknown passageway. Individuals who have dyslexia pause hundreds of times each day because the next moment is not clear. The supervisor must be aware of this fact.

If the supervisor takes time to shed enough light on these dark "unknowns," the apprehensive child will feel safe enough to move forward in confidence. If, however, the supervisor roughly or impatiently shoves the indecisive child forward, the youngster will be overwhelmed by panic and the ghost of impending failure. This child with faulty memory and incomplete perception will respond best to a guiding hand that reassures that all is well, but it should be remembered that he or she will freeze, panic, and rebel the moment that stress is felt too keenly. Fear is the constant shadow of individuals with dyslexia, no matter what the age—fear of failure, of being incompetent, of being rejected, of being criticized, of humiliation, of being impotent when others can do it well, of losing loved ones or cherished relationships, of dying, of being "dumb," and of not living up to the expectations of special persons in one's life. Such fears would freeze anybody.

This underlying aura of fear flavors every decision the child must make. Its aftertaste fills the emotions the way a bad smell fills a room. The haunting memory of other failures triggers faster heartbeat and physical constrictions that cause the chest to tighten, breathing to quicken, and blood pressure to soar. The frightened child is on guard, overly defensive, and on the verge of running away from the unknown. He or she wants to hide or escape. It is less painful to be scolded again for forgetting homework than to go through the agony of making another failing grade. It is easier to endure another reprimand for being lazy than it is to do one's best and still be criticized.

Older persons who have dyslexia often are criticized for "not taking that good job." They are subjected to comments such as, "Why did you quit your job? That's four jobs you've quit already this year!" What the critic does not realize is that invisible pain within the fearful worker finally became too acute to be endured. Those who have dyslexia are never fully free from uncertainty; however, if the right kind of supervision is provided early enough, most youngsters can learn to overcome this innate fear and develop coping strategies for stress.

Kinds of Supervisors

Supervision can come in a variety of ways. Individuals with moderate or severe dyslexia need a key person who is the main source of their supervision. For children, this usually is a parent, typically the mother. In single-parent families, the parent cannot always be available to supervise and keep the child on schedule, in which case, many children will turn to "substitute parents" for this help. In fact, virtually all persons who have dyslexia find someone on whom they can depend. Parents of such children often complain about the kinds of friends their youngsters prefer. It is natural for fearful, apprehensive, or insecure young people to seek out companions who do not judge, criticize, or scold. Persons who have dyslexia usually become attached to others who also have dyslexia because no one else is patient enough. When two or three such individuals form a group, they are developing their own community or substitute family where they feel welcome and free from the stress of judgment. Why should these children want to associate with people who continually nag, criticize, judge, scold, or otherwise make them feel like failures? Bonding to a group of companions who accept their type of thinking as normal is part of the process of finding a source of help that gives without always taking away. Occasionally, a child will find supervisory companionship in an older brother or sister. Sometimes grandparents, uncles, or aunts will fill this important role. Sometimes the supervisor is a scout leader, a coach, a church leader, a teacher, a school custodian, or a neighbor who operates a small business nearby. Many adults become surrogate parents for young people with dyslexia when they provide the patient, nonjudging guidance that is needed.

Providing Visible Structure

The most important type of supervisory strategy is something the person with dyslexia can see. Few individuals with dyslexia can develop full mental images just by listening or doing abstract thinking. They must see some kind of outline, sketch, graph, chart, or diagram before concepts begin to make sense. Even when they are good listeners and glean most of their new information through listening, they still need to encode it in some visible pattern that can be seen, pondered, touched, and examined over a period of time. Early in the nurture of a poorly organized child, parents and other supervisors must begin to develop visible structure clues and guidelines.

Color Cues

The right brain does not call things by name but recognizes them by shape, size, color, form, texture, place, and position. Long before children are ready to read words or interpret alphabet letters or numerals, they can follow right-brain structure. Poorly organized children who probably will be identified later as having LD must have a lot of right-brain structure in their early years. For example, specific places in their room must be coded. If the child shows good perception of color, then the room could be color coded. Bright red would show where socks and underwear always go, bright blue would show where pajamas go, bright yellow would show where shoes always go, and so forth. The child's socks would have bright red marks, the pajamas would have a bright blue patch, and his or her shoes would have bright yellow spots. Whatever the child is expected to organize and keep in place would be coded by visible color, which would not be named by the left brain but would be recognized and matched by the right brain.

Shape Cues

Some children do not respond to color cues. For example, from 3% to 7% of all boys are "color blind." If this is the case, other types of right-brain structure cues are possible. Some parents use geometric shapes as markers. Shoes go where the child sees a square, books go with the circle, and pajamas go with the triangle. Many families follow through by coding tools and equipment in the same manner. The child learns to match the shape of the tool with the hook or drawer that has a small matching shape in clear view. It is much easier to guide disorganized children through the chore of cleaning their rooms or putting tools back in the right place if the supervisor uses right-brain cues: "Now, John, let's find everything that looks like a hammer. That's good. Now let's find everything that looks like a nail. Do you remember where the hammers go? Look for the hammer drawer (or hook). That's right. Now do you remember where all nails go?"

Some creative children like to use animal cues. Shoes go in the bird drawer, books go on the elephant shelf, and pajamas go with the kangaroo. Socks and underwear go inside the dinosaur drawer. These kinds of structure cues greatly reduce stress in the lives of poorly organized children and their families. The child is trained to look for how things are alike and different, how certain things belong together in categories, how specific cues show the right place, and how to follow instructions. The key to effective supervision is to give visible guidelines for poorly organized youngsters because they cannot work structure out for themselves.

Lists and Outlines

As soon as children can read simple words, the supervisor starts making written lists and outlines. Each task to be done is written or printed on a list and clearly numbered. The child learns where the list always will be. Once the child is told where his or her list will be, that place stays the same. When the supervisor says, "Jay, go look at your list," Jay does not have to wonder where it is. Written lists remove nagging from the relationship between supervisor and child. When adults try to supervise orally, they inevitably end up in shouting matches with the forgetful child. "Jay, I told you to feed the dog." "No, you didn't." "Yes, I did! You never listen to a word I say!" This kind of verbal argument could have been avoided by posting a simple list:

1. Feed the dog.

2. Water the dog.

3. Wash your hands.

Supervisors of children who are disorganized must be prepared to split hairs. Most adults make the mistake of underestimating the intelligence of such a child who is loose and poorly organized. As noted previously, persons with dyslexia often are much brighter than average. They do not score well on standardized tests, but they are quite intelligent. It is just that this intelligence is loose, poorly organized, and often beyond their reach when organized, left-brain work is involved. This underlying intelligence fosters a lot of splitting. Supervisors of students with dyslexia often become intensely frustrated by the tendency to quibble because the child invariably splits hairs over tiny details that the busy supervisor has forgotten to mention. This frequently occurs because the supervisor assumes that the child will use common sense in interpreting what was said. A simple statement such as "Feed the dog" includes a lot of assumed material that the supervisor did not think it was necessary to say.

The following dialogue is typical of the splitting that occurs when supervisors take shortcuts:

SUPERVISOR: Jay, don't forget to feed the dog this evening.

JAY: OK.

When the supervisor comes home from work at 5:30 P.M., the dog has not been fed.

SUPERVISOR: Jay! I told you to feed the dog when you got home from school! You don't ever do anything I say!

JAY: No, you didn't.

SUPERVISOR: I certainly did! This morning I told you to feed the dog when you got home from school! Don't tell me I didn't tell you!

JAY: That's not what you said. You said to feed the dog this evening. It's not evening yet. Evening starts when the sun goes down.

This illustrates the hazard of giving oral instructions. Obviously, the best way to reduce or eliminate the problem is to make a specific, detailed, in-sequence list:

1. Feed the dog when you come home from school.

2. Check the dog's water.

3. Close the garage door so the dog can't get out.

The supervisor need only ask, "Jay, did you do everything on your list?" This places the responsibility back on Jay and avoids nagging and yelling over what was said that morning. If Jay has chosen not to look at the list, then he is responsible for the consequences. He cannot wiggle out of responsibility by splitting hairs over what was or was not said.

Memory Guides

As children move upward through school grades, they must learn to handle a multitude of memory tasks. Each new year introduces still more things to be remembered. Homework materials must arrive at home. Finished homework must be handed in to each teacher to receive a grade. Long-term assignments such as book reports, science projects, and term papers must be done on a schedule. Many youngsters do not go directly home from school. Our society includes several million "latchkey children" who are left alone early in the morning and late afternoon by working parents. Millions of youngsters take music lessons, have gymnastics training, and/or participate in sports after school. Teenagers often work part-time before and after school. Many youngsters attend religion classes on certain evenings of the week. From kindergarten upward, life becomes increasingly complex for today's children and families. It is imperative that children who lack organizational abilities be taught how to keep their duties and obligations in order.

Calendars

In Chapters 1 and 2, the poor sense of time and chronology that complicates life for children with dyslexia was discussed. These children have no internal awareness of events in sequence or of how one event relates to a series of others. They literally must *see* time in order to deal with it successfully. Dyslexia requires early use of a personal calendar. As soon as children become involved with day-to-day activities, they must start seeing their days, weeks, and months represented on a calendar. Before they can read the names of days and months, they need right-brain symbols. For example, each day could be a certain bright color. On the blue day, they take lunch money to school. On the red day, they have a music lesson after school. On the green day, they ride in the carpool to church or religious center for youth activities. On the yellow day, they take gymnastics lessons and so on. As soon as the children begin to work with letters, words, and numbers, these are added to the calendar. The supervisor takes a few minutes each day to go over the week's calendar with the child. This continual, consistent repetition begins to build a foundation for helping him or her think in terms of time and how events are related. He or she begins to see how one event comes first, another comes next, another occurs later, and so forth. By the time the child has seen his or her life represented in this calendar form for several years, a lifelong organizational skill has been established.

Daily School Log

Most students carry bookbags, which offers supervisors a way to help youngsters with dyslexia stay organized. Each evening, the supervisor should guide the student in making a simple log (list) of everything that must go back to school the next day. Everything means everything—nothing is assumed. Together, the child and the supervisor check the list: pencils, tablets, art supplies, erasers, or whatever the student needs to do his or her work properly. Does the child need new supplies? Have teachers announced that certain things will be necessary for upcoming assignments or projects? Does the student have all assignments finished? The supervisor and student go over the log together before bedtime. Next morning the supervisor issues reminders: "John, go over your log again. Don't forget anything that needs to go back to school." If John protests that he does not have time, the supervisor reminds him that he is responsible. He is not to call from school saying that he left something important at home. Again, the log becomes the source of pressure. If John chooses to take shortcuts, then he must face the consequences. If it was on the log, then the log will be the final authority.

Children with dyslexia must live by lists and calendars all their lives. They have no choice but to encode their responsibilities in a visible form because they cannot handle the stress of responsibility from memory. Early in their lives, they must develop habits of organizing activities, responsibilities, and choices around some kind of calendar or visible list. Successful persons with dyslexia carry pocket reminders everywhere they go. They have a multitude of organizational options:

1. Developing ways of making quick notes of whatever must be remembered;

2. Keeping lists of words they cannot spell but must write frequently;

3. Keeping lists of phone numbers, names of people they often see, clues about finding locations, birthdays, and anniversaries;

4. Learning to keep track of money by developing a budget log listing how much they have spent and how much is left;

5. Carrying small calendars showing long-range schedules such as coming holidays and vacation times.

These supervisory strategies are essential for individuals with dyslexia of all ages. The human supervisor of childhood gradually changes to the written supervisor that reminds at a glance. If these kinds of organizational strategies are taught to these persons when they are children, they can be free from much of the stress and uncertainty they often deal with at every turn.

BECOMING INDEPENDENT

As children who have dyslexia become adolescents and young adults, they go one of four ways. Most gradually will replace parent supervisors with a close friend, usually someone they are dating. As a special friendship or romantic relationship develops, these teens become dependent upon this new important person. Girls often become new supervisors for boys who have dyslexia. Occasionally, a nondisabled boy becomes the supervisor for a girl with dyslexia of whom he is fond. These relationships tend to become intensely emotional and usually are lopsided. The relationship actually becomes a parent–child situation with the supervisor taking the place of mom or dad. Although romance often is the basis for their relationship, these partners find themselves in conflict when one person gives advice and instructions while at the same time being the object of romantic affection. The partner with dyslexia often resents the parental role of the other, but he or she cannot get along without this help, which causes stress. Not many teens are mature enough to comprehend all of the elements in these complex relationships. The strong bonding that occurs in romantic partnerships is in conflict with the nurturing bond that exists between parent and child. When a person with dyslexia falls in love with someone who does not have dyslexia, it is difficult for them to work through the stress and frustrations that emerge from their unequal needs unless they are willing to receive counseling.

Marriage

When persons with dyslexia marry, they usually choose spouses who can fulfill the role of supervisor. The nondisabled spouse keeps the budget, makes the lists, manages the money, takes care of all the family details, reminds the partner when and where to be, and so forth. The supervisory spouse writes all the letters, pays the bills, plans for gifts and birthday celebrations, keeps the family on schedule for holidays, and stays in touch with important relatives. Obviously, this is not an equal relationship. The nondisabled adult must be both a marriage partner, with all that implies, and the parent who makes lists for the child. Solid, comfortable marriages can develop between an adult with dyslexia and someone without it. However, the spouse with dyslexia must be able to delegate the organizational chores to the other without feeling threatened or diminished. Meanwhile, the supervising spouse must be able to accept this dual role without complaint or criticism. Most marriages that include a spouse with dyslexia, however, are marked by conflict, resentment, and misunderstanding. Someone must be the organizer and manager of time and schedules.

Staying with Parent Supervisors

Not all young adults with dyslexia are ready to become independent of parents or childhood supervisors. In fact, many U.S. families still have adult children living with parents long after school years are over. In most instances, this continuing dependent relationship occurs because the child with dyslexia was not prepared over the years to become an independent adult. The steps in teaching visible structure described earlier in this chapter were not taken during childhood and early adolescence, and the level of fear was not reduced through careful teaching over a long enough period of time. In many families, it was easier for adults to do all of the planning and make all of the decisions without doing the work of teaching the child how.

It requires never-ending patience for parents to prepare a child with dyslexia for adulthood. These children are like all others in that they mature at different rates. Many adolescents with dyslexia are late developers, reaching their late teens or early 20s with the physical maturity of most 14-

year-olds. Young men with dyslexia often do not shave daily until age 21, nor have their voices fully changed until age 22. When their high school peers were dating and practicing romance, these late bloomers had no interest in such activity. As children, they were too immature to fit in with classmates in kindergarten and elementary school. In early teens, they were too immature to take part successfully in middle school and high school social life. As young adults, they are several years behind schedule in being ready to live alone without supervision. They therefore continue to live with parents who do not know how to help them other than to provide safe shelter. Members of this population struggle to find jobs at which they can make an independent living. When they work, it is usually for minimum wage, which does not provide enough net pay to support them separately.

Living Alone

Some adults with dyslexia live alone. They have managed to develop simple lifestyles in which they avoid anything that requires complicated planning. They seldom have many friends; they pay for everything in cash because they cannot handle the paperwork of banking; and they are socially isolated, self-contained, and alone. They live on the edge of boredom, and they are often intensely lonely, but they choose this solitary life because they can manage it without complication. Their social lives are restricted to only a few activities: playing an occasional game of pool, going to the park on their days off, attending movies, eating simple meals at the same fast-food restaurants, and watching television. They do not read, and they often do not have a telephone. In most cases they have chosen to be celibate. They are suspicious of strangers who show interest in them, and they avoid crowds as much as possible. Contact with family is carefully controlled and limited. If they attend religious services, it is to sit at the back so as not to call attention to themselves because they feel too illiterate to read from the Bible or follow words in a hymnal. These loners sometimes are mentally ill to some degree. The Menninger Foundation has documented a correlation between dyslexia and certain forms of mental illness that emerge during the early teens but subside in the early 20s (Jernigan, 1985). Sometimes these individuals develop enough courage to enroll in a course to upgrade literacy or job skills. Mostly they spend their lives off to themselves, attracting little attention and managing their meager resources in frugal ways. They do not view themselves as being worthy of anything better. They exist at borderline poverty levels, yet they do not question that position in life. Early in their lives, they came to believe that such a simple place in life was all they deserved or should expect.

Few of these people had much stimulation as children. Their own parents often were not well educated. Childhood for them was largely without emphasis upon learning. If these solitary adults ever thought about more education, they concluded that it would be beyond their ability. We have no idea how many intelligent, potentially creative individuals with dyslexia have fallen through the cracks.

Adults with Dyslexia in Prison

Since the early 1970s, many studies have been done of the learning patterns and levels of literacy among men and women in prison (Brier, 1989; Jordan, 1995; Payne, 1994; Pollan & Williams, 1992). A startling fact has emerged regarding learning disabilities among adjudicated delinquents and convicted felons. Approximately three out of four adolescent and adult males serving time within our penal systems show significant signs of dyslexia. The average level of literacy skills among this prison population is below fourth grade. Virtually none of these males serving time were identified as having a learning disability during their school years—most were evaluated for the first time as they entered the prison program. The shattering truth is that many males with dyslexia in our culture forfeit their freedom through crime.

There are myriad reasons for this problem. A majority of these incarcerated males with LD came from impoverished economic lifestyles where basic needs were not met during childhood and adolescence and in which education was unimportant. There often was no stable supervisory parenting during the formative years. The critical factor in their becoming involved with criminal activity, however, was their lack of literacy skills. They could not compete with better-educated individuals in the job market, did not have the personal skills to deal successfully with marriage, could not handle the reading and writing requirements of society in order to establish stable lives, and had no valuable parenting models to follow in their efforts to be fathers and husbands. They entered their teens and young adult years mostly illiterate, insecure, unstable, and unskilled. The question must be raised: How many of these men could have been saved had their dyslexic patterns been identified and supervised when they were open to teaching and guidance? Society has paid a staggering price in the loss of these young men who otherwise might have been guided toward productive lives.

Controlling and Manipulative Lifestyles

If most persons listed the least desirable habits in people they meet, high on that list would be the tendency to control others. At first glance, persons who are habitual controllers usually seem insensitive, self-focused, and determined to have their own way. Beneath this surface lies fear, which is the driving force behind the need to control. Many children and adolescents with dyslexia develop strong control strategies that they use to avoid much of the pain that comes through failure. These young controllers emerge into the adult world with consummate skills in manipulating and dominating others.

How do these individuals stay in control of others? A controller is a specialist in gathering and storing information about others. He or she spends extraordinary amounts of emotional and mental energy collecting bits and pieces of data about everyone he or she knows. This information is stored away for future use, the way a squirrel stores away nuts for the coming winter. All kinds of tidbits are gathered about all kinds of people: who they know, what they do, how much they earn, how much they spend, where they go, what they read, who are their friends, where they work, on and on and on. The controller constantly sniffs out new data, always alert for more information that can be stored away for future use. This cache of saved information is the currency that controllers use in future negotiations to gain their way over the will of others.

Controllers never "clean out" their old data files. A skilled controller can call up old facts that have lain dormant for many years, waiting to be used. In collecting these details about others, controllers ask endless questions that seem trivial because to them any piece of information might come in handy someday. Controllers go through life rummaging in the lives of others in their quest for bits of informational treasure. Some controllers have no subtlety or finesse. They blurt out blunt questions with no regard for the embarrassment this might cause. Others are quite subtle and charming as they cast their nets for whatever bits of data they might snare. This information-gathering process that might later empower the controller is a lifelong habit. It often is a compulsion because it is fueled by fear. If the controller has no way to make others do his or her bidding, then he or she is without power, status, authority, and social strength.

Quiet Controllers

Many people who are quiet controllers go steadily about their business, often with such subtlety and charm that others do not realize what they are doing. Quiet controllers are subtle manipulators. They do not shout or bully others openly, but instead use a variety of quiet techniques often based upon flattery. Quiet controllers are skilled at developing a sense of trust, masking their real intent of manipulating others to get their own way. When others are under their control, quiet controllers feel safe.

For example, if someone else makes a suggestion, the quiet controller smiles and agrees that the suggestion is a splendid idea, but would it not be better to do things another way? Then the controller lays out a plan supported by bits of information he or she has gleaned. The plan is stated in terms of calm reasoning as to why everyone should agree.

This quiet controller finally wears down all resistance and others give in, often without being aware that they are being used. Quiet controllers go through life getting their way by wearing others out. They frequently use guilt as a soft club by gently reminding, "Remember all the things I've done for you when I wasn't feeling well? Don't you think you could agree with me this time?" Others seldom realize that the quiet controller rarely lets anyone else have his or her own way. Over time, the quiet controller wins, no matter how long it takes or how many new arguments must be invented to sell that person's opinion. The control technique involves not just wearing others out, but also demonstrating superior knowledge.

Overt Controllers

The overt controller operates quite differently. This type of controller blusters, shouts, and intimidates the way a playground bully controls less aggressive playmates. The overt controller never listens to the explanations of others but interrupts and overwhelms them through strong argument. If anyone disagrees, the overt controller becomes huffy or angry, repeating in a loud voice that his or her decision is the best one. This type of controller wears down opposition so that others finally give in just to stop the argument. He or she is so aggressive that others back away because the fight is not worthwhile. As a child I learned a bit of wisdom within the farm community in which I grew up: "A dog can whip a skunk, but it ain't worth it." In working with many fearful, struggling students who are overt controllers, I have learned what that rural wisdom meant. Aggressive overt controllers are determined to win no matter how harshly they must bully others to get their way.

Whether persons with dyslexia use the quiet approach or the aggressive style to manipulate, many develop deeply imbedded controlling habits early in life. The driving force behind insatiable need to control is fear, as was stated earlier. The fear that overwhelms these individuals is based upon incomplete perception of what is happening in their environment. The moment strong uncertainty is felt, most of them pull back. Supervisors and instructors must keep in mind how strongly these persons need to feel safe. The moment they sense the risk of failure, they tend to freeze under waves of panic that often escalate into overwhelming fear.

Controlling Others to Avoid Stress

Staying in control of people and situations requires constant investment of mental and emotional energy. A quiet controller spends extraordinary amounts of time peering ahead while planning and scheming to get his or her own way, which means that the energy invested in controlling is not available for more productive work. Quiet controllers use this habit as a means of avoiding stress. If they can stay in charge and set the agenda, they can avoid tasks or situations in which they feel unsafe.

Ray is one of the most successful quiet controllers I have ever known. We met when he was a child, and I have followed him closely into his middle 30s. In spite of my affection for Ray, I recognize his deep habits of controlling every situation in which he finds himself. He has severe (deep) dyslexia at Level 8. At age 34, he struggles to read extremely slowly at fourth-grade level. His spelling skills are at the upper third-grade level, and his arithmetic skills are at the lower fourth-grade level. Listening comprehension is poor because of auditory dyslexia, and Ray also has Irlen syndrome. All his life, he has misunderstood words and misinterpreted much of what he hears. He could not cope with classroom vision tasks until he was fitted with prism lenses that were colored by the Irlen procedure. He is a deeply sensitive person with genuine concern for others, up to a point. His goal has always been to become a counselor so that he can help others through their own difficult years, but he is motivated toward this career because it would give him power over others. Ray, a charming man with a soft and gentle voice, is an unusually patient person who rarely shows anger, but he is one of the most self-focused, successful quiet controllers I have ever observed.

To understand why persons like Ray develop such strong controlling habits, we must keep in mind how difficult it is for him to comprehend new information. In earlier chapters, the factor of perceptual speed—how rapidly or slowly brain pathways can process language information—was discussed. Ray ranks at the 5th percentile of the adult population in perceptual speed. This means that 95 out of 100 others his age listen better, understand new meaning more quickly, and absorb new information more effectively than he can. To be in the bottom 5% in perceptual speed is a major handicap for anyone. This extremely slow processing rate makes it impossible for Ray to keep up with a news broadcast, take part in rapid conversations, read printed material quickly, recall specific information rapidly, or use correct names for things and people without feeling ignorant or "dumb." From early childhood, Ray has struggled to comprehend new information. His world has always overwhelmed him by a rush of new data to be absorbed, understood, and responded to rapidly. In the 25 years I have known him, I have spent many hours calming Ray's fears and helping him fill in gaps that constantly occur in his understanding. I never have become fully adjusted to the surprising gaps in understanding I stumble across in this gentle but fearful man.

Ray is a powerful quiet controller. It is his way of maintaining a sense of safety and security. If he loses control and begins to feel unsafe, either he leaves that situation or he exerts whatever effort is required to take control on his terms. He never raises his voice or becomes rude. He is a talented con man who spends much more time and energy staying in control than he spends trying to master new skills or overcoming a portion of this learning disability.

Balking

In any situation that presses Ray to accept another person's way of doing something, he balks. Balking is a major strategy that allows persons like Ray to gain control. In Chapter 1, the characteristics of hyperactive behavior that advertises its presence through aggressive, intrusive activity were reviewed. When a hyperactive or aggressive person balks, it is like a freight train slamming on its brakes. Sparks fly, voices screech, and the world knows that the person with ADHD has refused to cooperate. When a quiet, passive person like Ray balks, it is not seen so clearly. In fact, part of his controlling technique is to camouflage balking so that others do not see it. If the quiet controller can mask his or her underlying intentions of taking charge, he or she can gain control much more easily than if others are aware of what is taking place.

Smiling

In any situation that forces Ray to face new information, his first response is to smile. On the surface, a smile is seen as a friendly response, but this is not true for the quiet controller. Ray's smile is part of his strategy to disarm others and cause them to drop any defensive feelings they might have. As he smiles, he congratulates the other person for having good ideas. His wording of this praise is significant: "I really like your idea. I thought of that myself not long ago, and it is a very good idea." Then there is a pause accompanied by a thoughtful look. "But I've been thinking. There might be an even better way to do this." The smile, the kind and gentle voice, and the sincere expression by now have stolen the other person's heart. Ray already is in control. He continues to talk quietly, giving careful strokes to make the other person feel proud for having had such a good idea. Before anyone is aware, he has changed the agenda. He is skilled in working this con, which he learned early in his school experience. It seldom takes him long to have groups of experienced leaders eating out of his hand. Before they know what has happened, others have handed control over to this smiling, pleasant man, and Ray is again off the hook for taking any risk that might lead to failure. He thinks of himself as an accomplished leader. One day he told me his definition of leadership: "A leader is a person who gets everyone else to do the work." This warped principle has guided Ray through the dangerous places his severe LD has presented all his life.

Walking Away

Occasionally, Ray's controlling techniques fail to work, especially when he is contending with an overt, aggressive controller. He never has developed strategies to take control away from those who raise their voices and demand loud debate. In those situations, Ray simply walks away. If he cannot take control through his gentle techniques, which work for him 95% of the time, then he refuses to participate. Like most controllers, Ray is careful to choose his power contests. He wins control often enough through quiet manipulation to give aggressive persons their 5% of victories. I have watched numerous times as he has graciously smiled and walked away, leaving the aggressive adversary sputtering because the argument died before it started. Yet even in walking away, Ray controls. Robbing an aggressive person of the argument is Ray's quiet revenge, which is another form of taking power into his own hands.

Claiming Helplessness

Another strategy often used by quiet controllers is the appearance of helplessness. I frequently have seen Ray take charge by showing an innocent-appearing expression of being helpless; yet, I never have known him to ask for help directly. Ray never asks anyone for help, but instead trusts his controlling skills to gain that help without having to humble himself enough to ask. He discovered how to work his charm with classroom teachers when he was in elementary school. Primary dyslexia made it impossible for him to master basic skills in reading, phonics, and spelling, but he never was held back in school because he was illiterate. To this day, I could hold in one hand all of the written work he ever produced. He conned his way through 12 years of elementary and secondary school, then into college, without turning out more than a handful of written papers. His technique was to charm his teachers through his quiet, gentle, helpless smile and melt their hearts with his sweetness. How could any adult be so callous as to force this wonderful, struggling person to do academic work that clearly was beyond his ability? Classmates—always girls—and teachers did his work for him year after year.

During his senior year of high school, Ray proudly showed me a written book report on which the teacher had printed a large, red A. The paper contained fewer than 50 words, widely spaced and written so large that each sentence filled three lines. Ray had carefully enlarged his normally small handwriting into huge letters that quickly filled the page, then he finished writing on the back of the paper, creating the illusion that he had written a page-and-a-half book report. As I scanned this work of which he was so proud, I was amazed. He had conned his English teacher into accepting work that would not have passed for a third-grade language assignment. Ray's charm had worked again, and he was in control.

I grieved as I saw him reach age 30, still illiterate, still unable to write coherently, yet having made As in several college courses. Unfortunately, Ray has conned himself most of all. At age 34, he firmly believes that he should be hired for an administrative job because he has attended college even though he cannot do any kind of literacy work. This self-defeating lifestyle of manipulating, conning, and controlling others as a defense against pain and failure frequently is seen in intelligent individuals with dyslexia who have become quiet controllers.

The High Cost of Controlling

I wish that Ray's story had a happy ending, but, at this time, it does not. In spite of his charm, gentleness, and intelligence, he has not learned to deal with his invisible fear. His most urgent need is to feel safe and that means control. Developing better literacy skills is too threatening for his sensitive spirit. He habitually finds ways not to accept responsibility. His con habits are stronger now than they were years ago because he thinks they have gained him so much. Ray does not realize that by gaining control of every situation, or walking away when he cannot control, he has cheated himself of knowledge. He has no idea how to be an independent person. His lifestyle has enslaved him to depending on others. Beneath his charming surface is a hollow man without the strength to do useful work for himself.

DEVELOPING SELF-ESTEEM

Personal success rests upon a foundation that must be established during childhood if an adult is to build a stable, productive life. Each person must have a positive self-image so that he or she believes in his or her worth. Self-esteem must be strong enough to give persons sufficient courage to risk failure in order to find success and to like themselves. What one thinks of self determines how hard each individual is able to press toward success. Low self-image is like a strong hand on the shoulder that drags the person back when opportunity beckons. Low self-esteem whispers, "You can't do that! No use to try! You would only mess it up like you do everything else!" Negative self-image continually tells the self, "You're too ugly. Nobody cares for you. You're a loser. No one is going to give you a chance. You might as well forget about success. It is not meant for you."

During the four decades I have worked with the LD population, I have posed a question to persons with dyslexia of all ages. After we know each other well enough to be comfortable together, I ask, "When you look at yourself in the mirror, what do you see?" My question is meant as a metaphor, of course, not a physical act of staring at one's own face in the mirror. After more than a quarter of a century of asking this question, I still am astonished by the almost universal fear these individuals have of "looking at themselves in the mirror." Eight out of 10 persons to whom I have posed this question have given me this kind of reply: "I don't look at myself in a mirror" or "I can't stand to look at myself in the mirror." Only a few have enough courage and positive self-esteem to face themselves squarely without flinching or avoiding eye contact with self.

Professionals and parents who spend their lives with those who have dyslexia see certain causes for low self-esteem in this intelligent population. These sensitive individuals grow up under the shadow of judgment and criticism. Their mistakes continue day after day, year after year, and their best intentions usually are tarnished by failure. Their goals and ambitions are not realized because their dreams often lie beyond the limits imposed by their learning disability. Their plans continually fall through when they take shortcuts and try to ignore their perceptual boundaries. Their comprehension of family standards and cultural taboos often is incomplete or faulty. These acutely sensitive persons are especially vulnerable to certain factors that are seldom all that critical for nondisabled peers.

Guilt

A majority of the children, adolescents, and adults with dyslexia that I have known have suffered from unresolved guilt. Occasionally, I have met individuals so intensely guilt-ridden that they have become neurotic. Usually the level of guilt is more a nuisance, like a low-level toothache that never quite goes away. This pervasive guilt comes from several sources, all of which stem from the person's failure to live up to some goal proclaimed by society or family. Specific sources of guilt are seen in many persons with dyslexia when they fail to cope effectively with society's expectations.

The family of a child with dyslexia need not be religious to instill the concepts of guilt and sin. Most parents and members of the extended family hold certain strong beliefs as to what is right or wrong. Sometimes this is expressed through racial bias that teaches a young child not to associate with certain groups or through religious bias that forbids mixing with different religions. A majority of children with dyslexia grow up hearing religious teachings that implant strong, vivid mental images of God's wrath or punishment for certain activities. Most children gradually work out their own interpretation of religious teaching as they begin to read for themselves and develop broader understanding of truth and religious doctrine, but those with dyslexia cannot do so for themselves. Few readers with dyslexia can study the Bible or other scriptures for themselves to find out what sacred writing actually says about specific issues. The tone deaf barrier of auditory dyslexia creates continual misperception that makes it even more difficult for struggling listeners to remember accurately what they hear in sermons, church school lessons, and family discussions of religious issues. I seldom have met a person with dyslexia who had accurate or fluent knowledge of what his or her religion truly teaches. This special population often lives at the level of superstition, growing up with a primitive, incomplete understanding of religious doctrine or scriptural truth. It does not matter in what religion the child is receiving instruction. These youth cannot go to printed source materials and find out what the word of God or church history says, so they must rely upon others to interpret religious matters for them. This is especially true when youngsters who have dyslexia attend private church schools where truth and morality often are interpreted in strictly fundamental ways. It is too easy for misinterpretation to occur as issues of right and wrong are presented by adult leaders.

Shane is typical of many men with dyslexia that I have known. I first met Shane when he was a child. At age 10, he had primary (deep) dyslexia at Level 8. It was impossible for him to read, spell, do math computation, or maintain central vision without a great deal of supervision. He grew up in a strongly religious home where Christianity was interpreted in a strictly fundamental way. When his problems were identified, he was enrolled in a private school sponsored by a fundamental church where issues of right and wrong were spelled out in a rule book for the students. Shane could not read the rule book, nor could he read the Bible, which was quoted throughout the day by his instructors. I saw him periodically through his middle and high school years. Then he disappeared. He unexpectedly reappeared one day and was one of the most troubled and desperate young adults I have seen. His handsome face was consumed by grief and his athletic body was slouched and disheveled. This attractive young man in his early 20s fell into a chair in my office and began to sob his heart out. After half an hour of crying, he looked around my office where he had been many times. Finally he dried his tears and said, "It is always so peaceful here. I always feel so safe." Like many others through the years, Shane had "come home" to a sanctuary where he knew that he would not be judged or criticized.

I finally learned that Shane had attempted suicide a few days before that visit. It was his third suicide attempt since his 16th birthday. He hid his face in shame as he blurted out his story. He could not look me in the eye. He tried to tell me what was causing his deep grief, but he could not choke out the words. Finally I took him in my arms and said, "You are about to die from guilt, aren't you, Shane?" He clung to me and sobbed, "How did you know?" I replied, "You are feeling terrible guilt because you believe you have sinned." He put his head down and sobbed, but he nodded yes. "This is all about sex, isn't it, Shane?" I asked. Then it all came gushing out. For the next 3 hours I listened to his torrential confession of guilt. What a miserable sinner he always had been! What a dirty hypocrite he had turned out to be! Now there was no hope of salvation because God could not love anyone as dirty as he. This litany of guilt went on and on until Shane was exhausted. Then I asked what his awful secret sin had been all those years. "I want to have sex with girls," he blurted out. "But that's a sin. The Bible says a man will go to Hell if he thinks about having sex with girls. But I can't help it. It gets so strong sometimes I jerk myself off. Then I want to die because that's a sin and God hates any man who does that to himself. I can't go on living like this. I'm so dirty and filthy. I can't do anything right. I've disappointed you and if my Mom had any idea, she would throw me out of her house."

When the storm finally was over and Shane was calm, we carefully reviewed his concepts of sin and evil, right and wrong. Like so many other men with dyslexia that I have known, he had locked onto several misunderstandings of what his religion taught or meant regarding sexuality. This misperception had colored his entire life. His naturally strong sexual drive had overshadowed everything else, creating a strongly neurotic condition that made it impossible for him to function successfully in school or on a job. He could not date successfully because of his "terrible secret." He isolated himself from normal social life because of his belief that inwardly he was filthy for thinking certain things about girls. He began to drink heavily and take drugs to escape his haunting guilt. He began staying up all night because he was afraid to go to sleep. While asleep, he frequently had erotic dreams he thought would doom him to Hell. He had tried many times to read the Bible, but he could not find the scriptural passages that deal with morality and sexuality. He had driven himself into the emotional corner of believing that he was vile as a man, filthy in his Creator's eyes, and unfit as a member of society. This extreme level of emotional suffering had gone on for several years.

Eventually I asked Shane this question: "When you look at yourself in the mirror, what do you see?" His reaction was astonishing. "I have never looked at myself in a mirror!" he exclaimed. "How do you shave?" I inquired. "I hold a towel over my face," he said. "I use an electric razor and I feel where it is on my face. If I have to see part of my face, I move the towel just a little. I have no idea what my face looks like. But I know I'm very ugly." I gazed in awe at this handsome young man who could easily have become a fashion model. "What does your body look like?" I asked, referring to his athletic build and obviously good muscle tone. "I have no idea," he replied. "I work out and stay in shape, but I don't know what my body looks like. I can't look at myself. I am too filthy and ugly."

This story is an extreme example of guilt, of course. But most individuals with severe dyslexia harbor some kind of unresolved guilt that partly disables their ability to function well in society. Few adults with dyslexia that I have known have described themselves realistically or accurately. Virtually all these individuals put themselves down when they talk about physical appearance, attractiveness, level of appeal to others, and how righteous they might be. Those who listen to the secret stories of persons with dyslexia hear a litany of guilt from sin, inadequacy, failure, and unworthiness. This underlying sense of guilt is like smog over the landscape of a beautiful city. The natural beauty of the person is at least partially masked by a dark cloud that blots out his or her personal worth. After King David's tragic experience with Uriah and Bathsheba, he wrote these poignant words in Psalm 51: "My sin is ever before me." This is often true with those who have dyslexia. Their perceptions of right and wrong, adequacy and inadequacy, holiness and unholiness, being worthy and unworthy often are skewed and incomplete. They enter their adult years carrying unresolved burdens of guilt that never have been discussed or fully examined with someone they can trust.

It is critically important that supervisors of children with dyslexia take great care to make issues of religion, sin and righteousness, and morality fully clear. It requires much patient teaching and reteaching to help them comprehend the full message without omitting essential elements that change the meaning. Whatever the child comprehends, that is what he or she believes to be the truth. When overly sensitive youngsters like Shane misperceive such vital issues as normal sexuality, that misunderstanding sets into motion lifelong consequences that can disable the person emotionally and spiritually. This adds enormous stress to the already stressful life of growing up with dyslexia.

Personal Appearance

Few people would win the prize at a beauty contest. Most of us, of whatever age, must make the best of the physical endowments we inherit. How one's body is shaped, the characteristics of eyes and ears, the structure of one's face, the quality of one's teeth, all of these factors are part of one's self-image. The level of a person's self-esteem is closely tied to personal appearance. This is especially critical for individuals with dyslexia. These sensitive persons must deal continually with the risk of failure and the stress of probably making a mistake within the next few minutes. If the body is not attractive, it becomes all too easy to slip into the pit of low self-esteem that is so difficult to escape. Young people who do not have dyslexia may have trouble with poorly aligned teeth, slightly crossed eyes, severe acne, large ears, obesity, and so forth. Thoughtful parents do what they can to overcome these physical differences as children mature. If a child with dyslexia also has physical problems that diminish appearance, self-image suffers heavily in a culture that emphasizes good looks.

I remember many highly intelligent, overly sensitive youngsters with dyslexia whose parents did not have the insight to recognize the importance of their child's physical appearance. For example, countless times over a 10-year period I had to calm Mark down when he became enraged over his "crooked teeth." This physically attractive boy did have poorly aligned teeth that could have been corrected easily through orthodontal care. But his father saw no need to spend money for that kind of thing. The boy grew up watching his dad drive new Cadillacs and park expensive boat-and-trailer rigs in the driveway, but there never was any money for Mark's dental care. At age 36, Mark is still angry over his "ugliness" that he blames on his father's ignorance and stubbornness. It has colored all of Mark's self-image and self-esteem. His self-image is that his mouth is "ugly" and that his smile is offensive to others. In reality, he is a strikingly good-looking man, but his inner view of himself is the opposite. A lack of parental concern for this boy's physical appearance instilled a lifelong attitude of being "ugly" and unattractive, which made it much more difficult for teachers to reach Mark on an academic level.

Another person with dyslexia whom I know, Jill, always has been overweight and chubby. Performing in school was very difficult for her, but her learning disability was not identified until she was 15. By then, her parents had concluded that their daughter was "just fat and lazy." Discovering that she had a brain-based learning dysfunction did not change their attitude. During her critical teen years, Jill became very obese, which fulfilled her parents' claim that she was just a "fat, lazy slob." In the 15 years I have known her, I have never seen Jill look anyone in the eye. When she talks with me or anyone else, her eyes look elsewhere. She looks at me frequently with rapid, darting glances to see if I am listening as she talks. When her eyes contact mine, she blushes deeply and immediately turns her head. Her self-esteem is so low that she cannot tolerate the normal interaction that comes with eye contact between friends. After working at a series of low-paying childcare jobs, Jill met a man who liked her and wanted to know her better. She was astonished that any man could be interested in her at all, given her obesity. As the friendship progressed, she joined a weight reduction club and eventually lost 100 pounds. As her physical appearance improved, she began to use makeup attractively and dress in better fashion; however, her self-image remains low. No matter how good Jill looks, she cannot make eye contact as she talks with friends. There are too many ghosts from the past, too many voices still criticizing her appearance, to let her believe that anyone could ever find her attractive or interesting.

It is of critical, lifelong importance that children with dyslexia be encouraged to look their best and make the most of their attributes. The brain-based deficits that make life so complicated need the best possible packaging to allow these individuals to overcome their limitations and successfully enter society. It is a tragically false economy for families to save a few dollars during childhood years by not providing orthodontal care, acne treatment, or good-grooming instruction. Self-esteem is already too easily fractured in these young persons. To face life with deficits in physical appearance in addition to the underlying cognitive deficits is too much for many fragile ego structures. Of all our children, the ones with dyslexia are the most urgently in need of support in developing strong self-image and positive self-esteem.

The Impact of Chronic Failure

The most destructive factor in our society for the self-esteem of persons with dyslexia is chronic failure. To have dyslexia in U.S. society is to risk failure at virtually every turn. This failure can be those invisible moments when the memory "shorts out," but the person recovers quickly enough so that no one else notices the loss. Inwardly, however, the person feels the discordant twang of near failure. Failure can occur as the individual starts to write. Suddenly the mental image is blank and the pencil will not begin its task of encoding. The fingers are stuck while the memory searches for lost data, such as a number, the spelling of a familiar word, the beginning letter of one's own name, or which direction to turn the pencil in making the needed written symbol. Failure can occur momentarily as the person turns a corner and suddenly loses body-in-space orientation. The mental images of north, south, east, and west vanish. Awareness of which is left or right disappears, and the dyslexic person freezes, not knowing at that moment which way to turn. Again, these invisible stumbling points may not be observed by others, but inwardly, the person with dyslexia once again has failed to carry out a normal procedure.

Speaking is filled with hazards for individuals with dyslexia. The tongue may catch on a certain word or string of syllables, causing another "tongue twist" moment when the flow of articulation gets stuck. The needed word may be lost altogether, creating another moment of awkwardness when the speaker cannot continue his or her flow of speech. When dyslexia is below Level 5, these chronic "blips" usually are managed well enough so that no one else notices or pays attention. But when these dyslexic patterns are above Level 6 in severity, the moments of stumbling, reversing, or losing one's body in space becomes obvious and embarrassing. When dyslexia is above Level 7, the person is being corrected continually by others or scolded impatiently by a tone of voice that implies, if it does not say, "Why can't you ever get it right? How many times have you been told how to do it right?" Over the years, this chronic smog of failure engulfs the developing ego structure of the person, blocking out the warmth of praise and admiration required for healthy self-esteem to develop.

No Stories to Tell

I became painfully aware of the lifelong effect of chronic failure during a counseling session with Aaron, who was 19 years old. He had never been able to attend a full year of school because of extreme school phobia. Chronic failure during his childhood, along with harsh scoldings and punishment from his father, had created a neurotic personality structure too fragile to cope with group participation. Three times he had erupted into a violent frenzy at school while trying to defend himself. Three times he had been committed to mental health facilities for treatment of pervasive personality disorder. None of the mental health professionals recognized the severe dyslexic patterns in his language skills.

I met Aaron when he was 17, and he opened himself to me for the first time in his life. He trusted me to be gentle with his disabilities and not to criticize his weaknesses. He shared extraordinary poetry and song lyrics he had composed during his years of isolation from kids his own age. When he was 19, we began talking in-depth about his secret thoughts regarding himself and his failure to relate to the outside world. At that time, he was living alone in an apartment that was funded through a program for adults with disabilities. I asked Aaron if he ever visited places where he could meet young adults his own age. He said that he had gone to a few singles bars, and occasionally he had gone to church. But it did not work, and he had decided never to try it again. "Why not?" I asked. Without hesitation, he responded with one of the most profound statements I have ever heard a person with dyslexia make: "Because I don't have any stories to tell."

Those eight simple words gave me a tremendously important piece to the puzzle of dyslexia. After working with this special population for more than 30 years, I finally understood a major reason why self-esteem is so difficult for persons with dyslexia to develop. Chronic failure makes it very difficult, often impossible, for them to develop good stories to tell. I had not thought about that before. What do we all do when we get together? What happens at Sunday School or at the barber shop or when friends meet in the supermarket? What takes place when neighbors meet over the back fence or in the hallway or in the parking lot? What goes on continually where we work and when we travel? What is happening in those moments before the worship service starts or the concert begins? We tell stories. All kinds of stories. Most of our stories are good. We chat on and on about the little things that have happened, what our children are doing, the victories we have achieved, the problems we have solved. We gossip about people we know. We complain about our jobs or how we wish things were better where we spend our days. We confide little things about our lives. Sometimes we tell difficult stories about sorrow or misfortune. We spend a great deal of our social time telling stories.

Persons who have severe dyslexia, and even many of those with moderate dyslexia, often do not have good stories to tell. Aaron explained it so clearly, "Sure I have stories to tell. But who wants to hear my stories about getting kicked out of school, or being committed to the mental hospital three times, or being put on drugs to make me calm, or how my dad yelled and cussed me out? What kind of girl wants to go out with a guy who tells stories like that? And you know the weird sex fantasies I have a lot. I sure can't tell those stories to decent people. And nobody wants to hear my stories about being afraid all the time and being paranoid about strangers. I sure don't have any good stories to tell about school. Who wants to spend an evening listening to my stories about flunking third grade and being kicked out of elementary school? You're the only person I ever met who will even listen to my stories and not think I'm crazy."

Developing Good Stories to Tell

Aaron's case is extreme, of course, but his chronic failures at school, at home, and in society are a mirror of what most persons with dyslexia experience to some degree. It need not be this way. Children with dyslexia who are blessed with patient, observant parents do develop good stories to tell. Students who are fortunate enough to spend years with patient, flexible teachers develop anthologies of good tales about ways in which they succeeded within the school environment. They did not make top grades, but they were given opportunities to earn praise, which is what good storytelling is all about. Athletes who have thoughtful, caring coaches develop many good stories about athletic success and sports achievement. Individuals with strong right-brain talents for drawing, painting, crafts, and tool handling emerge into their teens and early 20s with good stories to both tell and show. Young adults who meet caring romance partners who accept left-brain limitations without rejection have many good tales of love and warm friendship. Good scout leaders, caring 4-H Club leaders, patient bosses, and many more supervisors, friends, and other adults can help the person with dyslexia develop good stories, not bad ones. The key is patient leadership. When these people are patient, thoughtful, and careful to make things clear, bright youngsters like Aaron do indeed develop a repertoire of good stories.

Building a Positive Self-Image

Positive self-image develops in persons with dyslexia through "baby steps" over a period of time. Those who are not troubled by left-brain limitations judge success by long strides forward, but people with disabilities gain success a little at a time. Children who are fortunate enough to have compassionate, observant parents make progress in small steps all of their lives because self-esteem is continually supported and nurtured. Language gaps are gently supplemented, not criticized. Directional confusion becomes part of a funny family game as everyone thinks of ways to help the child with dyslexia master left and right, north and south, east and west. All kinds of memory tricks are developed through rhymes and simple ways to keep things straight. Dyslexia is handled with a good sense of humor, not with scoldings and punishment when awkwardness or forgetfulness occurs.

Every "baby step" of progress is praised, the way star pupils are praised for outstanding achievement. Moments of fear that cause the child to freeze are treated thoughtfully, not with criticism. Impulsiveness or lapses of good judgment are absorbed by the family as the child is guided through the family standards of right and wrong. The tongue twisters and malapropisms that all persons with dyslexia create are treated with delight, as the child makes a major contribution to the family's fun and joy.

Parents and relatives look for the natural bent and the underlying talents, and they help the child grow in those unique areas, even though standard left-brain skills remain difficult. Over a period of years, all of these "baby steps" carry the child through adolescence and finally into adulthood with a healthy ego structure, strong self-image, and positive self-esteem. This fortunate person enjoys looking into the mirror because the image looking back is good and worthy of praise. The individual who has good stories to tell is strong, intelligent, interesting, and alive with hope. It must always be remembered that the stories come slowly over time. It is incredibly difficult for a child with dyslexia to become a confident adult with good stories to tell unless a parent figure who knew how to reinforce that child's bent, instead of criticizing for deficits, provided long-term support. By the time I met Aaron, it was too late. I shall always wonder what eternal difference it could have made had I met him and his parents when he was a child. Perhaps those bewildered adult supervisors could have learned how to deal with his needs more positively. If that highly sensitive boy had learned a few good stories to tell along the way, his adult self-esteem could have been salvaged and restored.

Chapter 6

Developing Social Skills and Independence

This book began with a review of the history of our knowledge of left-brain causes for specific learning disabilities. Chapter 1 summarizes the milestone neurological discoveries since 1809 that support the concept that dyslexia and other types of LD originate in the left brain. In Chapters 2, 3, and 4, the often devastating consequences of visual dyslexia, auditory dyslexia, and dysgraphia were discussed. These forms of LD originate from anatomical differences in left-brain structure. For almost 200 years, attention has been focused on learning struggles related to language processing that is the major function of the left brain.

Professionals of my generation, who began working with people who were struggling to learn in the 1950s and early 1960s, were aware that many persons with dyslexia display irregular, often disruptive patterns of immature emotions and a lack of commonsense reasoning. In my first classroom teaching experiences with adolescents who could not read, I became clearly aware of an overlay of emotionality in many of these individuals that kept them in conflict with peers, parents, and leaders. I have met grandchildren of the first persons with dyslexia I encountered in 1957. This three-generational involvement has let me observe the impact of immature or negative emotions on the lives of those who have dyslexia. But in the early years of my professional experience, a well-defined paradigm of the emotional side of learning disabilities did not exist.

NONVERBAL LEARNING DISABILITIES

In 1971, Doris Johnson and Helmut Myklebust published their landmark analysis of what they called *nonverbal learning disabilities* (NVLD) (Johnson & Myklebust, 1971). They defined this dysfunction as the inability to comprehend the significance of what occurs in the social world surrounding the person. Johnson and Myklebust pinpointed several primary characteristics of NVLD. First they noted a major social deficit: the individual is *very poor at pretending.* When others are having fun with a make-believe episode, jokes are flying, everyone is laughing or giggling at silly words and ideas, and the group is having a wonderful time gently teasing each other, individuals with NVLD do not get the point. They are puzzled and out of the loop in this kind of pretend socialization. Second, individuals with NVLD *cannot anticipate.* A major part of socialization involves guessing ahead, predicting what will probably happen, speculating about what maybe lies ahead, and making small talk about what might be. Individuals with NVLD do not have the ability to look ahead or anticipate what might come next. Finally, NVLD makes it impossible for the individual to read nonverbal social signals: *facial expressions, hand gestures, body language, friendly touching, tone of voice.* Individuals with NVLD do not comprehend these paralanguage components of successful socialization. Johnson and Myklebust concluded that such persons fail to read nonverbal social signals the way individuals with dyslexia fail to interpret printed symbols on a page. NVLD soon came to be called "social dyslexia."

Right-Brain Influence

In 1974, a team of neurologists led by Daniel Tranel studied maladaptive social behavior and erratic school performance in patients who had sustained various types of injuries to the right brain (Tranel, Hall, Olson, & Tranel, 1987). These researchers adopted the term *right-hemisphere learning disability* to describe the poor socialization patterns of these individuals. Tranel's team concluded that right-hemisphere dysfunctions (lesions) contribute to chronic disturbances in social skills and emotional balance. Martha Denckla expanded the earlier concept of NVLD to include visual deficits as part of the social-emotional difficulties associated with NVLD (Denckla, 1978). In the late 1970s a new designation emerged: SELD (*social-emotional learning disability*) (Rourke & Finlayson, 1978). SELD refers to lifelong errors in social judgment. These individuals never learn how to "dance the tribal dance" that centers on reading social signals correctly and responding to others in socially appropriate ways.

During the 1980s, brain-imaging science made it possible to explore right-hemisphere structures in persons who display NVLD or SELD patterns. Drake Duane, then a neurologist at the Mayo Clinic, described *Right-Hemi syndrome* based upon new knowledge of right-brain involvement in social and emotional behavior (Duane, 1985). Right-Hemi syndrome describes individuals who may be well educated but who do not maintain eye contact while conversing, speak in a sing-song way, smother friends and relatives with inappropriate displays of possessive affection, trigger such strong feelings of dread in others that peers and relatives try to avoid them, are blind to normal social signals from others, and do not comprehend the issues of personal privacy and personal space.

Kytja Voeller, a psychiatric specialist on childhood disorders, described *Right-Hemisphere Deficit syndrome* (Voeller, 1986). Her study linked obtuse behavior and failure to interpret social cues to right-brain damage or dysfunction. The youngsters she studied could not express their feelings in typical ways, yet they seemed aware of emotions in others. Voeller concluded that right-brain differences relate directly to the ability to enter into appropriate social relationships. In 1988 Robert Joseph at the Neurobehavioral Center in San Jose, California, published a comprehensive review of what had been learned about right-brain influence on emotion, visual-spatial skills, body-image awareness, dreams, and awareness of social processes (Joseph, 1988). Joseph pulled together a large body of knowledge of how the right cerebral hemisphere determines how well persons interpret and interact with the social world around them. In 1990 Margaret Semrud-Clikeman and George Hynd reviewed the latest evidence that right hemispheric dysfunction is directly related to NVLD (Semrud-Clikeman & Hynd, 1990). This study covered a broad range of behavioral, emotional, and perceptual dysfunctions that have been linked to differences in right-brain structure and development. Denckla then estimated that 10% of all persons with left-brain LD (dyslexia, attention deficits, aphasia) also manifest NVLD and SELD characteristics (Denckla, 1991b). This means that in the general population, 1% of all children, adolescents, and adults manifest right-brain dysfunctions related to poor socialization skills and emotional control; however, within the LD population, 1 out of 10 also have NVLD and/or SELD.

Midbrain and Brain Stem Influence

Since the early 1970s, Antonio Damasio at the University of Iowa has researched the role of midbrain and brain stem functions in how humans perceive the world around themselves. In 1995, he reported how the midbrain and brain stem participate in memory, along with contributing to the emotional patterns in a person's behavior (Damasio, 1995, cited in Siegfried, 1995). Figure 6.1 shows the midbrain structures that largely control the emotional qualities related to memory of events. The *amygdala, hippocampus,* and *cerebellum* form a neuronal team in generating strong emotions and in controlling the expression of strong emotions. When these midbrain structures are incompletely developed or have been damaged, the individual exhibits erratic emotions that often surge beyond self-control. Impulsivity, excessive hyperactivity, outbursts of aggression and violence, and inappropriate social behavior are linked to deficits in these midbrain regions. As Denckla has observed, 1 out of 10 of those who struggle with left-brain learning have difficulty coping with emotions generated by the midbrain.

Figure 6.2 shows how the right brain, midbrain, and brain stem generate permanent memories that are linked to strong emotions. Emotional memories are developed through a 5-step neurological process.

1. *The eyes see an event.* For example, the eyes catch sight of a copper-colored snake crawling toward the person who is walking down a wooded path. This visual information is flashed to the visual cortex at the back of the brain.

2. *The visual cortex simultaneously sends the visual information to two regions of the brain.* At the front of the brain is the *prefrontal cortex,* where the brain starts the process of interpreting what the eyes see. Inside the midbrain is the amygdala, which is involved in generating emotion and interpreting emotional information.

3. *The amygdala signals the brain stem and cerebellum* to get ready to deal with an emotional situation. These emotion centers go on full alert, awaiting further instructions from the prefrontal cortex and the amygdala.

4. *The prefrontal cortex decides whether the visual image is safe or poses danger.* The prefrontal cortex does a rapid memory check of past experiences with snakes.

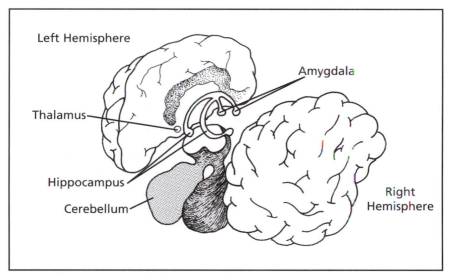

FIGURE 6.1. Strong emotions such as rage, lust, panic, excessive fear, hostility, excessive jealousy, impulse to hurt or kill, and extreme self-focus originate within the midbrain, also called the limbic system. Three structures within the midbrain (amygdala, cerebellum, and hippocampus) regulate and control strong emotions and dyslogical impulse. When socialization disorders occur, we find incomplete development of these midbrain structures.

5. *The amygdala sends the final signal to relax or run away.* If the prefrontal cortex decides that the snake poses a danger, the brain stem springs into action and the person dashes away to safety. If the prefrontal cortex decides that all is well, the midbrain and brain stem relax and that event is over. However, the person will carry such emotional memory tapes the rest of his

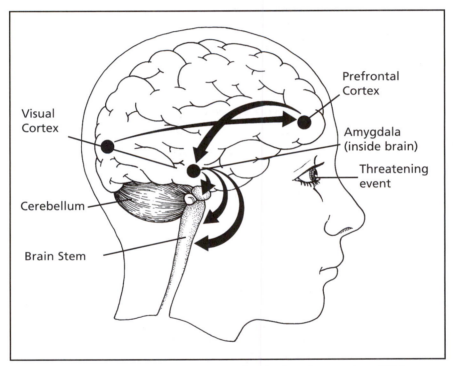

FIGURE 6.2. Three midbrain structures are involved in the creation of lifelong emotional memory: the cerebellum, hippocampus, and amygdala. When the eyes see a possibly threatening event, the visual cortex simultaneously relays that data to two brain structures—the amygdala within the midbrain and the pre-frontal cortex at the front of the right brain. The amygdala sends an alert signal to the brain stem to be ready to trigger the "fight-or-flight" response to danger. The prefrontal cortex reviews what the person has experienced in the past when this event has been encountered. If the prefrontal cortex decides that the event poses danger, a "red flag" signal is sent to the amygdala, which triggers the brain stem to go on full alert and either run away or fight to defend the person from this threat of danger. In extremely threatening events, permanent emotional memory is established. For the rest of the person's life, this event will trigger a phobic response unless the emotional memory is revised through desensitization.

or her life. The sight of a snake will continue to trigger this 5-step "fight-or-flight" cycle unless the emotions that drive the memory are modified through desensitization.

Impact of Emotional Memories

We all carry many emotional memories that color our lives. When danger-loaded memories are triggered by seeing a snake, or hearing certain "bad" sounds, or whiffing certain "bad" odors, the fight-or-flight cycle is set into motion. Blood pressure soars; breathing becomes rapid; armpits perspire; the mouth goes dry; and the strong emotions of fear, dread, and panic explode into action. When safety memories are triggered by seeing a loved one, hearing favorite sounds, or inhaling delightful aromas, the prefrontal cortex advises the midbrain and brain stem that all is well.

School Phobias

An active barrier to academic success for many persons with LD is the presence of frightening emotional memories of failures in taking tests, producing handwriting samples, doing reading, or working math problems. For many struggling students, the sight of paper and pencil triggers the 5-step emotional memory cycle. Test anxiety is a form of school phobia that engulfs students at exam time. Reading orally before the class often triggers the flight reflex that makes the student who is struggling want to run away from the event. Entering a school building often triggers nausea or deep anxiety for individuals who have hateful emotional memories of being in school. One does not need to have a disability to suffer from school phobia. Our current knowledge of how the midbrain and brain stem contribute to this crippling phenomenon takes away the blame. Being the victim of school phobia is not a personal choice, and the person with LD who also has school phobia is not just being immature. Right-brain, midbrain, and brain stem structures are active participants when negative emotional memories overwhelm the learning process.

Removing Negative Emotional Memories

One of the principal goals of effective teaching is to take away the fear of learning. Instructors of students with LD accomplish this renewal by following the kinds of strategies discussed in earlier chapters. For example, as Pete and Maria develop successful skills in controlling letter reversals and spelling more efficiently, they become more self-confident and less afraid of classroom learning. The more they succeed, the less they have to worry about triggering emotional memory cycles that used to torment them so acutely. As Andrew learns to write legibly, he is set free from old phobic reactions that used to cripple his performance. As Wayne becomes skilled at keyboard writing, he no longer feels afraid of the writing process. As Shane learns wholesome concepts about spiritual issues related to his sexuality, he is set free from the dreadful phobias that almost cost him his life. Those who teach and counsel such individuals have the opportunity to undo old emotional damage by replacing fear with strong self-confidence and positive self-esteem.

The Impact of Social Disability

In viewing the life of a person with dyslexia, we would probably conclude that if we had to choose between success in school or success in life, it ultimately would be more important for one to be socially successful. It is possible for an illiterate person to earn a living and be a contributing member to family and society, but it is virtually impossible for a person who is socially disabled to establish and maintain a successful life once he or she has passed beyond the shelter of the school years.

Social disability is a heartbreaking pattern for those who must live with such a person. The person who is socially disabled is oblivious to the protocols that must be followed if one is to love and be loved. Individuals with dyslexia and socialization disorders cannot read the subtle signals that tell most people how to respond to others. Persons who are NVLD or SELD do not see boundary markers that say, "Not just now. Give me some space." These individuals are self-centered in that their major concern is for themselves. They do not have the sensitivity to realize when they are being too overbearing or shrill or demanding. They are too socially unaware to recognize when their behavior has offended someone or when their habits are embarrassing, and they do not blend into the normal give-and-take that must occur in any successful relationship. They often display deep stubbornness that makes them impossible to influence, even when they are wrong and must change their ways, and frequently have poor manners that grate on the nerves of those who must share their space. They do not perceive how their decisions create problems for others, even when they spend impulsively or waste precious resources on trivial or immature things.

Persons with NVLD or SELD cannot accept or comprehend constructive criticism because they tend to be overly sensitive and too easily offended. They do not follow through on plans, do not see how poor punctuality affects co-workers, and cannot understand why they are unpopular on the job. They usually keep moving from job to job, unable to learn from their mistakes. Persons who are socially disabled and also have dyslexia are seldom sensitive to the needs of a spouse or children. Even though these adults who are NVLD or SELD may be affectionate and even good lovers, the long-range business of building a marriage and rearing children is beyond their understanding. Most have "tunnel vision," seeing only a few issues clearly and not comprehending social issues that also must be considered. As spouses they tend to be self-centered and blind to the needs of loved ones. As parents they tend to be overly demanding and narrow in how they discipline. As workers on the job, they tend to be stubborn and inflexible when it comes to following instructions. As citizens they generally are uninformed on issues that affect society. Teenagers with these disabilities tend to become strongly opinionated adults who harp on the same few issues over and over. As they leave their 20s and move on toward middle age, they settle into narrow, shallow lifestyles that become rigid and inflexible, which means that any spouse or companion must do most of the adapting and changing as time goes by. Persons with NVLD or SELD and dyslexia often are somewhat paranoid, never fully trusting anyone but themselves, and they frequently flare into angry confrontations when their points of view are challenged or criticized. To emerge into one's adult years as a person who is socially disordered is costly to everyone involved in that person's life.

Changing SELD

Is it possible to guide children with dyslexia in such a way that they will not become socially disabled? At the end of Chapter 1, the possibility of overcoming dyslexia if appropriate help is provided soon enough was discussed. If the dyslexic patterns are identified by age 7, and if good remedial teaching and home guidance are started at that point, 85% of these children can be taught to achieve academic success. At the same time, they also can be taught to relate successfully with their world and to stay in control of any SELD tendencies they might exhibit. The rate of success depends upon cooperation between home and school.

If dyslexic patterns are not identified until age 9, so that remedial teaching and guidance techniques are not begun until that age, there is approximately a 70% chance for successful remediation. In other words, 30% of the dyslexic/NVLD population is lost by waiting just 2 additional years. If dyslexia is not identified and treated until the early teen years, the rate for full remediation drops to 5%, and if the disability is not caught until the early adult years, only a few individuals can be helped. Early identification and treatment of left-brain LD and right-brain LD *can* change the academic and social patterns that characterize dyslexia, but as time goes by, this becomes increasingly difficult to do. Each passing year of academic failure and social struggle makes it less possible for deeply embedded patterns to be modified. Those who struggle with dyslexia along with SELD can and often do reach a point of no return.

SOCIAL DISABILITY PROFILE FOR INDIVIDUALS WITH DYSLEXIA

The syndrome called socialization disorder is composed of several overlapping factors, all of which interact like the roots of a tree to support the complex structure of social disability. By looking at each factor separately, we can see how NVLD and SELD personality styles develop. This also provides clues to help the person with dyslexia who also has NVLD or SELD change habits and grow a different way.

Self-Centeredness

The taproot of social disability is self-centeredness. This central orientation of self-focus supports the rest of the SELD structure. Extreme self-centeredness is described in psychiatric terms as narcissism. In ancient mythology, Narcissus was a handsome young man who could not take his eyes or thoughts off himself. He spent long hours gazing at his reflection in pools and mirrors, losing all contact with the outside world as he gazed at himself, loved himself, groomed himself, and thought only of himself. As the ancient myth goes, he eventually disappeared inside himself and was transformed into a lovely flower that looked at itself all day at the side of a pool. In modern terms, a truly narcissistic person would be mentally ill, incapable of normal emotional interaction with others. Persons with dyslexia and SELD are not mentally ill, except in isolated cases when true mental illness does emerge, but they are self-centered. Their primary concerns are "What do I get out of this situation? What is here for me? What can my friends and family do for me? What can I get for myself out of this new job? What does my roommate owe me for all I've done?"

This type of thinking dominates the waking hours of most persons with SELD who have dyslexia. They simply do not see the needs of others. When they occasionally do recognize that someone else has a need, the tendency is to do something impulsive for that person at the moment, then get back to the business of satisfying self. It is impossible for such a person to keep his or her attention focused very long on others.

Joe is a striking example of this socially disabled, dyslexic self-centeredness. I met him when he was 9. He was so frustrated in an elementary school classroom that he was having tantrums and disrupting everything the teacher tried to do. We formed an immediate bond because I was the first adult ever to give this frustrated child the quality of attention he was struggling to find. He loved me intensely in his self-centered way. As his guide and counselor, I was able to absorb his self-centeredness so that he felt great joy when we were together. His family could not help me with Joe's dyslexic tendencies because their deeply embedded family style was one of confrontation. The relationship between mother and father was based upon competition to see which adult could outsmart the other. This often-fierce rivalry was absorbed by the children, who carried this competitive spirit into their sibling relationships. The family environment included finding fault with one another, seeking ways to dominate one another, and never failing to remind one another of past mistakes. Joe entered this socially combative arena unable to cope. To survive, he had to become a little gladiator, slashing his opponents as they slashed him. Having dyslexia in that intelligent but verbally aggressive family was an emotionally abusive environment for such a sensitive child.

Professionals who work with students with dyslexia see a critically important survival paradigm: If such a person can find two sources of positive support, then he or she can change from being socially disabled toward being an outgoing, socially successful person. If the home cannot give such support, but the child can receive that support at school and from some other important source, the negative influence of home can be overcome. If the school cannot provide positive support, but the child can find it both at home and from another important source, then the child also can overcome the negative influences of the classroom. Unfortunately for Joe, he was isolated from positive change both at home and at school. The stubbornness and self-centeredness of his parents kept them from agreeing upon the best school placement where his academic and emotional needs could be met. If one parent suggested one place, the other disagreed.

Joe went through school in a learning environment that matched his home life in terms of competition, criticism for failure, and lack of support for positive self-esteem. At home he was regarded by parents and siblings as a problem child; at school he was regarded as a "lazy, disruptive boy" who would not try. His relationship with me was the only positive oasis in his emotionally arid life, but it was not enough to prevent him from becoming socially disabled. To survive, he had to be self-centered. To be thoughtful of others at home or school was to open himself up to criticism and ridicule.

In his teens, Joe wrote many pages of poetry. The spelling had many dyslexic patterns and the language skills were primitive, but the poetry was warm and beautiful. However, it was self-centered material. He was madly in love with many girls, but in a self-centered way. It was impossible for him to understand when I explained the give-and-take required in love. He developed the habit of buying each new girlfriend a single rose, which he presented over a candlelight dinner at a luxurious restaurant. At first, the girl was overwhelmed and delighted; however, within a few days or weeks, Joe would be telling me about how still another girl had rejected him for "some jerk not nearly as smart as I am." I would read a series of new poems he had composed, dyslexic spelling and all, which he sent to the former girlfriend, reminding her of what she had forfeited by refusing his love. It was impossible to make a dent in Joe's narcissistic patterns. He could not comprehend what I said about turning his attention from himself to others. "But I am one of the most thoughtful guys in town!" he would shout. "What do you mean, I am self-centered? I buy them roses. I take them to the nicest places to eat. I treat them like royalty!" "Yes, you do," I replied. "But why do you do all these things?" "So they will like me!" he exclaimed. He still could not recognize his self-centeredness in all those relationships.

Joe's social disabilities reached a peak in something he did one day. He brought me a set of photographs he had taken. As he proudly watched me look through the stack of pictures, he kept asking, "How do you like my photography? Don't you think I'm good with a camera?" I was astonished as I kept turning to the next picture. Every shot was of Joe. He had used three rolls of film to photograph himself. By setting the timer, he could settle into a new pose before the camera snapped yet another picture. Joe had brought me 108 snapshots he had taken of himself, and he could not comprehend why I was not delighted. He was baffled by my questions: "Why did you take pictures of yourself? Why not take pictures of others?" He slammed out of my office in a rage. "There you go, criticizing me! You're just like my parents!" After his first year of college, Joe took a vacation trip with a friend. When he returned, he showed me a lot of snapshots of his trip. I soon realized that every picture was of Joe. "Where is your friend?" I asked. "Oh, I threw away all the pictures he was in," Joe said, with a shrug.

Persons who are socially disabled and also have dyslexia do not always take pictures of themselves, but their lives are centered upon themselves. They are rarely aware that this is so. In fact, most persons with social disabilities that I have known think of themselves as thoughtful, considerate, generous people. Their blind spot is that they cannot see why they give gifts, do courteous things, or remember birthdays, that everything they do is designed to get something back in return. Their generosity is a means of receiving praise and satisfaction for themselves. If they do see a real need in others, they immediately turn that need back toward themselves. For example, if a person like Joe sees a friend crying, he or she may take the friend into a warm embrace. However, instead of listening to the friend's need, the person with SELD would say, "I know how you feel. Boy, have I cried a lot myself. Why, last week I cried when a girl broke up with me. You know, there sure are a lot of immature girls in this town. They just aren't mature enough to appreciate a guy like me. Yeah, I've cried a lot myself. My mom and dad make me cry a lot, the way they criticize me all the time. You ought to be at my house and hear them yell all the time." By this time, the friend with the problem has pulled away from Joe's embrace. The reality soon becomes clear that he is not really interested in the friend's problems. All he can think about is himself. And Joe faces yet another situation in which he is pushed away by someone who needed more than he could give.

Self-centeredness is common in children. In fact, one of the earliest habits, or social milestones, children must learn is how to share playthings in a group. Teachers and parents are delighted when youngsters learn this important social lesson of looking beyond themselves with playmates. The child with LD often has much difficulty acquiring this important social skill, but it can be taught if adults begin soon enough. Self-centeredness can be turned around along with reversed letters and scrambled sequence if addressed soon enough. It is critically important that children with dyslexia and SELD have models at home and at school of caring, sharing, thoughtfulness, and consideration of others. Adults cannot model concern for others if they themselves are self-centered. Children like Joe must have at least two instructional sources if these deep-seated tendencies are to be altered, and they must see these models day after day, over a period of years. Joe should have had several years of clear demonstration of unselfish affection in order to change his self-centered bent.

Learning not to be self-centered involves certain basic concepts, including how to read body language and emotional signs. This requires the same kind of careful coaching that goes into teaching phonics and reading when a child cannot "hear" the sounds in words. As children with dyslexia comprehend literacy skills, they also can master social awareness skills, if the instruction begins soon enough before habits and attitudes are set too deeply to be changed.

Noticing Others

Self-centeredness is constantly looking at self and paying attention to self. Social awareness is looking at others and paying attention to others. The first step is to change the point of focus from the self to someone else. Over a period of time, the child with dyslexia is taught what to do when he or she comes into a room. Adults explain, "Joe, don't wonder what everyone will think about you. That is a self-centered thought. Instead, look at other persons and speak to them. Look for signs that tell how they are. Is Mary happy this morning? How can you tell? Does her face show it? Do her clothes show it? Is Robert unhappy this morning? How can you tell? How does his face show it? How might his clothes show it? Is Mrs. Jordan happy today? Does she feel well this morning after her cold last week? How can you tell? Why don't you ask her if she feels better today? Did Jason have fun over the weekend with his dad? How can you tell? Listen to what Jason is saying. Is he telling happy stories about what he did with his dad? Or is he not talking about it at all? Look at Janice, the new girl in the class. Has she been crying this morning? How can you tell? Do her eyes look sad? Is there something nice you can say to let her know you are glad she is in your class? Remember how Robert is always losing his things? How can you tell if he has his pencil ready for class? Can you help him look for his pencil before the teacher asks him about it?"

These are the kinds of "baby steps" parents and teachers must take to help children with dyslexia learn how to turn their attention away from themselves. Some homes and classrooms have a natural climate of thoughtfulness where children are immersed in caring, thoughtful attention to others. Some children are sensitive enough to follow models and learn to behave that way. Others must be guided step by step, the way they must learn the multiplication tables. Children with SELD who also have dyslexia often come from homes and classrooms where this model of specific, long-range thoughtfulness is not demonstrated or taught. It takes many years of careful nurture with daily practice before the natural bent toward self-centeredness is changed in them.

Reaching Out to Others

During the past 38 years, I have worked one-to-one with more than 10,000 people with dyslexia of all ages. One of the most difficult skills for them to learn is how to reach out to others. Most must exert a great deal of conscious effort just to get through each day successfully. During academic years, their energies go into doing their best in difficult studies, keeping up with volumes of homework, dealing with the trauma of flunking tests and making low grades, absorbing criticism without being too badly hurt, and so forth. Although they seldom have much emotional energy left over for others, they must learn to become socially thoughtful persons, at least to some degree. These people must see the model of reaching out before they can claim it for themselves. From their early years, these children must see generous social attitudes demonstrated. If the family has a negative attitude concerning helping others, this lack of generosity is quickly absorbed by the children. If parents complain about having to be generous, then their children will have trouble being generous.

The lesson of reaching out to others was vividly implanted in my mind at the age of 7 by a single action of my father's. I have only a few clear memories of him. He was stricken with cancer before I started to school, which was toward the end of the Great Depression. Like so many other parents of the late 1930s, mine were out of work, and our family faced the terror of no income with three children to feed. My father's medical needs were supplied by the Veterans Administration (VA), but he had to live at a VA hospital to receive treatment for the malignancy. My mother moved my sisters and me into a very humble apartment in an impoverished neighborhood, while she tried to make ends meet on an income of $24.00 per month. I vividly recall that day when my father came home for a brief visit from the hospital. We were in the tiny backyard near the alley that the apartment faced, enjoying this rare family time together, when a shabbily dressed, very dirty man came along and asked for something to eat. As a 7-year-old, I had only a primitive notion of how scarce food was for our family, but I knew that we had to be very careful, that there were no treats and no extra helpings. I knew that things were bad and my mother cried a lot. As the shabby man stood there asking for food, I saw my mother shake her head. Later, I would realize how little she had for her own family, let alone anything to share.

My attention was suddenly drawn to my father's face. My father smiled at the stranger and asked him to sit down and rest. Then he turned to my mother and said, "Could you fix one of your egg sandwiches for this good man?" My mother's egg sandwiches were among the wonders of the world when I was a child. It was an exceptional treat when we got to have one of her creations with a fried egg, a slice of cheese, and toasted bread. I remember that scene as my dad rubbed the pain in his amputated leg, chatted with the stranger who had no place to go and nothing to eat, and showed me what it meant to reach out to someone beyond ourselves. I have never forgotten the gratitude as that stranger thanked my mother for her gift. An egg sandwich never brought more joy than hers did that day. As I have reflected on that scene so many times, I am so grateful for the gift my father gave me that day. He demonstrated what it means to reach out to others instead of feeling sorry for ourselves. That experience set into motion a lifelong pattern I have followed to this day.

Youngsters with LD often find it hard to reach out to others. Yet they can learn to do so if they see the model and are taught the skill. The crippling limitation of being socially disabled is not having the ability to reach beyond oneself, except for selfish purposes. This deeply important social skill can be taught if persons in the child's life do not wait too long. Reaching out to others can be demonstrated along with phonics, spelling, and math practice, and the child can learn what it means to attend to the world beyond self. For example, he or she can be taught to notice what others need: "Look at Mark. Why is he frustrated? Is there something you can do to help him find his eraser? Look at Sue. She can't get her pencil to draw that circle. Can you help her do it so she can finish her picture? Look at Joe. He can't see his math book under his jacket. Can you help him find it? Look at Mrs. Jordan. She dropped part of the math papers by her desk. Can you help her pick them up? Look at Mr. Jones, the custodian. He can't get all of his stuff through the door. Can you help him by holding the door open?"

These small steps in reaching out to others soon turn the self-centered bent another way. The child learns that helping someone in need brings its own burst of joy, its own rewards—that he or she does not need something in return. The act of being generous is a social skill, part of the "tribal dance" one must learn. Children with dyslexia can learn this skill, even when their own emotions are exhausted, if modeling is begun early enough.

Self-Pity

One of the most unattractive ingredients of SELD is self-pity. The "poor little me" syndrome is a major reason why persons who lack social skills are unattractive. Of course, many who do not have dyslexia also bog down in the swamp of self-pity. At times it feels good for any of us to "have a pity party," but the person with good self-image and social skills soon laughs and gets back to the business of being mature. It is especially easy for a child with dyslexia to develop self-pity. The refrain often sounds like this: "Nobody else has to do this much work. Why do I have to work so hard all the time? Jason makes good grades and he doesn't have to work all the time! How come my brother gets to ride his bike and I have to finish this homework? How come I don't ever get to play? I have to work all the time! It's not fair! How come I have some old learning disability? I didn't ask to be born this way!"

All of this is true, of course. It is not fair to be born with dyslexia. It definitely is not fair for your siblings to get to play when you have to keep on with unfinished work. It is not fair to have to go to tutors or special classes or summer school, never to have your papers on the bulletin board with gold stars, never to make top grades when you know that you studied harder than the star of the class. It is not fair when adults say, "If you just tried harder! I know you can do it. You just won't try!" It is not fair to be smarter than a friend, yet he or she can read better and make better grades. It is not fair always to lose your words and get tangled up trying to tell stories and look dumb every time you answer in class, never to finish a test first, never to get all of your work done so that it has to be taken home. It's just not fair!

The antidote for self-pity is a good sense of humor, which is not easy for the child with dyslexia to learn. How do you laugh about making poor grades? Where is the funny part of feeling "dumb" all the time? What is there to laugh about when you get lost turning corners and can't remember where you leave things, when you can't spell your own name, when you get things backwards or read "Altus" when the sign said Tulsa?

Wise parents and teachers help these children learn to smile instead of lapse into self-pity. OK, so it's not very funny when all of these dyslexic things happen, but let's see how we can make the best of it. It helps to start with the really funny things that come along. For example, most individuals who have dyslexia create marvelous tongue twisters that can be a lot of fun for the family. Relatives of these people actually can be proud of verbal slips that turn into famous family sayings. One day Keith was explaining why he wanted to be alone for a while. "I just need to be synonymous," he said, and his family had a wonderful new way of talking about privacy. There was no criticism or embarrassment, just praise and good humor over this rich contribution to the family vocabulary. One day Judy said that she had three "sliver dimes" in her coin collection, and her family suddenly had a new Judyism. After that, they all looked for "slivers" when they counted their change. Alex became her "daddy's little gril" when she got her letters backwards, and that grew into her father's tenderest term of endearment for his precious daughter. Erin always said, "Mom, where is my tallow?" when it was time for her shower. Her family adopted the wonderful new Erinism as they used tallows after their baths. I knew that Stan had outgrown his self-pity when he brought me a wooden statue he had carved and painted so carefully. "This is my dyslexic sheriff," he explained with a smile. He showed me the word he had carved below the sheriff's left foot: WARD. "That's dyslexia for DRAW," he laughed. One day Chris left his mom a note: "My book is no my bed." From then on, the family had a richly funny phrase. When anything was lost, they always said, "Look no the bed."

These are the kinds of "baby steps" adults can take in disarming the trigger of self-pity and turning it another way. But this journey away from self-pity must begin early, before the emotional concrete hardens into inflexibility. I have seen many children with dyslexia reach adult years without a sense of humor. Overly sensitive, they are beyond the reach of others who would like to help them loosen up. A lifelong pity party is the reflexive habit of blaming others instead of taking responsibility for oneself, of saying, "It is not my fault." This point of view makes excuses for self and places the blame on others: "I inherited this problem from my dad, so it's his fault I'm dyslexic." "I had lousy teachers who didn't like me, so I never learned to read." "My math teacher was too lazy to do her job, so I never learned my times facts." "They didn't like me in junior high school, so I dropped out when I got old enough." "My boss worked me too hard, so I just quit. I won't work anyplace I'm not treated with respect." This litany of self-pity goes on and on until the person finds himself or herself in the position of being a loser. If children with LD are not taught how to take responsibility and laugh at their mistakes, they gradually settle into the self-pity swamp, where they become encased in an attitude that is offensive to others and degrading to themselves.

Stubbornness

Persons with social disabilities usually are stubborn. Their interpretation of events has a bullheaded quality, and their approach to life is single-minded. They view life through the lens of self, conclude that whatever they think is correct, and then cling to that opinion, no matter what.

Earlier in this chapter I described Ray's tenacious preoccupation with being safe, of how he guaranteed his safety by always being in control. For many persons with SELD, being safe is guaranteed through being stubborn, which is a fiercely loyal protection of self. New suggestions are met with disbelief: "If I didn't think of it, it isn't important to me!" New ideas are dismissed with scoffing: "That's the dumbest thing I ever heard!" Skepticism frequently is displayed: "That won't work." End of discussion.

These individuals often dig in their heels and refuse to budge, which generates all kinds of friction and conflict. A parent who has social disabilities sees no value in the opinions of children or spouse, and any effort to bring up new ideas within the family is met with sarcasm and hostility. The stubborn person with SELD maintains control through verbal browbeating, nagging, threatening, and refusing to listen to anything new or different. If a new idea is brought into the relationship, it is pounded into the ground by verbal attack and belittling comments until the other person backs off.

This stubborn characteristic is especially detrimental in a culture where change is so prevalent and frequent. In Chapter 1, the workplace of the 21st century was described. Most workers will change jobs or occupations several times before retirement. During the 1990s, more than half of all families in the United States will have moved their place of residence several times. In most occupations, new technology makes old job knowledge obsolete within 5 years unless the worker continually learns and grows. Persons with dyslexia and SELD manifested by stubbornness do not adapt to such changes. They cling to whatever point of view they brought into adult life, and they fight to keep it that way. They tend to move from job to job, never understanding why boss after boss fires them or lays them off, but believing they are being strong in defending a principle. They cannot see the role they play in making it impossible for them to get along with others. Stubbornness locks the door against letting anything new come inside, freezes marriage into a one-sided relationship that gradually squeezes the life out of the spouse, and builds a wall between parent and child so that no communication can occur. Stubbornness drives wedges between coworkers and colleagues, creating division that eventually causes a work group to fall apart. The stubborn person, who does not see the situation realistically, is soon left behind as society moves forward and new technology makes old ways obsolete.

Stubbornness begins as a defense strategy based upon fear, as was shown in Chapter 5. Youngsters freeze when they are too afraid or too unsure to step ahead. If adults push the fearful child, he or she balks and sometimes lashes back. This is defensive behavior that thoughtful adults try to understand. Why is this bright child refusing to cooperate? Is the child afraid? If so, what is causing the fear? Thoughtful parents and teachers find ways to help stubborn youngsters release the fear so that progress can occur.

Children with LD are afraid of many things. Virtually everything they attempt poses a high risk of failure. Adults who work with children who have dyslexia recognize how often they freeze and feel immobilized. This defensive behavior protects the child from too much failure, because it is better to be scolded for not trying than to face the scolding that comes from failure. Stubborn habits thus are established early.

Unfortunately, not all parents and teachers know how to deal successfully with childhood stubbornness. Some adults, having a mindset that "No child is going to get the best of me," continue to push too hard. The contest of wills then is on. W. Hugh Missildine developed the concept of the "Over-coerced syndrome" (Missildine & Galton, 1972). He described this pattern as the ultimately stubborn child who digs in the heels and refuses to budge when adults press for obedience. The more adults press, the more the child refuses. These extremely stubborn children are believed to have been pushed too hard too many times while they were afraid. As a result, they have the automatic habit of digging in the heels in stubborn resistance when any adult pressure is felt or anticipated.

The person with dyslexia and SELD fits this pattern of extreme stubbornness even when there is no reason to display such an attitude. For the person, it is an effective form of control. Those around him or her either give in and do things his or her way or pay a heavy emotional price.

Because this kind of stubbornness originates in childhood fear, it is possible to avoid the problem by guiding children to learn better ways to deal with their fear. The process must begin early. Adults must recognize the signs of fear and quietly, thoughtfully discuss it with the child. "What exactly is causing you to be afraid, John?" "I don't know." "Are you afraid because it's dark?" "No." "Are you afraid because Daddy is not home yet?" "Yes," John blurts out. Or he may only nod his head. "OK. I'm glad to know how you feel. Come sit in my lap. Let's talk about it. Did you know that Daddy called while you were outside playing? Did you know that he asked how John is this afternoon? Did you know that when the big hand gets to six and the little hand is at nine, Daddy will be home?" As John quietly hears all of these facts, he relaxes and is no longer afraid. Now he is ready to eat supper and be ready to give his father a big hug at 9:30. This is the way thoughtful parents walk children through the moments of fear that spring up.

Teachers work in similar ways to disarm fearful students at school. Because handwriting is so difficult for him, John freezes when the class is asked to write the alphabet. He stares out the window and will not lift his pencil. The teacher quietly watches for a while, then comes over to his desk and bends down. "You know, John," she says quietly. "I wonder something. Has your pencil forgotten how to write A?" John nods. "Well, that's no problem. Here, let me help you teach your pencil how to write A. Pick up your pencil. That's right. Now I'm going to hold your hand around your pencil. Let's teach your pencil to write A. Oh, yes, that's very good. Now see if your pencil remembers how to write B." And John is at work without being afraid of failing.

It takes great courage for a fearful person to move ahead. "What if I fail? What if I don't know how? What if I look dumb? What if someone laughs at me or criticizes me?" All of these questions must be put to rest before fear can relax and progress can occur. The stubbornness part of SELD is born from this kind of self-questioning. Children can learn how to turn such questions into forward steps if they begin early and are taught how over a period of time. Stubbornness must be faced in so many areas: how one dresses for school, doing chores instead of playing, tasting new food, meeting new people, giving up worn-out clothes and toys, letting Mom rearrange the furniture, sharing things with others, letting brother or sister use your stuff, and so forth. Wise parents and teachers guide youngsters through these developmental steps, one at a time. Over a period of years, stubbornness is replaced by courage and willingness to try because fear has been removed through understanding, not by nagging, yelling, or criticizing.

Arrogance

Perhaps the most offensive SELD characteristic is arrogance. This often is the last straw in causing relationships to break apart. Self-centered persons frequently can be charming, and self-pitying persons often attract sympathy by appearing cuddly and needing lots of hugs. The arrogant person, however, is abrasive and cold in his or her display of superiority: "I am the best. I am the smartest. If you want to know, just ask me. Anyone who disagrees with me is dumb and stupid." An arrogant attitude places others in the embarrassing position of not being bright or competent. The arrogant person with SELD brags and struts with no regard for the feelings of others, and controls and dominates any conversation by a nonstop monologue about self: "I did this. I saw that. I said such and such." The opinions of others are dismissed with a condescending tone because they do not matter. This social bully intimidates others to get his or her own way.

Social Misfit

The person with SELD displayed through an arrogant attitude quickly becomes labeled as a "know-it-all" and is mocked behind his or her back. Yet, he or she is blind to this social reaction. Such a person is a social misfit, unable to fit successfully into groups. Because he or she cannot find acceptance in the usual social ways, the person often tries to develop his or her own controlled group. It is interesting to watch such an individual work out strategies for gaining a network of followers. Relationships are based upon the pretense that this person is special and that he or she has something unique that others do not have. Highly charismatic persons successfully manage for years in such an arrogant role. Within the group, there may be intense loyalty that defends the arrogant leader and explains away all of his or her rudeness.

Using Others

This type of leader views others with contempt, but strokes and grooms them in ways to make them feel important. The person with SELD seeks others who are vulnerable, who need to be associated with someone who represents power. These power groups are seen at every level: the school playground, large-city street corners, corporate boardrooms, religious organizations, the world of politics, and colleges and universities. Arrogance uses others, devalues their worth, degrades their dignity, and stifles their growth. Such persons are among the least loved of all members of society, but they never understand why. They are blind to the offensive impact of their behavior on others.

Attitude of Superiority

Of all the elements of social disability, arrogance is one of the most difficult to change. The example of Joe's behavior discussed earlier in this chapter demonstrated much arrogance. He truly thought that he deserved special treatment because he was bright. He used our friendship to brag to friends that he was "Dr. Jordan's special friend." Joe could not keep from making cutting remarks whenever he observed a mistake or weakness in others, and he could not keep his tongue from saying "I told you so" in a manner that triggered anger in others. His car was better. His all-weather coat cost more. His gold chain was more valuable. His dad made more money. Girls liked him better than they did other guys. Some day he was going to have his doctorate and make a lot of money. Joe never comprehended how this arrogant litany provoked others and made him the target of ridicule. He had no friends and he never knew why. It was impossible for him to accept any level of constructive criticism. His reaction would be, "There you go, criticizing me like my folks always do!" When the root of arrogance is not changed during the formative years of a child with SELD, it becomes an obnoxious weed that makes the person offensive and unable to fit into normal society. The depth of loneliness is incredible when the person stops pretending and actually looks for companionship, but he or she cannot understand why.

Reducing the Arrogance Level

How does an arrogant person learn to be humble? In most instances it seems impossible, once the characteristic becomes deeply embedded. To be arrogant is to be blind to others, seeing only self. How does one see others when one has no social vision? As with all other SELD characteristics, the key to change is beginning the process of teaching good social skills early. This transformation from being egocentric to recognizing the worth of others starts with "baby steps" that show the child how to look at others realistically. For example, Joe blurts out a judgment, "Jack is dumb! He's really stupid!" He should be guided through a discussion. "No, Joe. Jack isn't dumb. He is just as intelligent as you. Have you ever noticed that certain things are hard for Jack to do? Have you ever noticed how hard he struggles to write well? Watch how hard he must work to write as well as you do." "OK, but I'm better than he is at writing." "That's right, Joe, you are. But Jack is better than you at math. Have you ever noticed that every person is best at something, but nobody is best at everything?" "Well, OK, but it's still dumb the way Jack writes." "No, Joe, we aren't going to call anyone dumb. Do you want people to say you're 'dumb' because you can't remember your multiplication facts?" "No, but that's different!" "No, Joe, it is not different. Writing is easier for you than it is for Jack. But math is easier for him than it is for you. We aren't going to call each other dumb, Joe. That is not acceptable."

This kind of patient teaching bears good results over a period of time if the arrogant child receives this model from at least two sources. If Joe sees this thoughtful model in one person while he continually sees an arrogant, sarcastic, overly critical pattern in others, he will not change his bad habits. If two important people in his life demonstrate patience and kindness, there is enough outside strength to help Joe understand the social-emotional need to treat others as he would have them deal with him.

Unfortunately, the Joe whom I have described did not have this kind of patient guidance during his formative years. He followed the stringent, overly critical models of his home and the school he attended. His close, supportive relationship with me was not enough to change his bent toward being arrogant. Had either his home or school presented him with a nurturing, caring model and example, he and I could have replaced his arrogant spirit with a much better attitude of tolerance and compassion.

Immaturity

Most persons with dyslexia who have SELD are immature. Although they may reach physical maturity ahead of schedule, they remain behind schedule emotionally. They are impatient, flashing into anger at the least irritation. They are impulsive, making decisions and taking actions without thinking of consequences. They rarely fear physical danger, which deprives them of the warning signals most of us hear. Because they behave much less maturely than their peers, they are seen as misfits. They have short attention spans, becoming bored too soon to enjoy social activities. They are shallow spiritually because they have no patience for developing a deeper understanding of faith or religious teaching. They are materialistic, wanting all kinds of nice things without having the income to afford them. They are jealous, which makes them impossible partners in romantic relationships or friendships. They are insatiable, never achieving full satisfaction, no matter how much attention or affection they receive. They thus burn out personal relationships by being overly demanding and possessive. They are insecure, always fretting over little issues that most people shrug off. These immature individuals clamor, fret, fuss, beg, demand, accuse, blow up, have tantrums, waste what they have, and live dangerously.

Intelligence Far Ahead of Maturity

In evaluating the learning patterns of people with dyslexia, professionals usually find wide differences between their highest areas of ability and their lowest areas of performance. For example, most persons with dyslexia are quite intelligent. Mental age is usually higher than chronological age, but reading is well below mental age and work stamina age is far below mental age. When the person with dyslexia also has SELD, emotional maturity age also lags far behind the level of intelligence. The following profile provides a good example:

Mental age	16
Chronological age	12
Reading age	8
Work stamina age	7
Emotional maturity age	6

In a quiet, one-to-one situation, this student who is LD displays the mental ability expected of most 16-year-olds, although his age is only 12. However, in his seventh-grade classroom, his reading skills are stuck at a third-grade level. As the teacher works with his group, the youngster, who also has SELD, begins to fidget, squirm, and interrupt as a 7-year-old child would do. Compared with his classmates, this boy is immature and disruptive, never keeping his attention focused on the task. He reacts to stress as if he were 6. He flares too easily, whines too much, complains too often, argues too frequently, and wheedles to get out of work. He bursts into tears at a certain point of frustration. He is like an overwhelmed 6-year-old child trying to cope with middle school expectations.

Immaturity in Adults

Older persons who have SELD have the same kind of wide disparity between their highest abilities and their level of emotional control. Being immature means that they cannot cope with life at their age. Young adults who have SELD do not carry out responsibility. They cannot be depended upon to keep promises, show up for work on time, help out when they agreed, pay their share of expenses, pay bills on time, save money instead of spending, or deny themselves immediate pleasure so that something better can be enjoyed later. They give in to whatever whim or impulse bubbles up at the moment. If they have $50.00 to pay on the rent, they may spend it all for beer or a good time on Saturday, then be in trouble for not having rent money on Monday. If they promise to meet someone at a certain time, they may not show up or bother to call. Something else more immediate came up and they forgot their appointment. If they have a job interview at 9:00 A.M., they may oversleep and not wake up until noon, but they do not understand when someone else always gets the job. In the workplace they look for the easy way out and try to avoid doing whatever the boss assigned.

If these individuals get married, they are like disorganized children playing house. If a child is born to the marriage, the parent unfortunately is no more able to cope than a 12-year-old would be. Most of the cases of child abuse occur when such adults try to rear children. The crying of the child, the normal mess of changing diapers, the need to earn a steady income to provide food and medical care for the baby are too much for the adult with SELD. Without warning, he or she bursts into tantrums and tries to make the baby stop crying. A great deal of physical abuse toward the spouse or mate also often occurs. All their lives, these individuals have thrown tantrums, slammed doors, squealed tires, and gunned their car at 100 miles an hour when they are angry. They carry these habits into marriage, onto the job, or into any relationship.

Replacing Immaturity with Maturity

How do parents and teachers tame this kind of explosive emotional immaturity? Is it possible to turn this response a different way? If the process begins early, immaturity can be modified enough to give the person with SELD the basic social skills of self-control. When a child throws a tantrum, adults face certain choices. One reaction would be to fly at the child and spank, slap, or otherwise punish physically. This often stops the tantrum, but the adult has stooped to the child's emotional level. In effect, the adult's tantrum has won over that of the child. Peace may have been restored, but the child now has experienced the model of hitting when one is angry. Occasionally it will be appropriate for a supervisor to shock an angry child into breaking the tantrum. Sometimes one firm swat on the bottom is appropriate at the moment. However, the *habit* of hitting the child who is having a tantrum is not the way to teach mature behavior to these youngsters.

For children to behave with maturity, they must see it demonstrated every day. They must see what it means to have patience, to forgive, to maintain self-control, and not to hit back. Adults must demonstrate persistent patience over a long period of time. This does not mean that they should not be firm or decisive. However, the adult stays in charge in a way that guides the child through the moment of immaturity, followed by a discussion. "John, why were you so angry?" "He got my toy." "But you have a lot of toys. Just look at all of the toys you have to play with." "I want that toy. He can't have it!" "No, John, that is not how we do with our toys. We have to share. Did Jim jerk your toy away from you?" "No, but I wanted it next." "You mean that you were not playing with it when Jim took it?" "No, but it's mine! I want it. He can't have it!" "No, John. It is Jim's turn to play with the toy. You have another toy to play with. Later on Jim will let you play with his toy." If this type of patient rehearsal does not work, then John is firmly taken away from the situation. He may be taken to his room if he is at home or to a different part of the classroom if he is at school. The supervisor must not let him have his way. Over and over during his developmental years, John receives this kind of firm, reasonable guidance. The adult gives him something else to do, whenever possible, but the child's temper does not prevail. His tantrum does not make Jim give up the toy because John demands it.

As these children grow up, thoughtful parents and teachers should require certain amounts of responsibility from them. Parents can make written lists of chores and guide the child in doing everything on the lists. Teachers should write lists of assignments and show the child how to do every task on the lists. As parents and teachers work together, the child begins to understand that a certain amount of structure must be followed. He or she may not like structure but will learn to accept it. Sometimes a reward is the right way to motivate a child to finish responsibilities. Other times, taking away a privilege is the only discipline he or she will understand. Supervisors may have to ground the immature child if certain rules are ignored or disobeyed. Over a period of time, this type of structure instills a sense of responsibility within the child's emerging set of values.

Dyslogic Behavior

In the mid-1970s, John Wacker intrigued the clinical world when he published a monograph entitled *The Dyslogic Syndrome* (Wacker, 1975). After many years of struggling with his daughter's SELD, he outlined for the first time a pattern of irregular behaviors seen in many adults with social disabilities. Earlier in this chapter, the variety of research concerning right-brain lesions, midbrain differences, and brain stem influence on emotional memory and emotional control was reviewed. Incomplete cell development and other forms of neuronal difference produce a type of illogical, eccentric behavior in a certain number of young people (Right-Hemi syndrome). In Chapter 1, Barkley's research of oppositional defiant disorder was reviewed. Wacker pioneered the concept of the *Dyslogic syndrome*, which now is seen as a brain-based problem that partially blocks a person's ability to live by commonsense reasoning or logical thinking. Persons who display Dyslogic syndrome also display the symptoms of Oppositional Defiant Disorder.

Irrational Decisions

Dyslogic behavior is very upsetting to anyone involved in the life of the person who displays it. As the name implies, the individual with SELD does not do things in a normal, logical way. Decisions are unpredictable and irrational. For example, the person may suddenly sell his car for $300 after working 18 months and making $1,500 in payments. A girl with dyslogic behavior may drop out of school within a semester of graduation to work part-time for minimum wage. She got bored with school and wanted to start her career. It makes no sense that she now is earning $65 a week at a fast-food restaurant. A boy with this disability may suddenly quit his job 2 days after being promoted to assistant manager. "I just got tired of it," he explains. "How are you going to keep up your car payments and your insurance?" his father asks. "Oh, it will work out," he says as he dashes off to a party with his buddies.

Unfortunately, these types of people often marry others with the same disability, which creates a marriage not based on any structure or logical foundation. They run up debts on charge accounts, buy expensive items on impulse, party all night and sleep all day, do not clean the house or do dishes. They fight all the time, yet they are extremely jealous if one spouses flirts with another person.

It is impossible for parents to reason with young people who display this syndrome. They do not think in a logical way. They have no regard for tradition that expects everyone in society to be responsible. They have no intention of "dancing the tribal dance," yet they demand to have all the comforts modern society offers. They want their parents to give them money, pay their bills, or bail them out of trouble, but they refuse to work things out through counseling. These young people are too loose to establish productive lives. They do not follow guidance and cannot live by a schedule. They get themselves into astonishing, difficult situations with no plans for getting out because they live by the impulse of the moment.

Reducing Impulsivity

Is it possible to turn such oppositional, impulsive behavior another way? Because dyslexia is a left-brain condition, some who have it gradually outgrow enough of the LD pattern to become successful later on, although they must always deal with poor spelling, poor math computation, and faulty reading. Some are too severely handicapped ever to attain literacy skills, but they can become successful adults with the right kind of guidance during their formative years. Those who display the Dyslogic syndrome present an even more difficult problem. If this syndrome is caused largely by lesions within the right-brain hemisphere, then the disruptive, illogical behavior that results is beyond the reach of counseling or advice. If it is caused by neurological dysfunction, then the dyslogic person has little control over the disruptive, oppositional behavior that makes his or her life so unstable.

Firm Guidance with Structure

If dyslogical behavior is recognized early enough, it can be modified somewhat, although the person will always be prone to impulsive decisions and irregular behavior. If firm behavior modification is begun in childhood when the person is still teachable, it is possible to implant enough awareness of cause and effect to enable him or her to succeed by early adulthood. However, it is impossible to erase dyslogical thinking patterns altogether. The key is to maintain very tight structure over a period of years so the oppositional youngster is kept within certain boundaries. Every fence, every restriction, every adult limitation is clearly labeled and the reasons why are made clear. "No, Jason. You may not ride your bike over to Allen's house." "Why not? Jim gets to ride his bike anywhere he wants!" "No, Jason. Your brother does not ride anywhere he wants, and you know that. The reason you may not ride your bike to Allen's house is that you don't pay attention to traffic. Until you learn to stop and look carefully, you may not ride your bike that far. And that is how it is going to be."

No amount of complaining, threatening, or fussing changes the rule. So long as Jason's behavior is illogical or exposes him to danger, then his behavior will be supervised and controlled. As he matures, he is held responsible for paying for things he breaks. He must apologize whenever he is rude. He must face up to the part he plays when things get out of hand or he creates difficulty. He is not allowed to get away with blaming others, demanding his own way, saying hateful things out of spite, acting out jealous feelings, having money to splurge on whims, and so forth.

Step by small step, Jason learns certain lessons as he grows up. If he is immature, he will be disciplined like a younger child. If he creates an expensive loss of some kind, he must pay for the damage. He must earn a certain amount of money before he can make certain purchases. Whether he likes it or not, he learns that there are limits. He learns that there are laws governing society, and there are police officers who enforce those laws.

His parents must not take his side against teachers, unless a certain teacher was clearly unfair. They must teach him that a family must maintain a certain level of courtesy and mutual respect. Beyond a certain point, they must not give him money or pay the bills he accumulates. He learns that he cannot get away with using people, and that he must give a certain amount if he hopes to receive. These basic social lessons can be learned if adults do not wait too late. However, because the underlying cause for this irregular behavior lies within the brain structure, Dyslogic syndrome is impossible to change completely.

BECOMING INDEPENDENT

Being independent means that people can handle life alone without help. They can make personal decisions without a supervisor, plan ahead and work toward goals, and make choices based upon commonsense reasoning. They can work to establish a more comfortable life, with occasional help from others. Being independent means that they may turn to friends or parents for opinions but do not require the approval of others to know what to do. As adults, they must "cut childhood roots" to a certain degree and replant their lives with new concepts that do not depend upon what mom or dad say or do. They must be able to read all of the signs and do what they say without having to ask an interpreter for help. An independent person still enjoys talking things over with a trusted advisor, because being independent includes knowing the value of wisdom. Being independent means one can make decisions, change plans, establish new values, and start on new journeys without needing the help of anyone else.

It is difficult for persons with dyslexia to reach this level of independence. As demonstrated in Chapter 5, many persons with dyslexia marry someone who becomes the "parent" or "supervisor" to keep life structured. Most adults who have dyslexia feel more comfortable and a great deal safer if someone is nearby, ready to help when things are not clear. It actually is not necessary for such a person to become fully independent. One need not be totally alone and independent in order to have a satisfactory life. However, a certain degree of independence must be achieved if the man or woman is to become a fulfilled adult with positive self-esteem and a good self-image.

Certain basic skills must be mastered if those individuals with dyslexia become independent of their parents or other caretakers as they enter adulthood. As discussed in Chapter 5, people with dyslexia tend to go one of four ways as they leave their teen years. Most find a partner who provides enough support and structure to make the transition into adulthood successful. Others are not ready until much later to leave home and establish a life for themselves. Some drift out into the world as loners, living alone with little or no contact with society beyond a few narrow areas. Some become involved with illegal activity to the point of becoming wards of the court. This group includes many persons with Dyslogic syndrome and Oppositional Defiant Disorder who cannot manage the rules of society successfully.

Time Awareness

In earlier chapters, I discussed the lifelong problem persons with dyslexia have with time concepts. Few of them ever develop a clear, sustained mental image of time segments and how they occur in sequence. This means that as adults they must live by visible time schedules that provide a structure they can follow. Most of these individuals will need two forms of time chart—a pocket log they carry at all times and a larger calendar on which they jot down appointments and dates. Each person gradually refines these visible time reminders to fit his or her individual style. The pocket log must show time in weekly and monthly segments. Pages are arranged so that each week is divided into days, and each day is divided into hours. Space is provided to write appointments for each hour of each day. The adult who is dyslexic then learns to follow this guide.

Most individuals will develop their own "shorthand" symbols or codes for writing essential information. These personal codes are their lifelines, keeping them anchored in the stream of events as they move through time. Without this daily log, adults with dyslexia forget appointments, overlook important family events, and miss opportunities. At home or on the job, individuals who have dyslexia keep a calendar that shows long-range obligations such as birthdays, future appointments, and deadlines. The importance of training children to use these time-awareness procedures cannot be emphasized enough. When they are prepared to keep track of time, they have taken the first step toward becoming independent. It is a tragic mistake for adults to allow young people with dyslexia to drift into adulthood without this kind of careful preparation.

Living Skills

No person—with or without dyslexia—can become independent until he or she knows how to do such basic chores as simple housekeeping, cooking, laundry, and shopping. Parents must use the developmental years of childhood and adolescence to teach young people to live alone some day. If reading ability is too limited to permit them to cook from a recipe, adolescents with severe dyslexia can learn to prepare nutritious meals in a microwave oven. Parents should spend the high school years training teenagers with dyslexia to shop for food items that can be prepared without needing a recipe. Junk food items must be avoided and balanced eating habits established. The variety of foods available today allows for quick and simple microwave cooking. Potatoes can be baked in a few minutes, fresh vegetables can be steamed, and even eggs can be prepared, using certain utensils. A teen should not become an adult who knows only how to pop corn or warm up a frozen prepackaged dinner. Being independent means knowing how to prepare nutritious meals even when reading skills are limited.

It is equally essential that persons with dyslexia know how to keep house well enough to avoid living in squalor. All young people should be taught to make a bed, do laundry, clean up the apartment once a week, do dishes or use the dishwasher, and clean the bathroom occasionally. They must be able to invite friends over without being ashamed of their place. Becoming independent in personal affairs instills an important sense of pride in young people who have dyslexia. Keeping house adequately is as important as earning a living or finishing an education. Their self-esteem is greatly enhanced when they can keep their own place without needing help.

Managing Money

Probably the most difficult task for youngsters with dyslexia to learn is how to manage money. Individuals with poor arithmetic skills often struggle with the addition and subtraction involved in writing checks and keeping a checking account untangled. At times, these persons need help with their bookkeeping, but they must learn how to handle money for themselves. This process should begin by the early teen years.

Wise parents open a checking account for the child with dyslexia when he or she is 14 or 15. The teenager is paid a certain monthly "salary" that includes school lunches, fees for classes, a certain amount for clothing, and any other fixed expenses. The parent develops a simple budget showing what must be spent, when it must be spent, and how much money will be left after all bills are paid. The ideal system shows the youth how to write checks for school lunches, clothing, and any other purchase where a check is appropriate. The parent supervises this procedure, helping the teen learn to write a check successfully. The youth should not be expected to balance the checkbook alone. When the bank statement arrives each month, he or she watches while a parent reconciles the account. If the teen takes a part-time job, those earnings are deposited in the checking account, as well as in a savings account, if that is appropriate. The point is to guide youngsters with dyslexia step-by-step as they handle their own money. Over a period of several years, the teenager learns how to be independent in this area. The parents no longer have to do all of the work or make all of the decisions. If the child is also immature and impulsive, this self-control system is ideal for teaching the results of impulsive behavior by showing what happens when the account is overdrawn or when lunch money is spent for something else. The teen is responsible, not the adult. This kind of planning prepares the young person with dyslexia to step out into the adult world ready to handle simple money management.

Holding a Job

It is almost too late if a young person with dyslexia has not done some kind of work until after high school. Holding a job involves far more than earning money or putting in a certain number of hours during the week. It requires a certain level of social skill, including the ability to get along with co-workers, to follow instructions, and to please a boss. Many teens with dyslexia must learn these skills over a period of time, beginning in the early teen years or even before. If a child with dyslexia also demonstrates immaturity, social disabilities, or Dyslogic syndrome, it will be very difficult for him or her to master job skills. Youngsters who display obvious immaturity or oppositional attitudes may not be employable if they cannot fit into a job situation successfully.

As soon as a youth with dyslexia is capable of carrying out job responsibilities, he or she should begin part-time work. This usually requires a great deal of patient help from parents. Occasionally these youngsters are self-assured enough to find jobs on their own, but often parents need to walk them through the steps of locating possible jobs, interviewing with the employer, filling out necessary forms, and having dependable transportation. Parents must be willing to be available to these new workers, talking things over to make sure they are handling the job expectations well enough and helping them interpret workplace situations accurately. Occasionally they must step in as advocates if they realize that dyslexia has caused the child to misperceive something important. It is essential to give teens this kind of sheltered experience rather than assuming that they should wait until they are older to begin the work process. The sooner they enter the world of working and earning wages, the better prepared they will be to become independent as they finish school.

Dealing with Problems

Parents and teachers often do not realize that young people with dyslexia need a great deal of coaching over a long period of time in how to handle conflict effectively. More mature individuals work out their own ways of resolving conflict without needing outside help, but many do not. Fear is a major factor in the way a person with dyslexia faces an adversary or deals with a situation where he or she would rather not stay. Every worker will meet someone on the job who makes life miserable. The easy way out is to quit. Young people with dyslexia who feel a lot of fear must learn how to cope with those feelings without running away or giving up. Parents do not always know from the surface behavior what is bothering their child. What appears to be anger may actually be fear. What appears to be "leave me alone" behavior may actually be gnawing fear that the individual does not know how to express. He or she may be overwhelmed by humiliation and unable to express it in words or may feel too intimidated or threatened by a bully to say anything at all. Parents must be alert for signs of drawing back or wanting to quit.

Adults must be patient, not critical, until the issues are out in the open. Teens with dyslexia must learn to work through these issues while they still live at home. Waiting until adulthood to do so may be too late. It is impossible to become independent if one cannot handle conflict or deal with problems without help.

Chapter 7

Adults Who Have
Overcome Dyslexia

As shown in earlier chapters, not all persons with
dyslexia are able to overcome their problems and
become successful. Many are too scarred by childhood experiences to have the necessary courage or inner
strength to overcome their disabilities. For many, life circumstances overwhelm their ambitions, crushing hopes and
dreams. Yet many who are dyslexic do break through the
barriers that block their way. As they pass through their
teens and enter early adulthood, they find ways to compensate, bypass their learning disabilities, and achieve victories
that may have seemed impossible in early years. How does
someone overcome such a deep-seated, life-saturating condition? Why do certain individuals emerge from years of
struggle and near failure as happy creative adults while
classmates and peers with the same kind of disability do
not? We have examples of intriguing success stories told by
victorious adults as they reflect on hurdles they have
crossed—stories that are greatly encouraging to reflect on.
In Chapter 5, I described the experiences of Jay, the emotionally scarred man with LD who had no stories to tell. It is
only appropriate to counter this with some exciting victory
stories from adults who overcame their language disabilities
in remarkable ways.

A strong controversy exists among professionals as to
whether we may discuss learning disability, dyslexia, or dys-
functional language development in historical figures. Issues

of the *Journal of Learning Disabilities* have reflected the wide differences of opinion surrounding this issue. Volume 4, Number 1 (January 1971, pp. 34–45) presented a forthright article by Lloyd J. Thompson, MD, from Chapel Hill, North Carolina, entitled "Language Disabilities in Men of Eminence." Thompson discussed the findings of his research concerning handwritten documents, diaries, publications, and personal interviews of relatives of such historical persons as Thomas Edison, Harvey Cushing, Woodrow Wilson, Auguste Rodin, and Albert Einstein. Thompson presented his theories regarding what causes dyslexia, to which he attributed the language disabilities of most of his men of eminence.

A few years later, Volume 20, Number 5 (May, 1982, pp. 270–279) of the *Journal of Learning Disabilities* presented an article by Kimberly A. Adelman and Howard S. Adelman. These specialists in learning disability refuted Thompson's earlier opinions on the basis that he did not have clear-cut clinical evidence of dyslexia in his subjects. As these publications show, equally thoughtful points of view exist on both sides of this issue. Regardless of whether the posthumous labels of dyslexia or language disability are applied, there is clear evidence of struggle with language skills in the lives of such persons. It is helpful to see how persons of historical significance overcame their language-processing disabilities enough to achieve success.

THOMAS ALVA EDISON

Like many individuals with dyslexia through the years, Thomas A. Edison barely survived the first years of childhood. His mother, Nancy Edison, was 37 when he was born. She had already lost three children through miscarriage, and she was determined that this last child should survive. He was somewhat deformed at birth, with an overly large head, and his early motor and language skills were very slow to emerge. Physicians of that day advised his parents that the child had suffered from "brain fever" and would always be an "invalid." It is recorded that relatives, friends, neighbors, and professionals of that day advised Nancy Edison to "put him away" and not to hope that he would ever be "normal." When Edison was sent to school, he was diagnosed as "mentally ill" because he could not do the academic work expected at that time. Mrs. Edison became enraged over that diagnosis. She withdrew her struggling son from school and vowed to teach him at home by herself. When Edison was 7, he contracted scarlet fever, which set into motion the gradual deafness that destroyed his hearing by early adulthood.

During Edison's childhood, adults labeled him as "backward" and "addled." He strongly resented such labels, and he turned to his mother as his main source for knowledge. Mrs. Edison, who was a former teacher, developed ways to help her son learn. Mr. Edison became strongly disappointed in his "retarded son" and refused to pay for extra things, so mother and son were on their own to devise an educational program the best they could. From time to time, Edison returned to public school, but he could never fit into a classroom structure. In his later years he wrote, "I remember I used never to be able to get along in school. I was always at the foot of the class. . . . My father thought that I was stupid, and I almost decided that I was a dunce" (cited in Thompson, 1971).

Throughout his developmental years, Edison listened as his mother read to him. Through listening he absorbed great quantities of literature, history, science, philosophy, the Bible, and whatever else Mrs. Edison could supply. This home-school education nurtured the boy's hunger for knowledge, but he did not develop traditional literacy skills. In his biography of Edison, Josephson described the boy's literacy skills as follows: "Her son never learned how to spell; up to the time of his manhood his grammar and syntax were appalling. We see that he was hard to teach. Whatever he learned, he learned in his own way. In fact, though his mother inspired him, no one ever taught him anything; he taught himself" (Josephson, 1959).

At age 19, Edison wrote a letter to his mother:

Dear Mother. Started the Store several weeks. I have growed considerably I don't look much like a Boy now- How all the folk did you receive a Box of Books from Memphis that he promised to send them-languages. You son Al. (cited in Jordan, 1989b).

Edison kept a diary for most of his adult life. As he grew older, he developed a simple writing style that allowed him to express his thoughts clearly, but he always used simple words and short sentences. He avoided words that he could not spell.

At age 67, Edison wrote an essay that revealed his deep, often bitter feelings toward public education:

> I am frequently asked about our system of education. I say that we have none. Our system is a relic of the past. It consists of parrot-like repetitions. It is a dull study of twenty-six hieroglyphs. Groups of hieroglyphs. That is what the young of this present day study. Here is an object. I place it in the hands of a child. I tell him to look at it . . . . Why should we make him take impressions of things through the ear when he may be able to see? . . . It is of the utmost importance that every faculty should meet the environment. What is the use of crowding the mind with facts which cannot be utilized by the child because the method of their acquisition is distasteful to him?
>
> I like the Montessori method. It teaches through play. It makes learning a pleasure. . . . That system of education will succeed which shows to those who learn the actual thing—not the ghost of it. I firmly believe that the motion picture is destined to bear an important part in the education of the future. (cited in Jordan, 1989b)

The fertile mind of Thomas Alva Edison, which gave the world so many life-changing inventions, realized the value of multisensory learning for children. He had achieved his knowledge by developing multisensory techniques and strategies that allowed him to connect several sensory pathways at the same time. He realized that rote memory was not the best way to teach children, especially those who struggled with the traditional method of silent learning.

Edison's writing displays numerous signs of dyslexia. What was the key to his success? Early in his life, he became angry, and his anger became the primary drive that allowed him to conquer his language disabilities. Edison's intuitive mother was able to channel that anger in productive ways so that her son did not waste his potential just being angry. He learned to move ahead in spite of being rejected by his father and being hideously labeled by his school. For Edison, anger turned the right way was the key to future success. In his later years, he no longer needed that anger to drive him forward, but it was the essential ingredient that kept him moving ahead during his difficult formative years.

GEORGE S. PATTON IV

George S. Patton IV, the famous general of World War II, had a most unusual childhood. His father was a strong, domineering man who reared the family in isolation on a ranch. The Patton children were forbidden to mix with other youngsters, and they did not attend school until their teen years. George Patton III strongly believed in the oral learning tradition. He thought that no child should learn to read until after age 12. The Patton children were immersed in oral reading. Adults in the family took turns reading aloud from the classics and the Bible. George S. Patton IV spent his first 12 years in this isolated environment, absorbing oral literature the way he breathed air. He had an extraordinary memory for what he heard. After hearing an adult read or deliver a speech, he could recite it almost word by word without ever having seen the printed text. Patton developed a grand style of oratory, strutting about the ranch shouting long poems and literary passages by the hour. He brought great pride to his father, who probably had a reading disability himself and therefore had no regard for traditional literacy skills. By his 12th birthday, Patton had the literary education of an adult, all of which was learned orally.

At age 12, Patton was sent to a private school designed to prepare him to enter the U.S. Military Academy at West Point. At that time he could not read—he was an authority on world literature and he could write in a unique script, but he *could not read.* Entering the private preparatory school was a deep shock to his self-esteem because suddenly he was transplanted from a home environment where he was adored as a "genius" to a school environment where he was regarded as ignorant. He compensated by getting information from classmates and quickly placing himself in the good favor of his instructors by keeping every rule better than anyone else. In the prep school, and later at West Point, Patton astonished his peers and leaders by his remarkable auditory memory. He could hear a lecture or sermon once, then repeat it verbatim days later.

Patton never became a fluent reader, so he compensated through his oral retention skills. He developed irritating show-off habits of overwhelming his critics by his phenomenal memory. He was an avid student of the Bible, military history, poetry, and certain areas of literature, but his reading was always slow and labored. When he commanded armies during World War II, he was often seen alone, laboriously working through the Bible or some other reading material by muttering it aloud to himself as he slowly sounded out the words.

How did this brilliant man who apparently had dyslexia succeed? Critics have been harsh in describing Patton's arrogance and often haughty behavior. His enemies delighted in reminding the world of his famous outbursts of temper, as when he slapped a young soldier across the face for refusing to join the front lines in combat. Those who regarded Patton as a friend, however, recognized that he had an extraordinary drive to succeed. He was a proud man who strongly held to certain principles. He had an abiding religious faith, which he was not ashamed to proclaim. He never resolved certain hostile feelings toward military leaders who made his life difficult, and he had a constant need to prove that he was as good or better than anyone else. Pride, ambition, and a brilliant capacity to absorb what he heard gave Patton the ability to overcome the language-processing difficulties that embarrassed him so deeply during his adolescent years.

WOODROW WILSON

It seems incredible that a person with language disabilities could become president of a prestigious university, and then president of the United States, but that is the story of Woodrow Wilson. At the beginning of the 20th century, Wilson was president of Princeton University. This man who had been a child during the Civil War, was elected president of the United States in time to guide the country through World War I.

Like so many others with dyslexic-like patterns, Wilson had been taught at home during his early school years. There he listened to many hours of oral reading from the Bible and classical literature, but he did not learn the alphabet until age 9 and did not learn to read until age 11. He never did well in school. Those who have researched his life report that he was always considered to be a "mediocre student." He tried to avoid subjects that required abstract reading, excelling instead as a public speaker and in student debates. During his early adult years, he became known as an orator.

Tommy, as Wilson was called by his family, was ill much of his life. As a result, he did not finish high school, and his college studies often were interrupted. He became fatally ill toward the end of his term in office as U.S. president. This lifelong illness, along with his language-processing problems, often forced him to drop out of school or change his plans. A major influence during childhood that enabled him to deal with these enormous problems was his father, who was a minister. The Reverend Wilson spent long hours reading Scripture to his son, discussing doctrine, and helping him develop a deep sense of right and wrong. As an adult, Wilson carried this spiritual attitude into his career. He exhausted himself working for world peace and was a major force behind the creation of the League of Nations following World War I. In fact, he no doubt shortened his life as he pressed for his ideals of peace and world brotherhood. Wilson always needed help to express his ideas in writing. His outstanding speaking skills masked the underlying struggle he always had with reading and spelling.

What was the secret of this man's success? There is no evidence that Wilson was angry or that he sought to vindicate himself before his critics. His motivation came from those deeply held spiritual values his father had helped instill. He overcame his language handicaps and poor health in order to make the world a better, more peaceful place for future generations.

ALBERT EINSTEIN

Of all the famous people within the last century, perhaps it is most surprising to find that Albert Einstein was considered to have a language disability. His son, Albert Einstein, Jr., gave a thoughtful summary of his famous father's early years: "He was even considered backward by his teachers. He told me that his teachers reported to his father that he was mentally slow, unsociable, and adrift forever in his foolish dreams" (cited in Thompson, 1971). During his early years, Einstein had very poor speech, developing far behind the usual schedule in this area. His parents feared that this late-developing child was "dull." At one point, the boy was dismissed from school and called a "dunce" by exasperated teachers. His speech was always slow and labored, which caused him to appear shy. In his later years as a faculty member at Princeton University, Einstein spoke softly and was difficult to understand. In fact, he lost three teaching positions early in his career because he could not communicate adequately during lectures.

At age 12, Einstein could barely read, and his speech was awkward and difficult to understand. Yet his brilliance began to emerge in his mastery of mathematics and physics, although he struggled to verbalize his astonishing mathematical concepts. His writings of that time are filled with poor spelling and dysgraphic patterns. His language skills were always poor, even while his skills in higher math soared beyond the understanding of all but a few of the world's scholars.

All his life, Einstein remained a private, very shy man who occasionally blossomed in a public way. He appeared in commercial advertisements during his tenure as professor at Princeton University, and his unique personal appearance became known worldwide.

How could such a shy, sensitive, language disabled man succeed? Einstein had to absorb enormous insults during the first third of his life. This gentle, compassionate person had no way to hold his own in a competitive world in which success was measured by how well one could "defend his own territory." This meek, soft-spoken individual saw within himself the ability to contribute new knowledge to the world, knowledge that would revolutionize civilization, but never let people know the emotional pain he endured before his intelligence was finally recognized. Einstein succeeded in spite of language disabilities because he had a new dream, one that he strongly believed had to be recognized by the critical world in which he lived. There was no anger or driving ambition behind this man's success—just enormous strength that gave him the ability to absorb insult and keep on trying until he finally caught the attention of others.

NELSON A. ROCKEFELLER

One of the most powerful political figures of the middle 1900s had severe dyslexia. Nelson Rockefeller was governor of New York for four terms, then was appointed vice president of the United States. He was a philanthropist who gave millions of dollars to improve the quality of life for people around the world. This talented, important man had a reading disability that was so severe he could not read speeches on television. In fact, he employed full-time assistants to be with him at all times to help him cope with language situations made difficult by his disability. In 1976, Rockefeller published a brief biography to promote a nationally televised program about dyslexia. His own words are the best way to understand how this courageous man finally won success:

> Those watching the Public Broadcasting Service program on "The Puzzle Children" [October 19, 1976] will include a very interested Vice President of the United States. For I was one of the "puzzle children" myself—a dyslexic, or "reverse reader"—and I still have a hard time reading today. But after coping with this problem for more than 60 years, I have a message of encouragement for children with learning disabilities and their parents. Based upon my own experience, my message to dyslexic children is this:
>
> - Don't accept anyone's verdict that you are lazy, stupid, or retarded. You may very well be smarter than most other children your age.

- Just remember that Woodrow Wilson, Albert Einstein, and Leonardo da Vinci also had tough problems with their reading.

- You can learn to cope with your problem and turn your so-called disability into a positive advantage. Dyslexia forced me to develop powers of concentration that have been invaluable throughout my career in business, philanthropy, and public life. And I've done an enormous amount of public speaking, especially in political campaigns for Governor of New York and President of the United States.

No one ever heard of dyslexia when I discovered as a boy, along about the third grade, that reading was such a difficult chore that I was in the bottom one-third of my class. None of the educational, medical, and psychological help available today for dyslexics was available in those days. We had no special teachers or tutors, no special classes or courses, no special methods of teaching—because nobody understood our problem. Along with an estimated 3 million other children, I just struggled to understand words that seemed to garble before my eyes, numbers that came out backwards, and sentences that were hard to grasp.

And so I accepted the verdict of the IQ tests that I wasn't as bright as most of the rest of my class. Fortunately for me, the school (though it never taught me to spell) was an experimental, progressive institution with the flexibility to let you develop your own interests and follow them. I had a wise and understanding counselor (Dr. Otis W. Caldwell). "Don't worry," he said, "just because you're in the lower third of the class. You've got the intelligence. If you just work harder and concentrate more, you can make it." So I learned through self-discipline to concentrate, which in my opinion is essential for a dyslexic. While I could speak French better than the teacher, because I'd learned it as a child, I couldn't conjugate the verbs. I did flunk Spanish—but now I can speak it fluently because I learned it by ear. My best subject was mathematics. I understood the concepts well beyond my grade level. But it took only one reversed number in a column of figures to cause havoc.

When I came close to flunking out in the ninth grade— because I didn't work very hard that year—I decided that I had better follow Dr. Caldwell's advice if I wanted to go to college. I even told my high school girl friend that we would have to stop dating so I could spend the time studying in order to get into Dartmouth College. And I made it by the skin of my teeth. I made it simply by working harder and longer than the rest—eventually learning to concentrate sufficiently to compensate for my dyslexia in reading. I adopted a regimen of getting up at 5 A.M. to study, and studying without fail. And thanks to my concentration and the very competitive nature I was born with, I found my academic performance gradually improving. In my freshman year at Dartmouth, I was even admitted to a third-year physics course. And in the middle of my sophomore year, I received two A's and three B's for the first semester. My father's letters were filled with joy and astonishment.

I owe a great debt to my professors. Most of all, however, I think I owe my academic improvement to my roommate, Johnny French. Johnny and I were exact opposites. He was reticent and had the highest IQ in the class. To me, he was that maddening type who got straight A's with only occasional reference to books or classes. He was absolutely disgusted with my study habits— anybody who got up at 5 in the morning to hit the books was, well, peculiar. Inevitably, Johnny made Phi Beta Kappa in our junior year, but my competitive instincts kept me going. We were both elected to senior fellowships and I made Phi Beta Kappa in my senior year. Johnny, of course, had the last word. He announced that he would never wear his PBK key again—that it had lost all meaning.

Looking back over the years, I remember vividly the pain and mortification I felt as a boy of 8 when I was assigned to read a short passage of Scripture at a vesper service—and did a thoroughly miserable job of it. I know what a dyslexic child goes through—the frustration of not being able to do what other children do easily, the humiliation of being thought not too bright when such is not the case at all. My personal discoveries as to what is required to cope with dyslexia could be summarized in these admonitions to the individual dyslexic:

- Accept the fact that you have a problem. Don't just try to hide it.

- Refuse to feel sorry for yourself.

- Realize that you don't have an excuse. You have a challenge.

- Face the challenge.

- Work harder and learn mental discipline, the capacity for total concentration.

- Never quit.

If it helps a dyslexic child to know I went through the same thing . . .

- BUT I can conduct press conferences in three languages

- AND I can read a speech on television—IF I rehearse it

six times, with my script in large type, and my sentences broken into segments, and long words broken into syllables

- AND I learned to read and communicate well enough to be elected Governor of New York four times

- AND I won Congressional confirmation as Vice President of the United States

then I hope the telling of my story as a dyslexic will be an inspiration to the "puzzle children," for that is what I really care about.

(Reprinted with permission from *TV Guide Magazine*. Copyright © 1976 by Triangle Publications, Inc., Radnor, Pennsylvania.)

What was the key to Nelson Rockefeller's success in spite of having dyslexia? He was fiercely competitive. Instead of getting his feelings hurt when adults and roommates criticized him, he was determined to show them that he was just as smart as anyone else. This overachievement brought him all kinds of honors that did not seem possible for a person with his disability. Rockefeller wanted to win badly enough to sacrifice pleasure, convenience, and comfort to reach his goals. The night he died of a heart attack, he was working on a publication that would share one of his main interests with the world.

STEPHEN J. CANNELL

Not everyone has heard the name Stephen J. Cannell, but millions of people around the world have enjoyed his television programs *The Rockford Files, Hardcastle and McCormick, Riptide,* and *The A-Team.* The writer and producer of these highly successful television shows has dyslexia. Cannell remembered his struggle in getting through school. "When I was in junior high school," he recalls, "people used to say to me, 'Stephen, can't you look at that word and see it's not right?' But every time I looked at the word, it looked fine" (personal communication, March 11, 1988). There were times when this kind of pressure from teachers and friends would get him down. Sometimes he thought he could not do anything right. "Dyslexics tend to be pretty poor students," he said. "But it has nothing to do with intelligence. The biggest problem with dyslexic kids is that they get down on themselves. They can feel that they aren't smart in some ways, that they're retarded, and of course they aren't."

Cannell recalled that when he was growing up, dyslexia was still a mystery. No one understood it well enough to explain the problem to the children who had it or to parents and teachers. Cannell, however, decided to be a writer, even though he could not spell well or write without mistakes. In order to accomplish his goal, he developed strict habits for studying. He was up early every morning, not allowing himself to sleep late or to put off the task of getting to his work. In college he did a lot of writing. He recalled that his professors would say, "Stephen, your writing is very interesting," but they would give him Fs because of poor spelling. Still, he knew that his ideas were good enough to put on paper. He developed a method for enrolling in college courses—he would ask each instructor what that person's policy was regarding misspellings. In this way he found professors who would overlook poor spelling and give him credit for the value of his ideas and concepts. One instructor became intrigued with Cannell's vivid storytelling ability and taught him how to express his ideas in clear writing. This polished his visual imagination, which can clearly be seen in the popular television shows he has produced.

Cannell is at work by 6:00 A.M. every day, working steadily at his typewriter until 11:00 A.M. "My secretary has learned to figure out my mistakes," he explained. "What happens is that I tend to mirror-read and reverse letters. I am absolutely unaware that I am doing it. It slows me down as a reader and makes me a horrible speller because no word really looks right to me." In discussing his problems publicly, Cannell hoped that he could be a good role model for youngsters with dyslexia. "I hope they are saying, 'Gee, here's a guy who couldn't even read and now he is making a living as a successful, famous writer.'"

What was the key to Stephen Cannell's ability to overcome his dyslexia? He developed strong self-discipline and learned to write at a keyboard, letting someone else worry about correct spelling, good grammar, and accurate punctuation. He learned not to feel sorry for himself. Cannell developed an attitude that let him turn loose the worry and frustration of having dyslexia and allow his mind to soar with ideas.

PHIL TROYER

Few people have ever heard of Phil Troyer. Dyslexia almost destroyed his life before he found a source of love, acceptance, and guidance in overcoming his deep fear of failure. Troyer published a novel (*Father Bede's Misfit,* 1986), a story about his own struggles to overcome his disability. Troyer was reared in a gentle Amish home. His father was a professor of English and dean of a well-known university who considered it a weakness for men to show emotion or affection. Troyer had severe dyslexia, but his childhood problems were not diagnosed. His family had no idea why he struggled so hard yet achieved so little in academic endeavors. This deeply sensitive boy, who grew up without enough support to develop good self-esteem, vividly recalled the crushing experience he endured being laughed at by classmates because he could not read, write, or spell. His parents and teachers were unsympathetic when he turned to them for help. He therefore grew up fearing that he was "dumb" and defective. He described his teen years as "insecure, lonely, and frightening." There was no help available to relieve this deep misery.

In his early adult years, Troyer discovered a small monastery in New Mexico where he was taken in by the compassionate monks. Father Bede became especially interested in him and helped him become part of the community. At the point of emotional breakdown, Troyer began counseling with a psychiatrist, who realized what the problem was and provided a diagnosis of dyslexia. As part of his recovery therapy, Troyer began to write. Over a period of time he produced a novel that is a slightly fictionalized version of his life, telling the story of a man with dyslexia who almost did not survive. Troyer then began writing a second novel about his reconciliation with his father, who learned to express his love for his son before his death.

How did Troyer overcome dyslexia? When he was at the lowest possible level of depression and confusion, a loving counselor and mentor came into his life and became a strong friend who believed in Troyer at a time when he could not believe in himself. An unexpected demonstration of love and confidence awakened the life that had almost slipped away through despair. With the support of this man and a loving community of dedicated friends, Troyer came back to life. With guidance and therapy he was able to rebuild his lost self-esteem and discover talent and intelligence within himself.

RICHARD YaDEAU

Richard YaDeau, MD, is a surgeon in St. Paul, Minnesota, and also director of oncology at Bethesda Lutheran Medical Center in that city. In 1985, he became president of a nationwide nonprofit health maintenance organization that brings medical care to many people, and he has guided the establishment of a St. Paul hospice program where terminally ill patients may die with dignity. YaDeau has vivid memories of a dyslexic childhood although his disability was not diagnosed until much later in his life. In spite of failing grades during his first 8 years in school, he was "socially promoted" each year, entering each successive grade without the literacy skills to do the work. Then he was denied admission into high school until his father begged school administrators to give his son a chance. Later YaDeau would say, "It made me angry that school officials kept flunking me for spelling and would not listen to what I had to say." Eventually he was admitted to Yale University, where he earned his undergraduate degree. He earned his medical degree from New York Medical College and also served a successful tour of duty as an officer in the U.S. Marine Corps.

Like so many other so-called late-blooming dyslexics, YaDeau proved that he was capable of completing a complex education if officials would give him the opportunity. He will never forget how his parents were advised to enroll him in a trade school because it was believed he would never be able to handle college studies. He was allowed to finish high school only because of his parents' constant pressure on school officials. Had school teachers had their way, he would have become an academic dropout in his middle teens.

What enabled YaDeau to overcome dyslexia? It was his parents, who intervened on his behalf when no one else believed in him. Through their persistent pressure, school officials reluctantly gave him a chance, even though they were convinced it would be a waste of time. As he finished maturing during his late teens and early 20s, this late bloomer began to prove to skeptical adults that he had the potential for college success. Once he had earned his professional credentials, he proved himself worthy of his parents' trust.

JOSEF SANDERS

One of the most courageous men I have ever known is Dr. Josef Sanders. Although he has dyslexia, he founded a highly successful publishing company, Modern Education Corporation, producer of excellent educational materials for more than 20 years. Like thousands of children with dyslexia, Sanders was almost a casualty in his early years. He has told his story in the following words:

> I was LD before it was popular to be LD. I was born prematurely and weighed only 3 pounds, 2 ounces. In those days, it was tough dealing with premature babies. My development was fairly normal until it was time to begin to speak. I began to stutter at age 3 and continued stuttering until age 5. I used my left hand more than my right hand, and my parents were told to tie my left hand to my side to force me to be right-handed. My kindergarten teacher discovered that I had difficulty concentrating, and I talked a lot in class. I was never a discipline problem, but I was always restless

in structured situations. I was told to wear glasses, but I hid them under my bed because I felt ugly wearing them.

By the time I was in second grade, my learning problems were becoming obvious. I had difficulty learning to deal with symbols, both letters and numbers. My writing was very poor, and I had trouble following the teacher's directions. During second grade I realized that learning was becoming very difficult for me and that I was not catching on like my classmates. My teacher that year was frustrated with me. That was the first time I perceived myself as not being as good or as smart as other students. The teacher tied colored yarn on my wrists so I could tell the difference between right and left. I had great difficulty copying from the board. I severely reversed words (was/saw, on/no), and I had a hard time with b, d, and p. I could not write the alphabet without melody (singing the alphabet song).

By the time I entered fourth grade, I was so far behind the others the principal called my parents in for a conference. They were told that I appeared to be mentally retarded, and they were advised to place me in a special school for mentally retarded children. I will never forget coming home from school and seeing my mother crying. I asked what was wrong, and she said that the principal had told her that I needed to go to Sunshine School. My first response was that it sounded like a nice place. Sunshine School sounded pleasant and pretty. I will never forget how this caused my mother to sob. Finally she told me that Sunshine School was for mentally retarded children. She explained that my school thought I was mentally retarded and needed special education. The tone of my mother's voice struck fear into me. Suddenly I knew why she had been crying. All at once I realized that I was a different student. That moment was a major turning point in my life. I felt like a lost child with no sense of direction.

A few days later, I discovered that I was a very fortunate person. My mother became intensely angry about what the principal had said. She vowed not to send me to that school for retarded children. She declared that she would work with me herself every day until I could read, write, spell, and do math like other kids my age. This was an awful, painful period for me and my family.

As I struggled with my learning disabilities, I learned to escape from school frustration by playing by myself and using my imagination. I would create my own toys. My parents had very little money, and they could not buy things for me. So I created my own playthings. I learned to be grateful for being able to create things for myself. If I had the choice of playing or studying with my mother, I naturally chose to play outdoors. I did not like school and could not concentrate longer than a few minutes at a time. Half an hour of study with my mother was like an overweight 50-year-old man trying to run the Boston Marathon. It was difficult and very painful. My mind would wander, and I would cause my mother to become so frustrated. I just wanted to get out of the kitchen and play outdoors. Mother made me read aloud to her every day, and I hated it. Reading aloud is still a traumatic experience for me. I had so much trouble reading aloud in class or with my mother, I developed psychosomatic illnesses. The thought of reading aloud made me want to die. I could not breathe. My heart made palpitations. I was overwhelmed by extreme fear. My eyes could not track along the lines of the page. I stuttered and sounded like a little child just learning to read in first grade. I hated those times in reading circle or with my mother when I had to read aloud because my disability was always "found out." I sounded so dumb! To this day, all of those old feelings come back if I am asked to read aloud in public. Recently I turned down a prestigious part in a worship service at my synagogue because of this old phobia toward oral reading. (personal communication, 1988)

Sanders struggled through high school, finally earning his diploma. He then joined the military service, where he began to discover new skills within himself. Like most low-birthweight boys, he was very late reaching important developmental milestones. Sanders is a classic example of a late bloomer who began to blossom during his early 20s. Eventually Sanders earned a bachelor's degree, a doctorate in educational psychology, and his credentials as a speech pathologist. He worked for several years as a highly successful speech therapist, then entered private practice, working with frustrated youngsters who were struggling with learning disabilities. In the 1960s he founded Modern Education Corporation and began to market helpful materials for the field of special education.

What gave Sanders the ability to overcome dyslexia? It was his unquenchable courage. No matter how difficult his life became through the pain of chronic arthritis, the frustration of having dyslexia, and the anxiety of surviving the uncertain economics of private practice and running a business, he never gave up. His deep religious orientation has given him a sense of purpose—he believes he is on this earth for a reason and that he will receive the strength he needs to function day to day. Sanders's courage has enabled him to overcome dyslexia.

HOW DO PERSONS WITH DYSLEXIA ACHIEVE SUCCESS?

These just-described examples of achievement by intelligent individuals with dyslexia contain important wisdom for those who struggle with learning disabilities. What does it take to cope successfully with the hidden disability called dyslexia? As we have seen in these brief glimpses into the lives of past and present persons with dyslexia, certain factors must exist to enable frightened, frustrated, and often overwhelmed individuals come to grips with their language problems. The following characteristics seem to be necessary to allow dyslexic strugglers to overcome their disabilities.

Anger

The role of anger in overcoming dyslexia must be understood carefully. Of itself, anger is usually a destructive force that distorts reality and blocks the person's ability to deal with issues clearly. To be angry is to be deeply upset; to feel anger is to have adrenaline pour into the bloodstream to trigger the body's defenses against danger. To feel hot anger is to see an enemy who must be attacked and conquered. Anger is an explosion of the emotions that usually destroys objective thinking and distorts the intentions of others. To stay angry very long triggers a cascade of destructive forces within one's body and personality. As a rule, therefore, it is wise to avoid becoming angry.

The kind of anger that actually helps individuals with dyslexia overcome their disabilities takes the form of righteous indignation. For example, being indignant over injustice can be a constructive emotion. Indignation played a powerful role in Edison's eventual victory. He would not accept the verdict that he was defective, retarded, or unworthy. His pride was wounded by his treatment by the schools of his day, and he vowed never to submit to that form of deprivation. Within Edison the young man was a burning indignation that smoldered like a carefully banked fire. He was angry at being treated in such a thoughtless fashion, and he simply would not permit it. This simmering resentment over the injustice of being wrongly labeled was the driving force that gave Edison the power to compensate for and eventually overcome the disabling effects of dyslexia. Although his writing always contained poor spelling and limited language expression, he honed his skills to prove to the world that he was worthy of respect and admiration. Without this fire of anger, Edison the right-brain genius would never have emerged, and the world would have lost his vital contributions.

Fortunately, Edison had the devoted support of a mother who believed in him and pledged with him to beat the odds. She molded his anger into a constructive force, helping him find strategies of success. With her assistance, Edison learned how to channel his anger and not waste his strength in useless battles against events and attitudes he could not change.

Edison's first motivation was to prove himself to a critical, skeptical world that did not care whether he lived or died. Unfortunately, many persons with dyslexia are taught to believe themselves to be undesirable and unattractive. Edison, for example, was rejected by his own father and pushed from the educational system of his day. He experienced failure at numerous jobs during his early years, but he learned how to turn his hostility into a strength. Constructive anger is essential for many individuals who are dyslexic. This kind of anger is often described by these persons as a motivating force for success. Those who overcome this disability do not allow their anger to make them overly bitter or resentful. Instead, they gain wisdom to reflect on early struggles with the eye of the philosopher—an angry one, to be sure, but not a bitter one. The *right form* of anger can help open the door to success for individuals with and without dyslexia.

Pride

Like anger, pride often is the downfall of those who feel its intoxicating power. In its usual form, pride does indeed make tyrants and arrogant braggarts of us all. Raw pride is an ugly force that steps all over others and brags of its own worth. Unrefined pride struts and postures and claims rights it does not deserve to have. In most religions, basic human pride is regarded as sin, an emotion to be avoided, not cultivated among our children. Pride is the root of all sorts of difficulties in human relationships, perhaps because a proud person seldom is attractive. Of itself, pride is to be avoided and brought under control.

Yet pride can be the key to success for many persons with dyslexia. For example, Patton overcame his disabilities through pride, even though he was not fully successful in taking the raw edge off that characteristic. History records many moments when he behaved in an arrogant fashion that disappointed his friends and created embarrassment for himself. However, Patton survived his reading disability exactly because of that strong confidence in himself. When pride takes the form of self-confidence, it energizes the person to keep on trying. Pride must exist *to a certain degree* before a healthy self-image can evolve. Being sure of one's own worth is vital if any kind of victory over adversity is to be achieved. This is especially true for individuals with dyslexia.

Often underlying the stories of successful persons with dyslexia is the quiet theme of pride. Conquering a language disability must involve a certain degree of pride because the struggling reader, speller, or writer must feel worthy of learning in order to do difficult work better. Overcoming the disabling aspects of dyslexia requires pride *in its positive form.* In Chapter 6, the unfortunate effects of arrogance and self-centeredness were displayed in Joe's pathetic story. Joe's kind of pride cannot help the person with dyslexia break free. But a quiet, calm, low-key pride continually reassures the person: "I am worthy of success. I am worth what it costs to overcome this present condition. I have a worthwhile contribution to make in the years ahead. I am valuable. I am intelligent. I deserve an opportunity to prove myself."

Faith

Having faith is such a simple thing, yet it does not always exist in the individuals who surround children with dyslexia. Several of the success stories in this chapter have included the element of faith: A mother believed in her child when other relatives did not, parents believed when school leaders did not, the person with dyslexia believed, even when everyone else did not. Struggling people believed beyond doubt in a Creator who had a purpose for their lives. Faith could be considered the most "blind" of all human emotions, for it knows even when there is nothing tangible to see or to provide a foundation for knowing. Faith is the most optimistic of all of our attitudes because it insists that substance exists where only emptiness appears. Faith is based on hope, and hope believes far beyond facts and solid data. Faith says that this struggling child is not mentally retarded even when all the standard test scores indicate otherwise. Faith looks beneath the surface of life and sees undeveloped potential that cannot be seen by casual observers. It could be compared to the person who, when all others see random bits and pieces, immediately perceives a finished mosaic. Critics see only useless fragments that should be swept away. Faith looks at a child with disabilities and sees beauty in the soul and strength in the unbloomed intelligence. Faith does not give up when leadership wants to end the relationship and send the struggler away.

Faith, that invisible, rather foolish, unscientific, often irrational force is absolutely critical if persons with disabilities are to overcome their struggles. Those of us who build our relationships upon faith continually hear suffering people say, "I could not have made it without you. You are the only person who still believes in me." We who do intervention counseling with individuals on the verge of suicide often hear, "You are the only reason I am still alive. If it weren't for you, I would not be alive today." It is impossible for a child to survive the earlier years of dyslexic struggle without someone's faith. Someone must be able to see beyond test scores or classroom behavior and recognize the potential that can be developed with patient care. That person must teach the struggling child that he or she is worthy of being loved, that he or she has value and why that value must be preserved for the future. Without hope, there is no reason to endure the endless challenges that must be overcome if individuals with dyslexia are to succeed.

Inner Strength

Persons who overcome their disabilities have an inner strength that does not always display itself on the surface. The stories about Wilson and Einstein tell of two men with language disabilities who at first seemed too weak to overcome their handicaps. They did not have the blustering self-confidence of Patton or the fiery anger of Edison. However, as their lives slowly developed, those two men demonstrated enormous inner strength that allowed them to overcome their language disabilities. Wilson was able to become a successful speaker who could convince world audiences of the merit of his concepts of peace. Einstein did not learn to speak or write fluently, but he manifested a relentless spirit that produced the revolutionary formula $E = MC^2$, which changed the course of human life forever. Individuals who overcome dyslexia must have an inner strength that is as tough as an old oak tree whose roots anchor it firmly against hurricanes and tornadoes. These quiet ones must absorb insult without breaking apart and must bend with the force of the "explosions" around them, then come back to a standing position still upright and intact. Overcoming life's extra challenges involves having an inner structure as tough as iron.

The quality of inner strength includes the ability to absorb enormous insult without retaliating. The teachings of Jesus include the fascinating concept of going the extra mile, doing more than is required, and surprising the adversary by unexpected acts of kindness. Adults with dyslexia often need this quality, this capacity to stand still in the face of powerful forces, to know not to fight every battle that comes along. A certain degree of meekness—that ability to turn the other cheek in the face of confrontation—is required at times. In their quest to overcome their disabilities, persons with dyslexia must control the urge to gain revenge. If they react to conflict on that level, they will be unable to overcome their limitations successfully.

Competitive Spirit

As was seen in the stories of Einstein and Wilson, not all individuals with dyslexia succeed through competition. Dr. Josef Sanders did not need to defeat his critics in order to climb to the top of his profession. On the other hand, individuals such as Rockefeller did find their victory through competition. For them, the urge to compete is the key to opening up the future. There is a heady quality in competition that triggers an adrenaline flow that kicks the person's skills into overdrive. Those who have such a spirit are lost when there is no challenge. They need a clearly defined adversary to overcome.

This spirit of competition can easily get out of control, of course. We all recoil from fiercely competitive people who thrive on challenge. Overly aggressive persons who live for competition are very uncomfortable to be with. Like prancing, high-spirited colts in a stockade, it is not safe to be in their presence. But the competitive spirit that enables adults with dyslexia to overcome problems is a more disciplined attitude that does not involve an intent to hurt or deprive others while achieving one's goals.

For competitive adults such as Rockefeller, the key difference is an underlying theme of thoughtfulness and concern for others. In Chapter 6, the unfortunate pattern called social disability was discussed. This includes self-centeredness, a universally unpleasant characteristic. The competitive spirit described in Rockefeller's account is a compassionate attitude, not an aggressive desire to dominate. Persons like Rockefeller need the challenge of someone such as his roommate, Johnny. The spirit of competition cannot see itself except by looking into the mirror of challenge. Once competitiveness sees its counterpart in the mirror, it is able to focus energy toward specific, well-defined goals. Without this focus through challenge, individuals with dyslexia do not have a clear enough vision to know how to move ahead successfully. As we have seen, certain individuals such as Albert Einstein are able to see themselves clearly without standing before the mirror of challenge. If so, then the spirit of competition is not part of their way to success. However, the competitive spirit may be essential for certain people who cannot define themselves any other way.

Self-Discipline

Every person with dyslexia needs to be self-disciplined. This characteristic is the glue that holds all the other ingredients of success together. Each person must learn how to say no to things that would distract them from their main goals. Everyone who succeeds must be able to start early, as Rockefeller and Cannell explained, instead of taking it easy. Those individuals with dyslexia who do succeed must be able to ignore pain, inconvenience, disappointment, frustration, depression, and all of the other voices that clamor for attention. Being self-disciplined means being able to make one's own plans, manage one's own time, meet one's own obligations on schedule, control desires that would eat up scarce resources, and so forth.

Cultivating self-discipline is probably the least appealing activity anyone is asked to do. If human characteristics were given colors, self-discipline would probably be dull gray. Staying in control of self is a parental role. One cannot romp as a carefree youngster and be self-disciplined. One cannot always take second helpings or have rich desserts or satisfy strong cravings the moment they arise. Self-discipline is like a parent having to say no to a clamoring child. Staying in charge of oneself is not always a pleasant activity. When everyone else is goofing off or out at the lake or on a holiday, self-discipline sternly says, "No, you have to stay home and work." Everyone gets tired of doing one's duty. Everyone wants to take a break at some point. The self-disciplined person must do duty and keep on with chores until important things are accomplished.

As Rockefeller so fluently explained, self-discipline is the structure that holds the dyslexic pieces in place. When the loose pieces of dyslexia are carefully organized into a solid mosaic, self-discipline is the glue that makes the picture stay together. Persons with dyslexia who fail are those who never develop the structure of self-discipline. They go through life with too many pieces missing from their mosaic. Those who overcome are the ones who learn how to say no when the inner self clamors for satisfaction.

Loving Support

No one has yet researched the effect of love upon the lives of individuals with disabilities, but it does not require validated studies to know that love is an essential element. Troyer's story brings this quickly to mind. As was described in Chapter 5, love definitely was missing from the life of Shane, the boy who was so defeated by guilt. Through the years, I have known many individuals with dyslexia who did not receive enough loving support to sustain them. Professionals who counsel persons struggling with this disability continually deal with torn emotions that destroy self-esteem because the person has no one to turn to for love and reassurance. Every success story is about loving support from some important source. I am always shocked to hear a sorrowing person with dyslexia say, "You are the only one who still loves me after the mess I've made of everything." When loving support is taken away by those who lose faith, there may be nothing left upon which the person with the disability can depend. Many attempts at suicide are triggered when the struggling person realizes that no one cares.

Loving support is always evident in the "victory stories" of individuals with dyslexia. As a rule, this support comes more from mothers than from fathers. I have seen many grandparents or an aunt or uncle assume this role also. Youngsters continually find loving support within their extended families of religious leaders, scout leaders, coaches, and teachers. Teenagers with dyslexia often form their own support groups, finding among their peers the non-judgmental acceptance they cannot find elsewhere. I frequently discover caring support behind prison walls where we least expect to find it. One often sees a bond of loving support within military units where men or women live in close quarters. It is impossible to overcome dyslexia if one is all alone.

As was seen in several of the stories in this chapter, the presence of loving support was a healing agent for an embattled child. To spend a day struggling through school, as Sanders described, is to suffer emotional bruises and wounds. To have dyslexia within a high-achieving family often inflicts battle scars upon the ego structure of the vulnerable child. To have dyslexia in a competitive world where everyone else earns praise is to expose oneself to constant danger of emotional injury. The vulnerable child must have a source of healing from day to day. Loving support is the healing medicine for these battle-weary strugglers.

A Friendly Advocate

Every individual, but especially someone who has dyslexia, needs a person to be on his or her side. This goes beyond loving support because it also involves playing the role of advocate, speaking out on the struggler's behalf, arguing his or her case when words fail. Someone must be there who believes, who cares, and who will come to the defense of the individual with dyslexia. This advocate usually is the mother, although when matters become serious, many fathers do step in for a while. Teachers frequently intervene on the behalf of a struggling learner, and school counselors are forever trying to change a teacher's mind regarding a low-achieving student. Individuals with dyslexia can often go awhile managing fairly well, if their lives are well structured. At some point, however, they will need a friendly advocate to speak for them.

As I look back over the past 4 decades of working with students with dyslexia, I remember many who failed. In almost every case, there was no one to intervene. In the highly competitive arena of fluent speech, the person with a language disability could not find the necessary words to defend him- or herself against articulate, aggressive authority. Occasionally, the stubbornness that can develop in some persons with dyslexia can defeat the efforts of friendly advocates. In most instances, however, failure occurs because there was no one to take a stand. Conversely, all individuals with dyslexia that I have seen succeed had that advocate. Sanders and YaDeau both described persons who took charge of their troubles and guided them safely through their crises. In both cases, parents played this role.

Courage

I have been astonished repeatedly by the level of courage I have seen in individuals struggling to learn. Like most people, I have needed a certain degree of courage in my own life, but I never have faced the enormous daily problems that most persons with dyslexia deal with in our society. It is impossible to survive with dyslexia in the Western world without courage. As children struggle through school years, they often do not realize that their level of struggle is unusual. They often assume that everyone must work just as hard. They are amazed when they learn that their classroom struggle is actually unique among their peers. How can a rational person face certain daily failure without becoming mentally ill? How can children with LD endure the constant threat of failure and disappointment without at least becoming neurotic? How do people who cannot read, write, spell, or do math computation survive mainstream education where busy teachers often have no idea how to meet their needs? Persons with dyslexia who succeed exhibit persistent courage and emotional toughness. They do not become neurotic or mentally ill. Those who do not possess enough courage will go under.

During the 1980s, the Menninger Foundation began to map certain forms of mental illness that often emerge during the middle teen years within the dyslexic population (Jernigan, 1985). It is not yet clear what the relationship with dyslexia actually is. However, it is known that eating disorders such as anorexia nervosa and bulimia appear more frequently within the LD population than among nondisabled students. Certain forms of adolescent schizophrenia also occur more frequently among struggling learners. None of this really should be surprising, considering that many children with dyslexia face the stigma of being called "lazy." They often are told by important adults in their life that they just are not trying hard enough. They hear smart-aleck remarks made by peers about "going to the dummy class" when they leave the classroom to go for special help. When an inflexible or incompetent psychometrist reports a low IQ score on a timed, standardized test, how does the dyslexic child handle the shocking conclusion that he or she is "moderately retarded"? When classmates win praise and have their better work displayed, how does the embarrassed child with dysgraphia cope? When everyone else is telling stories about academic victories, what does the struggling learner say? To survive 12 or 13 years in a generally hostile environment should produce several million mentally disturbed children, but it does not.

These children survive because they have courage. They have a built-in toughness that enables them to deal with chronic near-failure successfully, although not happily, not joyfully, and often with much pain. If they have courage, they make it through those destructive years with only old scars left to show their conflict.

No Self-Pity

A person with dyslexia cannot overcome the disability if he or she wallows in self-pity. To feel sorry for self is to turn inward: "Poor little me! Look at my misfortune! Life is not fair! Everyone else is to blame! Look, everyone, look at me! Poor, pitiful little me!" This cannot be within the vocabulary of persons with dyslexia, if they are to overcome their disability patterns. As described in Chapter 6, feeling sorry for oneself cripples the personality, leaving no strength for forward movement. Self-pity drains away vital emotional energy that is needed to sustain courage. Wallowing in the dark pool of self-pity submerges the person in a sticky emotional mess that quickly snuffs out any beauty. No one has much sympathy for someone who shows self-pity, but this is especially true for individuals with dyslexia.

The antidote for self-pity is a sense of humor, at least to some degree. No one can laugh very much at true misfortune, and there certainly is nothing to chuckle over when one is in pain. But the attitude of good humor must flourish strongly enough to enable a person to break free when self-pity reaches out to take control. As was shown in earlier chapters, parents and teachers must begin early in the life of a child with LD to teach survival skills, including avoiding self-pity. It is impossible to overcome dyslexia if this defeatist emotion is an active part of one's life.

Chapter 8

Looking to the Future

When I began working with struggling students in 1957, the word dyslexia was not included in most dictionaries. Only a few professionals and educators had heard the term, and it was generally regarded with skepticism and disbelief. As department chair at a major university during the late 1960s, I found that my research on dyslexia often was ridiculed by colleagues who were embarrassed to have that kind of "nontraditional study" conducted on their campus. That original hostility toward the issue of dyslexia began to change in the mid-1970s when P.L. 94-142 mandated that students with dyslexia "shall" be educated in the "least restrictive" and "most appropriate" ways. The Harvard studies of neurological differences of dyslexic brains brought this issue directly to the front lines of education, and the brain imaging technology of the 1980s provided the scientific foundation for the study of dyslexia and other types of LD. In 1985, Drake Duane was able to declare with confidence at a national symposium, "Dyslexia is the most thoroughly researched of all learning disabilities" (Duane, 1985). By 1990, only a few hardcore skeptics continued to insist that the issue of dyslexia was irrelevant.

Like my professional contemporaries, my career in dealing with this problem has consisted mostly of educated guesses and intuitive hunches. The techniques my generation used with the LD population from the 1950s into the 1980s were largely trial and error. Certain teaching strategies worked well in established left-to-right sequence, overcoming reversals, and building basic literacy skills, but we had no truly scientific foundation for what we did. For example, in the 1940s Grace Fernald pioneered the technique of using sand trays and cut-out sandpaper shapes for finger tracing of letters and words. This tactile–kinesthetic device became a stock-in-trade for educators around the world (Fernald, 1988). Between 1920 and 1940, Beth Slingerland developed diagnostic strategies that became the *Slingerland Screening Tests for Identifying Children with Specific Language Disabilities* (Slingerland, 1976). As we enter the new century, the Slingerland tests remain one of the most effective ways to identify dyslexia in the classroom. Anna Gillingham, a colleague of Slingerland, collaborated with Samuel Orton to develop the Orton/Gillingham Method for teaching literacy skills to persons of all ages who have dyslexia. This highly structured method has been incorporated into the *Writing Road to Reading* (Spalding & Spalding, 1957), a multisensory remedial program that continues to be one of our most effective vehicles for overcoming dyslexia. From the 1950s into the 1970s, Marianne Frostig expanded the remediation of perceptual deficits with her acclaimed visual–perceptual and visual–motor coordination strategies. At the same time, out of personal frustration concerning the education of her son with LD, Sally Smith launched a homeschooling program based upon her own common sense. Her concern for struggling learners led to the founding of the Lab School in Washington, DC. Smith and her colleagues have set worldwide standards of excellence for teaching those who are LD. Despite all this, we who pioneered diagnostic and remedial strategies had little scientific evidence to back our theories. We shall enter the 21st century able to give much more than hunches and guesses to future generations of persons with dyslexia.

BRAIN SCAN INFORMATION

As brain scan techniques become more sophisticated, it will soon become routine to check the central nervous system of children, adolescents, and adults with LD in ways that pose no threat to the soft tissues of the brain or to delicate structures of nerve pathways. Brain imaging technologies excite molecules within targeted brain regions. These excited molecules give off "echoes" of energy that create colored images on a screen. By studying changes in these color patterns, researchers discover how the person's brain processes language information. This is a safe way to study brain wave patterns that often reveal the potential for dyslexia within the left cerebral cortex (Jordan, 1995). Several new brain scan systems show great promise for giving specific information about how brains function. One technique, positron emission tomography, or PET scan, uses tiny amounts of radioactive isotopes to make brain centers "glow." The scanner then photographs different brain centers as they work. It is simple to compare nondyslexic brains with dyslexic brains doing such work as reading, spelling, listening, writing, and speaking. The PET scan pinpoints differences in brain structure that explain why certain students struggle with left-brain learning.

Another brain scan technology is based upon magnetic resonance imaging (MRI). MRI scans produce detailed images of the brain, pinpointing abnormalities and differences in brain structure where language processing and attention control occur. The MRI technology shows much promise for spotting neuronal differences related to learning disabilities. Still another brain scan method, brain electrical activity mapping, or BEAM, triggers selected activity within various parts of the brain. By exciting specific brain areas for very brief moments (1/1,000th of a second), it is possible to evoke a variety of responses such as surprise wave, recognition wave, selective attention wave, and sexual orientation wave. Researchers believe that, by the early 21st century, we will have the ability to map learning disability brain waves to guide us in teaching children with dyslexia in the most effective way. Experimental work already has shown the potential for designing remedial–tutorial programs according to what brain images reveal about the brain's structure. Individuals who have visual dyslexia would be given listening–speaking instruction rather than reading, persons with auditory dyslexia would be given a visual learning program with little emphasis on listening or spelling, and people with distinctive right-brain structures related to strong talent for keyboard use would be placed in computer-based programs.

These and other research methods will continue to open vast areas of knowledge into how the living brain functions or fails to function. By the late 1980s, it was possible to discover primary dyslexic markers in unborn fetuses through intrauterine technologies. In 1986, pioneers of fetal development such as Bruce McEwen at the Rockefeller University School of Medicine and Veronika Grimm at the Weizmann Institute of Science in Israel described future routine prenatal tests for dyslexia, the way we now test developing fetuses for Downs' syndrome and other genetic differences (cited in Jordan, 1989a). This kind of knowledge always holds double power, of course. In the wrong hands, this sort of expertise can become a tool used to weed out "undesirable" characteristics. However, the hope for future treatment of dyslexia is that detection of the pattern during fetal development will allow us to begin remedial steps early enough to avoid problems later on. The tragedy of dyslexia has been to discover it by accident after the child's self-esteem has been shattered through failure. In the near future, detecting dyslexia before a child is born will allow parents to prepare for remedial steps in language development from the time of infancy. The earlier dyslexia is identified, the more effectively it can be overcome.

IMPROVED PHYSICAL HEALTH OF INDIVIDUALS WITH DYSLEXIA

Researchers have focused much of their attention on the health patterns found in persons with dyslexia their DNA relatives. During their Harvard studies of dyslexia, Geschwind and his colleagues (Geschwind, 1984) gathered much information about health patterns in blood relatives of dyslexics, as was noted in Chapters 1 and 2. For example, relatives of persons with deep dyslexia tend to have overly sensitive digestive tracts with chronic problems related to how the body processes foods and beverages. There is a higher than normal tendency for stomach and duodenal ulcers, colitis, gastritis, and chronic bowel problems such as Crohn's disease. DNA relatives of persons with dyslexia have a higher than normal occurrence of autoimmune disorders such as lupus, arthritis, and fibromyalgia. Autoimmune disorders include problems involving basal metabolism, the endocrine system, and thyroid production; these cause the body to make itself ill. Persons with dyslexia and their relatives also have much higher than normal levels of chronic allergies—including asthma and respiratory problems—which leave the person open to infection that leads to frequent bronchitis and pneumonia. Another common problem is overreaction to food substances causing cytotoxic problems. These family members have more chronic health-related problems than the rest of the population (Jordan, 1995).

As this information becomes more generally known by health-care providers, counselors, and educators, future generations will receive more helpful nutritional guidance and health care. Parents will be counseled from the beginning that the health and nutritional needs of the child with dyslexia are different. Culprit foods and beverages that trigger digestive misery or allergic reactions will be eliminated from the diet. Parents and lunch-program supervisors will be alert for certain foods that often trigger cytotoxic reactions in learners with LD: *milk, caffeine, grape extract derivatives, white wheat products, salicylic foods* (tomato products, green peppers, strawberries, cucumber), and *chemical additives* (MSG, flavor enhancers, preservatives, dyes and color enhancers).

These food and beverage ingredients are not life threatening, nor do they necessarily promote hyperactivity. However, they often make life miserable for those who have dyslexia. In the next century, health-care providers and other adults involved with a person with dyslexia will be better informed about the domino effect that culprit foods and beverages often have on the classroom behavior of persons with dyslexia.

IMPROVED MENTAL HEALTH CARE FOR INDIVIDUALS WITH DYSLEXIA

For the past 30 years, I have been involved intimately with two generations of persons with dyslexia as they progressed from childhood through adolescence into adulthood. Professionals who have had this long-range involvement have seen within individuals with dyslexia lifelong frustration, anguish, and difficulty in coping with the emotional and spiritual domains of their lives. During the 1970s, researchers of mental health patterns of struggling learners began to map emotional differences related to dyslexia and other forms of LD. Through 2 decades of clinical practice with strugglers of all ages, I have been part of often-controversial efforts to improve mental and emotional health for individuals with LD.

Influence of Diet on Emotions and Behavior

During my years of private practice, from 1973 to 1990, I worked closely with a new branch of psychotherapy called *ecological psychiatry.* This specialized form of mental health care investigates the influence of diet on the emotional difficulties encountered in certain persons with dyslexia, Attention Deficit Disorder, dyslogic syndrome, SELD, and Oppositional Defiant Disorder. When every other form of therapeutic intervention fails to make a difference, a routine called *rotation diet* often breaks through the barriers to set the person free from tormenting mental anguish or violent behavior. In Chapter 1, I reviewed the research of Schachar and Wachsmuth (1990) as well as Barkley's (1990) evidence that ODD, CD, and MDD are related to ADHD. Also discussed were the brain-based causes of ADHD. Many individuals with these disorders respond well to rotation diet control that eliminates trigger foods and beverages (Jordan, 1995).

In 1993, a British team of researchers led by Christine Carter at Queen Elizabeth Hospital for Children in London provided new evidence for the impact of diet upon certain persons who struggle hard with life and learning (Carter et al., 1993). This team devised a Few Food Diet that is a variation of the rotation diet regimen developed by American researchers during the 1970s. Working with a large group of youngsters with severe ADHD, Carter's team corroborated the findings of earlier studies that when the digestive tract and central nervous system no longer are exposed to certain dietary agents, many out-of-control individuals settle into a reasonably normal lifestyle. Quality of learning and quality of living are significantly improved when culprit dietary factors are eliminated.

The issue of dietary influence in LD behavior is one of the most controversial topics of the past 20 years. A search of the professional literature reveals a great range of differing opinions and research conclusions on the issue of dietary reactions in individuals with LD. Like the issue of dyslexia itself during the 1950s and 1960s, there is no universal agreement regarding the role of food and beverage control for persons with LD. However, as countless parents, educators, and counselors know from firsthand experience, some of these individuals do better when cytotoxic agents are removed from their diets. As we enter the 21st century, the impact of diet on emotions and behavior will become more clearly defined and better understood. For at least some of these strugglers, changing food and beverage lifestyles makes the difference between success and failure. In many instances, the very survival of the distraught individual is at stake.

Mental Health Problems

In 1993, Deborah Huntington and William Bender reviewed several hundred studies done from 1965 through 1992 related to emotional development of youngsters with LD (Huntington & Bender, 1993). They explored research related to self-concept, attribution (assigning blame for failure to self or others), anxiety, depression, and suicide among adolescents with LD. They concluded that there is an alarming risk for severe depression and suicide among these adolescents. Huntington and Bender summarized what I have witnessed firsthand during 40 years of involvement with this special population. In looking to the future, these researchers propose that teacher training include specific instruction to equip classroom instructors to understand the symptoms of depression and the signals of potential suicide. Also, school counselors must be prepared for ongoing documentation of depressive behaviors in adolescents. Teachers and counselors must be fluent in recognizing emotional disturbances related to eating disorders, chronic depression, the desire to die, excessively low self-esteem, chronic lack of hope and joy, and other red-flag emotional states.

Chronic Depression

A decade ago, the Menninger Foundation in Topeka, Kansas, was among the first mental health institutions to recognize the fragile ego strength of many youngsters with dyslexia (Jernigan, 1985). Psychiatrists and psychologists at the Menninger Foundation began to document mental health tendencies within the dyslexic population treated at that institution. All new adolescent patients entering the Menninger Clinic for psychotherapy were screened for dyslexia. Jernigan developed sophisticated evoked potential EEG evaluation techniques that identified deep dyslexia in new patients. The foundation's researchers found a higher than normal incidence of anorexia nervosa and bulimia among these teens than among the nondyslexic population. This research also documented certain forms of psychotic illness that emerged as youngsters with dyslexia reached their middle teens. These psychotic breaks with reality tended to diminish and often disappear by the early 20s. The Menninger Foundation studies documented that certain adolescents with dyslexia go through a "twilight zone" of mental illness that stretches from about ages 15 to 25. These adolescents are much more likely to suffer from chronic depression and manic–depressive illness than the nondyslexic population. Figure 8.1 shows a manic–depressive mood scale developed as a result of the Menninger Foundation studies.

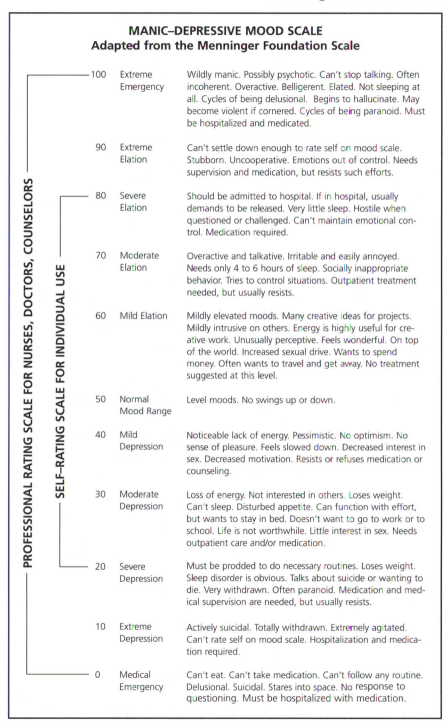

FIGURE 8.1. Self-rating and professional rating scale for identifying levels of severity in manic–depressive mood swings.

Aggression and Violence

In the spring of 1995, I encountered aggression and violence in a most unexpected place. One day I went to lunch at a hotel where I frequently enjoy an hour of private time over a sandwich and the morning newspaper. I know the restaurant staff quite well and enjoy hearing stories of the ups and downs of their lives. I settled into my usual place and began to read the paper. Suddenly I was aware of a difference in the atmosphere of the coffee shop. Clustered at the tables on the right side of the room were 20 or so men. Clustered at tables on the opposite side of the restaurant were 20 or so women. It was clear that they were members of a large family group with striking physical resemblances. Then I noticed that everything was too quiet for a public place. The wait staff— Glenda, Joanne, and William—were serving tables with eyes very wide, as if they were waiting for a bomb to explode. Without warning, two of the men leaped to their feet and began slugging at each other with their fists. Equally suddenly, several women rushed across the room to join the fray. Within seconds the most aggressive family fight I have ever witnessed was in full surge. In all my years of working in prisons, hospitals, and juvenile facilities, I never have witnessed such a violent outpouring of aggression. As tables fell and dishes crashed to the floor, William came to my table with eyes as big as saucers. "Hell done broke loose here!" he said.

This family storm lasted only a few moments. Then the combatants, whom I learned were brothers, settled back to their lunch, and the women, who were wives and sisters, returned to their side of the room. In excited whispers, the wait staff told me the story. This family group ("just like a warring tribe," Glenda said) had arrived the day before for a wedding. Within hours of their arrival, the hotel staff had to intervene to stop two family fights in the corridor. At dinner time the night before, the group decided they did not like the food. They trouped into the hotel kitchen, pushed the chef and his staff outside, and proceeded to prepare their own evening meal. I learned later that during the wedding reception in the hotel ballroom, another fight broke out. This time the hotel management called the police and evicted this warring tribe from the premises. The family was billed for hundreds of dollars in property damage.

As our global society approaches the 21st century, we are painfully aware of the increase of aggression and violence in our culture: bombings of public buildings, battered spouses and children, vandalism to schools and public property, drive-by shootings in normally quiet neighborhoods, ramming of vehicles on freeways, robbery and murder of tourists and foreign visitors. The list seems endless. Researchers and other people have wondered why. Could there be a link between genetics or brain chemistry imbalances and the rise of aggressive, violent behavior around the world?

In the 1950s, Konrad Lorenz aroused an outpouring of criticism when he argued that just as we have instincts for eating and drinking, so also do we harbor instincts for aggression (cited in Stolberg, 1994). As aggression increased around the world, some researchers began to search for the "crime gene." Others scoffed at such a notion. In Chapter 6, the concept of socialization disorders (NVLD and SELD) were discussed. There is much evidence that these forms of behavior originate within the right brain, midbrain, and brain stem when cell clusters are formed differently. Earlier in this chapter, I noted the frequent relationship between dietary intake and disruptive emotional and behavioral patterns. Is it possible to explain certain types of mental illness, aggression, and violence by looking for biological causes?

By 1987 researchers in the field of behavioral genetics were ready to declare that certain biological predispositions to criminal behavior are inherited (Gerelik, 1993, cited by Stolberg, 1994). Bouchard and Lykken at the University of Minnesota's Twin Research Center discovered that tendencies for aggression correlate as strongly in identical twins reared apart as in identical twins reared together in the same nurturing environment (cited in Stolberg, 1994). In 1987 the world was surprised by the results from a Danish study of male identical twins, the largest study of twins ever conducted. It revealed that when a male identical twin committed a crime, his twin was five times more likely than the average Danish man to commit a crime as well. When a fraternal twin committed a crime, his twin was three times more likely than other Danish men to break the law (Stolberg, 1994).

Jane Fullerton and Terry Lemons researched the increase of juvenile violence and aggression among young people in Arkansas who came under the jurisdiction of the juvenile courts. Statistics from the Arkansas Crime Information Center revealed a 6.6% increase in juvenile crime between 1979 and 1992. In a 3-year period from 1989 to 1992, there was an increase of 255% in violent and aggressive behavior in adolescent males, including a sharp rise in murder by juveniles (Fullerton & Lemons, 1994). A report published by Jeffrey Halperin and his colleagues at Queens College in New York (Halperin et al., 1994) concerned the role of serotonin (a major brain enzyme that regulates emotions and self-control of impulses) in boys who were aggressive and those who were not. This research team discovered that boys who displayed aggressive behavior responded differently to serotonin. Also in 1994, Sheryl Stolberg summarized research on the treatment of aggression in adolescents. She established a biochemical link in the brain structure of youth who were violent or overly aggressive. These individuals responded positively to Clonidine®, a drug designed to decrease symptoms of anxiety, impulse behavior, poor concentration, mood swings, and vulnerability to overstimulation (Stolberg, 1994).

As we enter the 21st century, we will better understand the mental health differences in many persons with LD. Ongoing research will provide the knowledge to recognize disruptive emotional patterns earlier in life, and more clearly in the classroom and in society as a whole. New medical technologies will provide tools for decreasing the often tragic results of outbursts of aggression and violence, unrelieved depression, and ruinous eating disorders that often accompany LD. Thoughtful educators will put into practice Huntington's and Bender's recommendations that classroom teachers and school counselors be trained in observing mental health patterns in adolescents who have learning difficulties.

In 1986, Bruce McEwen, a neuropsychologist at Rockefeller University School of Medicine, made a prophetic statement, "There is no such thing as a purely psychological process. Everything is a least party related to body processes" (cited in Jordan, 1989a). This concept of mental health care will release future generations of persons with dyslexia from unnecessary years of anguish and defeat. When body processes cause abnormalities in emotions and mental health, appropriate medical intervention is required. Those individuals with dyslexia who grow up in the 21st century will have access to sophisticated help.

CLASSROOM MANAGEMENT OF DYSLEXIA

My generation of educators began teaching in classrooms that contained virtually every variation of learning differences. The only separate classes available in those years were devoted to individuals with severe disabilities who could not function at all in mainstream placement. My first years of classroom teaching required me to meet the needs of youngsters with moderate mental retardation, children with emotional disturbances who disrupted class by temper tantrums and aggressive explosions, and even students with borderline psychosis who masturbated all day and could not take part in group activities. I also had students who could not read, write, spell, or do arithmetic without help. My early teaching years were saturated by pessimistic, often bitter comments in the teachers' lounge as I listened to veteran instructors tell their stories of the "ne'er-do-well kids" who could not learn, were impossible to teach, and were going to drop out of school anyway. Mainstream teachers 40 years ago carried such deep resentment over having so many strugglers in their classes that no child's needs were fully met.

Then came the educational trend of the late 1960s—establishing resource rooms or learning labs for pupils with special learning needs. I was among the pioneers who taught school districts how to develop those "pull-out" special programs for children with LD. Struggling learners went down the hall or outside to portable classroom buildings for special instruction, leaving mainstream classrooms free to do traditional teaching with no worry about accommodations. By the mid-1970s, every school district receiving federal funds had resource room or learning lab adjunct teaching.

Separate teaching for struggling learners never was universally accepted by educators. A remarkably intuitive school leader in Minnesota, Mary Lee Enfield, refused to acknowledge that children with dyslexia could not be well taught within the mainstream classroom. From 1968 to 1987, Enfield demonstrated how to keep these students in the mainstream classroom without neglecting their skill development. Following Orton's principles for teaching individuals with dyslexia, Enfield developed a three-part classroom system and showed hundreds of teachers how to use it effectively. Each teacher was supported by aides who tutored individual children with LD and small groups while other students worked at a faster pace in larger groups. Three principles for teaching students with LD were strictly followed:

1. *Direct Instruction.* Nothing was left to chance. Each step of what every student with LD was expected to learn was spelled out in outlines, lists, and visible step-by-step instructions. Those who listened well were given instructions and new material on audiotapes.

2. *Systematic Phonics.* In Chapter 3, I reviewed how to teach visual phonics to students with dyslexia by letting them see language sound patterns instead of trying to hear them. The Minnesota project developed clearly defined ways to teach word sounding and spelling patterns to these youngsters in the mainstream classroom.

3. *Multisensory Rehearsal While Learning.* The many ways in which multisensory learning can take place were described in Chapters 2 and 3. The Minnesota project made sure that every child with LD practiced seeing, saying, hearing, and touching simultaneously. Teacher aides and study partners guided them through this supportive program.

Full Inclusion

The Enfield method (Enfield, 1988) became a nationwide standard for many schools where pull-out or separate classes for students with LD were deemed inappropriate. The success of this Minnesota project was largely responsible during the early 1980s for the rising tide of dissatisfaction with the idea of separate classrooms for learners with LD. Many educators and other leaders began talking about including all students rather than excluding those with differences. In 1986, Madeline Will, then Assistant Secretary for Special Education and Rehabilitative Services in the U.S. Department of Education, proposed The Regular Education Initiative (REI) (Will, 1986). Will's plan would place all students with "mild disabilities" in mainstream classrooms. Educators who valued Enfield's successful treatment of dyslexia in the mainstream rallied to this possibility. REI soon came to be known as *inclusion*. As momentum grew behind this proposal, the rallying cry of *full inclusion* was born.

Full inclusion became the theme behind changes in landmark legislation related to learning disabilities. In 1975, P.L. 94-142 required all schools to provide the "least restrictive" and "most appropriate" educational environment for every pupil with diagnosed learning differences or special needs. This legislation was the legal foundation for requiring schools to provide separate educational environments when the mainstream was deemed too restrictive and inappropriate for meeting special learning needs. In 1990, P.L. 94-142 was revised and renamed the Individuals with Disabilities Education Act (IDEA, P.L. 101-476). Proponents of IDEA hailed this revised federal legislation that authorized full inclusion, insisting that it was undemocratic and unfair to exclude any student from mainstream participation, regardless of disabling condition. In less than 5 years, REI had bloomed into a trend to restore all students to the mainstream classroom, as it was when I began teaching in 1957.

The sometimes acrimonious debate over what is the most appropriate, least restrictive learning environment for students with dyslexia will continue into the next century. Those who appreciate the successful mainstream teaching of leaders such as Enfield vigorously support the concept of including all children—even those with severe disabilities—in mainstream classrooms where teacher aides provide support while allowing these children to be with same-age peers. On the other side of this issue are vigorous opponents. For example, the most influential group involved with learning disabilities, the Learning Disabilities Association (LDA), stated, "LDA does not support 'full inclusion' . . . or any policies that mandate the same placement, instruction, or treatment for ALL students with learning disabilities" (Gallagher, 1994, p. 19). In 1995, James Kauffman and Daniel Hallahan edited a comprehensive critique, *The Illusion of Full Inclusion.* These editors, and the authors of the chapters in this book, were sharply critical of reducing separate specialized learning environments and moving their students into mainstream classrooms. Edwin Martin (1994) noted the high rate of failure when adolescents with LD were placed in mainstream high school classes after spending several years receiving separate support in resource rooms and learning labs. Drawing upon data researched by SRI International, Martin concluded that 60% of the special education students who were placed in regular classes dropped out of high school because of failing grades in required courses they could not handle. Martin said, "To me, the data indicate that the prospects for inclusion are not encouraging . . . . for children with learning disabilities, the outcome data show high failure and drop-out rates" (Martin, 1994, p. 40).

Legal Issues in Mainstream Education

The controversy over the least restrictive, most appropriate educational placement for students with LD has created an industry devoted to interpretation of federal and state statutes governing special education. Peter and Patricia Latham, attorneys who founded the first 4-year college for individuals with LD, published *Learning Disabilities and the Law* in 1993. In this volume they reviewed the growing body of legal opinion and litigation related to the educational placement of persons with LD in our society. Currently, the myriad legal issues surrounding treatment of learning differences in this country have not begun to be resolved. Throughout the United States exist many legal firms who specialize in litigation between dissatisfied parents of children with LD and schools. The Americans with Disabilities Act of 1990 significantly increased the legal controversy by mandating the end of discrimination against individuals with disabilities in the workplace, public accommodations, education, employment, and professional licensing. As a result, litigation levels leaped dramatically as all public and private agencies were required to make their buildings accessible to everyone, regardless of type of disability. At the same time, employers were to include persons with all types of disabilities in their workforce if they could be accommodated reasonably in the workplace. Within colleges and universities debate raged over how to provide accommodations for students who needed special considerations. Should those who have dyscalculia be required to take college algebra if such a course was not vital to the student's major area of concentration? Should students with dysgraphia be permitted to write comprehensive exams on a word processor? These are examples of the kinds of questions that arose. Numerous court decisions laid fines and other legal discipline upon professors and schools who refused to comply. These legal and ethical issues surrounding learning disabilities will not be resolved any time soon.

Perhaps the most sobering and poignant warning about full inclusion came in 1991 from Larry Silver, widely regarded as a beloved "father" of the LDA. Silver, who has practiced child psychiatry for many years, has been a guiding voice for more than 30 years in helping our society learn good treatment of individuals with LD. Silver found himself feeling uncomfortable during the emerging discussion of REI, inclusion, and full inclusion. "Something bothered me," he stated. "This discomfort seemed to have nothing to do with the model as presented or with the arguments against it. This discomfort was deeper" (pp. 389–390). To illustrate his point Silver described an incident in New York City. As he walked down a street, he saw a homeless woman coming toward him. She was hallucinating and delusional. Suddenly he was back in the 1960s, when a dramatic change occurred in U.S. society regarding the treatment of mental illness. During Silver's early years of psychiatric practice, a point of view arose that too many mentally ill patients were being warehoused in too many mental hospitals, that they were isolated and often too far from home or family. A movement grew to "deinstitutionalize" these troubled, isolated adults. Well-meaning leaders promoted a plan to set up community-based mental health centers to care for the deinstitutionalized mental patients. In other words, these individuals would be mainstreamed so they could share the world instead of being relegated to separate support systems. Many of us remember when this concept was approved. Within a relatively short time, residential mental institutions were emptied of chronically ill adults, who were "sent home" to be cared for in their home communities.

Larry Silver drove home his concern in the following words:

> Something happened. The community could not handle the patients who were discharged to community services that did not exist. The concept failed. The most visible evidence of this failure is now seen in every city in this country: homeless people. Fifty percent of the homeless people are mentally ill. They left the institutions, but communities were not able to accept them. . . . I worry. I worry that we will see a new type of homeless—students with learning disabilities, wandering the halls. Students with learning disabilities walking to the office because they have misbehaved. Students who will give up on education and become school "pushouts," not "dropouts." Much as it happened in our cities, the quality of life in the classroom will continue to deteriorate for the regular students. (Silver, 1991, p. 390)

The debate over full inclusion will continue well into the 21st century. Models for successful mainstreaming of students with LD, like Enfield's program in Minnesota, will increase because numerous schools will provide the right kind of classroom support for mainstreaming students with perceptual differences. However, the very real probability also exists that many schools will not provide that kind of support. If so, those communities will see the fulfillment of Silver's premonition that in the wrong learning environment, mainstreamed adolescents with LD will become a new kind of homeless population. As of 1996, we do not know how accurate Silver's foreboding image might prove to be.

Instructional Materials

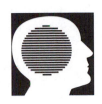

Source for Colored Page Overlays:

Irlen Institute
5380 Village Road
Long Beach, CA 90808
Phone: (310) 496-2550
Fax: (310) 429-8699

IRLEN DIAGNOSTIC CENTERS

ALASKA
Anchorage
(907) 345-0894

ARIZONA
Phoenix
(602) 274-2930
Tucson
(602) 364-5192

CALIFORNIA
Los Angeles
(310) 496-2550
Modesto
(209) 577-0880
San Diego
(619) 259-7329

San Francisco
(510) 729-7932

COLORADO
Boulder
(303) 499-0406

FLORIDA
Miami
(305) 595-5554
Orlando
(904) 383-1911

HAWAII
Honolulu
(808) 988-3060

ILLINOIS
Chicago
(708) 998-0966

KANSAS
Wichita
(316) 689-4233

KENTUCKY
Paducah
(502) 898-7144

MASSACHUSETTS
Boston
(617) 491-2088

MICHIGAN
Ann Arbor
(313) 663-5590
Detroit
(810) 524-9680

NEW YORK
New York
(212) 397-9620

NORTH CAROLINA
Greensboro
(919) 292-2131

OHIO
Toledo
(419) 843-7829

OKLAHOMA
Ardmore
(405) 226-8477

OREGON
Pendleton
(503) 938-3038

PENNSYLVANIA
Erie
(814) 833-2988

TEXAS
Baytown
(713) 428-7039
Dallas
(405) 226-8477
(214) 235-8457
Houston
(713) 771-3108
Laredo
(210) 717-3337

WASHINGTON
Seattle
(206) 562-8928

CANADA
Ottawa
(613) 230-3995
Regina
(306) 584-9124

Franklin Learning Resources, 122 Burrs Road, Mt. Holly, NJ 08060
1-800-525-9673   Fax (609) 261-8368

A Quick Guide to Electronic Book Features

PAGE NUMBERS	CATEGORY	SPELL CORRECTION	VOCABULARY ENRICHMENT ACTIVITIES	PERSONAL WORD LIST	SPEAKING CAPACITY	ADVANCED VOCABULARY	THESAURUS	DICTIONARY	GRAMMAR HANDBOOK	VOCABULARY BASE	BATTERY TYPE	PRODUCT DIMENSIONS (L x W x D)
	BOOKMAN SERIES											
3	MVS-840 (Speaking Desktop)	●		●					●	Varies	4 AAA	5-3/4" x 4" x 1"
4	MWD-640 (Desktop)	●		●					●	Varies	4 AAA	5-1/2" x 4" x 1"
4	MWD-440 (Pocket)	●		●				●		Varies	2 lithium	4-5/8" x 3" x 1/2"
	LANGUAGE MASTER SERIES											
7	LM-6000	●		●					●	110,000	4 AA	5-3/4" x 5-1/2" x 1-1/4"
9	LM-6000 SE*	●		●		●			●	110,000	4 AA	5-3/4" x 5-1/2" x 1-1/4"
10	LM-4200	●						●	●	83,000	4 AAA	5-5/8" x 4-1/4" x 1"
10	LM-3500	●						●	●	110,000	4 AA	7" x 5" x 1-1/4"
	SPELLING SERIES											
11	ACE-200	●	●							80,000	4 AAA	5-1/2" x 4-7/8" x 3/4"
11	SA-98	●	●							80,000	4 AAA	6" x 4" x 3/4"
	DICTIONARY COMPANION SERIES											
12	ES-90**	●		●				**		50,000	4 AAA	6" x 4" x 3/4"
12	SDC-300**	●		●	●			**		50,000	4 AAA	5-1/2" x 4-7/8" x 3/4"
	WORDMASTER SERIES											
13	WM-1055	●		●		●	●			83,000	4 AAA	5-1/2" x 3-5/8" x 3/4"
13	NCT-102						●			100,000	1 lithium	4-1/4" x 2-1/2" x 3/8"
	DIGITAL BOOK SYSTEM SERIES											
14	DBS-2 / DBS-2D	●		●						N/A	4 lithium/4A	See pg. 14
	ESL/EP FOREIGN LANGUAGE SERIES											
15	SM-1000	●		●					●	250,000	4 AAA	5-7/8" x 4-1/4" x 1"
16	SM-550	●		●					●	250,000	4 AAA	5-5/8" x 4-1/4" x 1"
16	SM-515	●		●					●	250,000	2 lithium	4-3/4" x 3-1/4" x 5/8"
16	FP-650	●		●					●	200,000	4 AAA	5-5/8" x 4-1/4" x 1"
16	FP-615	●		●					●	200,000	2 lithium	4-3/4" x 3-1/4" x 5/8"

*Contains a full array of special needs functions   **Hardcover Merriam-Webster Dictionary accompanies unit.

Checklist of Visual Dyslexia Symptoms

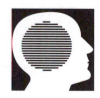

The following informal checklist can help parents and teachers identify visual dyslexia. It is important to withhold judgment until a definite syndrome of dyslexic symptoms has been identified in a student's behavior. If a significant cluster of perceptual errors appears as the adult studies a student's performance, then it is generally safe to conclude that visual dyslexia exists.

____ **Confusion with Sequence**

> ____ has poor concept of time
>
> ____ has poor concept of chronological order of events
>
> ____ cannot give day, month, and year of birth
>
> ____ cannot write months of year
>
> ____ cannot write days of week
>
> ____ cannot remember multiplication tables

____ **Difficulty Following Directions**
(This can also indicate Attention-Deficit Disorder)

> ____ cannot remember daily routines at home
>
> ____ cannot follow teacher's directions in classroom

_____ cannot comprehend instructions when given to a group; must have one-to-one explanations

_____ needs constant reminding of what to do

_____ **Faulty Oral Language**

_____ loses words and/or "goes blank" while telling, naming, describing

_____ can tell stories or give oral reports but gets details in wrong sequence

_____ has difficulty with correct sequence of events

_____ **Faulty Reading Comprehension**

_____ fails to identify main ideas

_____ tells story details out of sequence

_____ loses meaning of sentences or paragraphs before reaching the end

_____ fails to draw inferences from what has been read

_____ has difficulty recalling details when answering comprehension questions

_____ **Slow Work Rate**

_____ seldom finishes timed exercises

_____ easily frustrated when pressured for speed

_____ has a considerably slower work pace than classmates

_____ can do satisfactory work if given ample time and help

_____ will not use full time allowance on timed tests; guesses, marks items at random

_____ **Difficulty with Alphabet**

_____ does not know alphabet in correct sequence

_____ omits certain letters from alphabetic sequence

_____ mixes capital and lowercase letters

_____ mixes manuscript and cursive styles

_____ confuses similar letters

_____ writes certain letters backwards or upside down

_____ sings alphabet song or repeats rhyme to check sequence

_____ is not able to synchronize voice, finger, and eyes while checking work

_____ **Confusion with Symbols**

_____ writes capital *B* and *D* instead of lowercase *b* and *d*

_____ confuses symbols in reading, writing, and arithmetic

_____ cannot conserve the form in copy work (loses mental images as eyes refocus)

_____ confuses similar symbols

_____ b–d–p–q	_____ h–n
_____ h–y	_____ m–w
_____ r–n	_____ l–i
_____ r–c–s	_____ n–u
_____ f–t	_____ N–Z
_____ 3–E	_____ 6–9
	_____ +, ×, ÷

_____ **Errors in Oral Reading**

_____ reverses whole words

_____ reverses beginning letters

_____ transposes *l* and *r* in consonant blends

_____ substitutes similar letters or words

_____ transposes letters inside words

_____ fails to see small details in words

_____ fails to see punctuation marks

_____ omits endings

_____ telescopes (leaves out letters or syllables)

_____ perseverates (adds extra letters or syllables)

_____ **Errors in Spelling**

_____ transposes silent letters within words

_____ does not recall correct order of letters

_____ misplaces silent *e*

_____ **Errors in Arithmetic**

_____ reverses the process while working problems

_____ carries or borrows wrong digit

_____ cannot organize facts in story problems

_____ misreads signs (plus for ×, times for +, subtract for +)

_____ **Errors in Copying**

_____ loses place on board (far point)

_____ misspells on paper

_____ fails to observe capital letters

_____ fails to observe punctuation marks

_____ fails to space properly

_____ erases frequently

_____ overprints to correct mistakes

_____ reverses letters

_____ reverses whole words

_____ telescopes

_____ perseverates

_____ works unusually slowly

_____ tries to avoid copying tasks

Checklist of Auditory Dyslexia Symptoms

The following checklist can help parents and teachers identify patterns associated with auditory dyslexia. It is important to withhold judgment until a definite syndrome of symptoms has been identified.

____ **Confusion with Phonics**

    ____ cannot distinguish differences in vowel sounds

        ____ does not hear long vowel sounds

        ____ does not hear short vowel sounds

        ____ does not hear schwa vowel sounds

        ____ does not hear changes in vowel sounds

    ____ cannot distinguish differences in consonant sounds

    ____ does not hear differences between similar consonant sounds:

        ____ /b/ /d/   ____ /b/ /p/

        ____ /d/ /t/   ____ /g/ /k/

        ____ /m/ /n/   ____ /f/ /v/

        ____ /s/ /z/   ____ /th/ /f/

_____ does not hear the sounds within consonant clusters

_____ cannot interpret diacritical markings

_____ cannot interpret phonetic respellings

_____ **Confusion with Words**

_____ cannot tell when words are alike or different

_____ cannot hear or say rhyming words

_____ gives garbled pronunciation (echolalia)

_____ **Confusion with Spelling**

_____ writes very slowly

_____ depends upon memory tricks to recall spellings

_____ cannot apply phonics rules when spelling

_____ tends to spell phonetically

_____ breaks consonant clusters when spelling (transposes *l* and *r*—*paly* for *play, bran* for *barn, gril* for *girl*)

_____ confuses sounds of consonant letters:

_____ *c* for *k*	_____ *f* for *v*
_____ *m* for *n*	_____ *d* for *t*
_____ *s* for *z*	_____ *f* for *th*

_____ does not hear sounds of /m/, /n/, /l/, /w/, or /r/

_____ telescopes (leaves out sounds when writing words)

_____ perseverates (adds sounds when writing words)

_____ does not hear accent in words

_____ does not hear vowel sounds within words

_____ does not hear syllables within words

_____ does not remember different or unusual spellings

_____ cannot retain memory of basic spelling words

_____ asks speaker to repeat

_____ erases, marks over, crosses out

_____ tries to hide work while writing

_____ **Reinforcement While Writing or Reading**

_____ whispers while reading silently

_____ whispers while writing

JORDAN AUDITORY SCREENING TEST (JAST)

Auditory Profile

Check the areas in the Auditory Profile that show the items missed by the student. This will indicate specific speech sounds that he or she is not perceiving accurately. Some persons with auditory dyslexia make perfect scores on this test. Do not either eliminate or verify the existence of dyslexia based on the student's performance on the JAST alone. Other dyslexic symptoms must be obvious before this screening test can be considered reliable in predicting auditory dyslexia.

Initial Consonant Sounds

_____ /b/–/d/ Items 1 and 6

_____ /d/–/t/ Items 2 and 5

_____ /b/–/p/ Items 4 and 7

_____ /f/–/v/ Items 9 and 12

_____ /h/–/wh/ Items 11 and 14

_____ /m/–/n/ Items 13 and 28

_____ /y/–/w/ Items 16 and 21

_____ /d/–/j/ Items 17 and 20

_____ /s/–/z/ Items 19 and 24

_____ /k/–/g/ Items 22 and 25

_____ /r/–/l/ Items 23 and 27

Final Consonant Sounds

_____ /s/–/z/ Items 1 and 9

_____ /d/–/t/ Items 3 and 8

_____ /g/–/k/ Items 5 and 10

_____ /m/–/n/ Items 6 and 14

_____ /d/–/j/ Items 12 and 22

_____ /f/–/v/ Items 16 and 19

_____ /b/–/p/ Items 17 and 20

_____ /b/–/d/ Items 18 and 23

Name _____ Age _____ Grade _____

Dyslexia Symptoms _____ _____ _____ _____

  none   moderate   pronounced   severe

Directions: "Listen carefully as I say each set of words. Tell me if the words sound exactly alike, or if they are different." Mark each correct response *1.* Mark incorrect responses *0.* Mark *X* for any set of words the child does not respond to.

Initial Consonant Sounds

_____ 1. bed–dead
_____ 2. dime–time
_____ 3. look–look
_____ 4. back–pack
_____ 5. tam–dam
_____ 6. dill–bill
_____ 7. pane–bane
_____ 8. say–say
_____ 9. fat–vat
_____ 10. no–no
_____ 11. hot–what
_____ 12. vetch–fetch
_____ 13. mile–nile
_____ 14. where–hare
_____ 15. got–got
_____ 16. yet–wet
_____ 17. Dane–Jane
_____ 18. you–you
_____ 19. Sue–zoo
_____ 20. jot–dot
_____ 21. we–ye
_____ 22. cob–gob
_____ 23. rack–lack
_____ 24. zipper–sipper
_____ 25. goat–coat
_____ 26. might–might
_____ 27. lake–rake
_____ 28. noose–moose

_____ **TOTAL CORRECT**

Final Consonant Sounds

_____ 1. fuss–fuzz
_____ 2. caught–caught
_____ 3. bet–bed
_____ 4. red–red
_____ 5. muck–mug
_____ 6. hum–hun
_____ 7. give–give
_____ 8. clod–clot
_____ 9. his–hiss
_____ 10. bug–buck
_____ 11. seat–seat
_____ 12. mad–Madge
_____ 13. yes–yes
_____ 14. run–rum
_____ 15. pig–pig
_____ 16. safe–save
_____ 17. pub–pup
_____ 18. stub–stud
_____ 19. live–life
_____ 20. stop–stob
_____ 21. make–make
_____ 22. wedge–wed
_____ 23. rid–rib
_____ 24. love–love

_____ **TOTAL CORRECT**

0 to 3 errors—probably no disability, unless other symptoms are apparent in daily work

4 to 6 errors—probably moderate degree of disability, if other symptoms are apparent in daily work

7 to 10 errors—pronounced disability is indicated, especially if other symptoms are apparent in daily work; thorough hearing diagnosis is indicated to be sure the child is not partially deaf

more than 10 errors—serious problem is indicated if other symptoms are apparent in daily work; hearing diagnosis must be done to determine part that actual hearing loss may be playing in learning difficulties

Checklist of Dysgraphia Symptoms

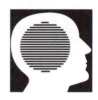

This checklist can help parents and teachers identify dysgraphia.

_____ **Difficulty with Alphabet or Number Symbols**

_____ does not remember how to write certain letters or numerals

_____ distorts shapes of certain letters or numerals

_____ has awkward, uneven overall writing

_____ has difficulty transferring from manuscript to cursive style

_____ continues to print manuscript style long after introduction to cursive style

_____ fragments certain letters or numerals

_____ does writing that resembles "bird scratching," is virtually illegible

_____ has difficulty distinguishing between capital and lowercase letters

_____ mixes capital and lowercase letters

____ Confusion with Directionality

____ writes certain letters, numerals, or words backwards (mirror image)

____ tends to write on mirror side (left side) of vertical midline when moving to next column

____ marks from bottom to top when forming certain letters or numerals

____ uses backwards (clockwise) motions when writing circular strokes in certain letters or numerals

____ continually erases or overprints to change what was written first

____ has writing that slants up, down, or wobbles up and down

____ Sentence Structure

____ composes meaningful content in spite of poor handwriting

____ transposes grammatical elements within sentences, but produces good overall meaning

____ tends to use fragments instead of complete sentences

____ Difficulty Conserving Form in Copying Simple Shapes

____ distorts simple shapes

____ fails to close corners

____ draws "ears" where lines meet or change direction

____ has difficulty reproducing simple designs from memory

____ work deteriorates toward end of writing exercise

____ has difficulty staying on lines when tracing

___ Tendency to Telescope

___ omits letters when writing words

___ omits syllables or sound units when writing words

___ runs letters and words together

___ runs words together (usually when copying)

___ Tendency to Perseverate

___ adds unnecessary letters or sound units to written words

___ repeats the same letters or syllables in written words

___ adds unnecessary sound units to spoken words

___ repeats syllables or sound units in spoken words

___ falls into parrotlike repetition of rhyming sounds during games or conversation

Checklist for Dyscalculia

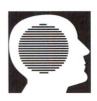

_____ cannot remember arithmetic facts or procedures

_____ reverses numerals while writing or copying

_____ gets numerals out of sequence

_____ must count fingers and whisper to do problems

_____ must use scratch paper to work out arithmetic processes

_____ does arithmetic problems very slowly

_____ cannot remember which direction to go in working problems

_____ cannot keep number columns lined up correctly

_____ does not pay attention to math signs, such as dollar signs, commas, decimals, plus and minus signs, greater and lesser than signs

_____ has messy, hard to decipher handwriting on math papers

_____ does constant erasing and changing

_____ shows much frustration while working problems

_____ needs continual one-to-one redirection

_____ cannot do math work without help or supervision

_____ finally learns addition and subtraction, but is lost with multiplication, division, and decimals

_____ does much better with a hand calculator

Resources for Help with Learning Disabilities

ORGANIZATIONS

Recording for the Blind (RFB)
20 Roszel Road
Princeton, NJ 20542
(609) 452-0606
(800) 221-4792

RFB is a national, nonprofit organization that provides taped educational books free on loan, books on diskette, library services, and other educational and professional resources to individuals who cannot read standard print because of a visual, physical, or perceptual disability.

The Orton Dyslexia Society
8600 LaSalle Road
Chester Building, Suite 382
Baltimore, MD 21286-2044
(410) 296-0232
(800) 222-3123

The Society is an international scientific and educational association concerned with the widespread problem of the specific language disability of developmental dyslexia. Local and state chapters serve as literacy resources for adults with dyslexia and those who teach or advise them.

Learning Disability Association of America, Inc. (LDA)
4156 Library Road
Pittsburgh, PA 15234
(412) 341-1515
(412) 344-0224 (Fax)

LDA (formerly ACLD), a nonprofit, volunteer advocacy organization, provides information and referral for parents, professionals, and consumers involved with or in search of support groups and networking opportunities through local LDA Youth and Adult Section chapters. A publication list is available. The Association also prints *LDA Newsbriefs*, a bimonthly newsletter for parents, professionals, and adults with LD. Available for $5/year by contacting LDA.

Children and Adults with Attention Deficit Disorder (CH.A.D.D.)
499 Northwest 70th Avenue
Suite 308
Plantation, FL 33317
(305) 587-3700
(305) 587-4599 (Fax)

CH.A.D.D. is a nonprofit, parent-based organization that disseminates information on ADD and coordinates more than 460 parent support groups. It also publishes a semi-annual magazine, *CHADDER*, and a newsletter, *Chadderbox*.

PUBLICATIONS

College Students with Learning Disabilities: A Handbook
LDA Bookstore
4156 Library Road
Pittsburgh, PA 15234
(412) 341-1515

Written by Susan A. Vogel, this publication is designed for students with learning disabilities, admissions officers, faculty and staff, and/or administrators. The handbook discusses Section 504 in regard to college admissions, program accessibility, teaching and testing accommodations, test taking, and self-confidence building strategies. Available for $5.80.

Peterson's Guide to Colleges with Programs for Learning Disabled Students
Book Ordering Department
P.O. Box 2123
Princeton, NJ 08543-2123
(800) 338-3282

Written by Charles T. Mangrum II and Stephen S. Strichart, this is a comprehensive guide to more than 900 two-year colleges and universities offering special services for students with dyslexia and other learning disabilities. The *Guide* is available for $19.95, plus $4.75 shipping and handling.

Unlocking Potential: College and Other Choices for Learning Disabled People: A Step by Step Guide
Woodbine House
5615 Fishers Lane
Rockville, MD 20852
(800) 843-7323

Written by Barbara Schieber and Jeanne Talpers, this is a comprehensive resource for considering, locating, and selecting postsecondary resources. This award-winning book teaches and assists readers throughout the entire postsecondary selection process. Available for $12.95 (paperback).

Schoolsearch Guide to Colleges with Programs and Services for Students with Learning Disabilities
Schoolsearch Press
127 Marsh Street
Belmont, MA 02178
(617) 489-5785

This guide lists more than 600 colleges and universities that offer programs and services to high school graduates with learning disabilities. It is available for $29.95.

References

Alston, J., & Taylor, J. (1987). *Handwriting: Theory, research and practice.* New York: Nichols.

American Psychiatric Association. (1980). *Diagnostic and statistical manual of mental disorders* (3rd ed.). Washington, DC: Author.

American Psychiatric Association. (1987). *Diagnostic and statistical manual of mental disorders* (3rd ed., rev.). Washington, DC: Author.

American Psychiatric Association. (1994). *Diagnostic and statistical manual of mental disorders* (4th ed.). Washington, DC: Author.

Americans with Disabilities Act of 1990, 42 U.S.C. §12101 *et seq.*

Ardrey, R. (1961). *African genesis.* New York: Macmillan.

Ardrey, R. (1972). *The territorial imperative.* New York: Macmillan.

Barkley, R. A. (1990). *Attention deficit hyperactive disorder: A handbook for diagnosis and treatment.* New York: Guilford.

Bastian, C. H. (1869). On various forms of loss of speech in cerebral disease. *The British Medico-Chirurgical Review, 43,* 209–236, 470–494.

Berlin, R. (1884). Uber dyslexie [About dyslexia]. *Archiv fur Psychiatrie, 15,* 276–278.

Berlin, R. (1887). *Einebosondere art der wortblindheit: dyslexia* [A special type of wordblindness: Dyslexia]. Wiesbaden: J. F. Bergmann.

Brier, N. (1989). The relationship between learning disability and delinquency: A review and reappraisal. *Journal of Learning Disabilities, 2,* 546–583.

Broadbent, W. H. (1872). On the cerebral mechanism of speech and thought. *Transactions of the Royal Medical and Chirurgical Society, 15,* 145–194.

Broca, P. (1861). Remarques sur le siege de la faculte du langage articule suivie d'une observation d'aphemie. *Bulletin Societe Anthropologia, 2,* 330–357.

Carter, E. M., Urbanowicz, M., Hemsley, R., Mantilla, L., Strobel, S., Graham, P. J., & Taylor, E. (1993). Effects of a few food diet in attention deficit disorder. *Archives of Disabilities in Children, 69,* 564–568.

Clements, S. D. (1966). *Minimal brain dysfunction in children* (Monograph No. 3, Public Health Service Bulletin No. 1415, NINDS). Washington, DC: U.S. Department of Health, Education, and Welfare.

Copeland, E. D. (1991). *Medications for attention disorders (ADHD/ADD) and related medical problems.* Atlanta: 3 C's of Childhood, Inc.

Critchley, M. (1970). *The dyslexic child.* London: Heinemann.

Denckla, M. B. (1978). Minimal brain dysfunction. In J. S. Chall & A. F. Mirsky (Eds.), *Education and the brain* (pp. 223–268). Chicago: University of Chicago Press.

Denckla, M. B. (1985). Issues of overlap and heterogeneity in dyslexia. In D. B. Gray & J. F. Kavanaugh (Eds.), *Biobehavioral measures of dyslexia* (pp. 41–46). Parkton, MD: York.

Denckla, M. B. (1991a). Academic and extracurricular aspects of non-verbal learning disabilities. *Psychiatric Annals, 21,* 717–724.

Denckla, M. B. (1991b, March). *The neurology of social competence.* Paper presented at the Learning Disabilities Association national conference, Chicago.

Denckla, M. B. (1993). The child with developmental disabilities grown up: Adult residua of childhood disorders. *Behavioral Neurology, 11*(1), 105–125.

Duane, D. (1985, November). *Psychiatric implications of neurological difficulties.* Symposium conducted at the Menninger Foundation, Topeka, KS.

Education for All Handicapped Children Act of 1975, 20 U.S.C. §1400 *et seq.*

Enfield, M. L. (1988). The quest for literacy. *Annals of Dyslexia, 39*(2), 219–225.

Evans, M. M. (1982). *Dyslexia: An annotated bibliography.* Westport, CT: Greenwood.

Fernald, G. (1988). *Remedial techniques in basic school subjects* (L. Idol, Ed.). Austin, TX: PRO-ED.

Fullerton, J., & Lemons, T. (1994, February 13). Special report: Filling the cracks in juvenile justice. *Arkansas Democrat-Gazette,* p. A22.

Galaburda, A. (1983). Developmental dyslexia: Current anatomical research (Proceedings of the 33rd annual conference of The Orton Dyslexia Society). *Annals of Dyslexia, 33,* 41–54.

Gall, F. J., & Spurzheim, J. C. (1809). *Untersuchungen uber die Anotomie des Nervensystems uberhaupt und des Gehirns insebesondere.* Paris: Treuttel & Wurtz.

Gallegher, L. N. (1994, May/June). Inclusion, reform, restructuring and practice. *LDA Newsbriefs, 29*(3), 19.

Geiger, G., & Lettvin, J. Y. (1987). Peripheral vision in persons with dyslexia. *New England Journal of Medicine, 316,* 1238–1243.

Geschwind, N. (1984). The biology of dyslexia: The after-dinner speech. In D. B. Gray & J. F. Kavanaugh (Eds.), *Behavioral measures of dyslexia* (pp. 1–19). Parkton, MD: York.

Goldscheider, A. (1892). Uber centrale Sprach-Schreib-und Lesestorungen. *Berliner Klinishe Wochenschrift, 29,* 64–66, 100–102, 122–125, 144–147, 168–171.

Grashey, H. (1885). Uber Aphasie und ihre Beziehung zur Wahrnehmung. *Archiv fur Psychiatrie, 16,* 654–688.

Grimm, V. (1986, November). *Neuroendocrinology.* Symposium conducted by the Association for Children and Adults with Learning Disability, New York.

Hallowell, E. M., & Ratey, J. J. (1994). *Driven to distraction: Recognizing and coping with attention deficit disorder from childhood through adulthood.* New York: Pantheon.

Halperin, J. M., Sharma, V., Seiver, L. J., Schwartz, S. T., Matier, K., Wornell, G., & Newcorn, J. H. (1994). Serotonergic function in aggressive and nonaggressive boys with attention deficit hyperactivity disorder. *American Journal of Psychiatry, 151,* 243–248.

Hammill, D. D. (1990). On defining learning disabilities: An emerging consensus. *Journal of Learning Disabilities, 23,* 74–83.

Harris, T. L., & Hodges, R. E. (Eds). (1981). *A dictionary of reading and related terms.* Newark, NJ: International Reading Association.

Hinshelwood, J. (1900). Congenital word-blindness. *The Lancet, 1,* 1506–1508.

Huntington, D. D., & Bender, W. N. (1993). Adolescents with learning disabilities at risk? Emotional well-being, depression, suicide. *Journal of Learning Disabilities, 26,* 159–166.

Individuals with Disabilities Education Act of 1990, 20 U.S.C. §1400, *et seq.*

Inhelder, B., & Piaget, J. (1974). *The early growth of logic in the child.* New York: Harper & Row.

Irlen, H. (1991). *Reading by the colors.* Garden City Park, NY: Avery.

Jackson, J. H. (1874). On the nature of the duality of the brain. *Medical Press and Circular,* p. 1.

Jernigan, S. (1985, November). *Measures of brain function: Understanding the influence of brain dysfunction on behavior and learning problems.* Symposium conducted by the Menninger Foundation, Topeka, KS.

Johnson, D. J., & Myklebust, H. R. (1971). *Learning disabilities.* New York: Grune & Stratton.

Jordan, D. R. (1972). *Dyslexia in the classroom.* Columbus, OH: Merrill.

Jordan, D. R. (1974). *Learning disabilities and predelinquent behavior of juveniles.* Oklahoma City: Oklahoma Association of Children with Learning Disabilities.

Jordan, D. R. (1989a). *Overcoming dyslexia in children, adolescents, and adults.* Austin, TX: PRO-ED.

Jordan, D. R. (1989b). *Jordan prescriptive/tutorial reading program for moderate and severe dyslexia.* Austin, TX: PRO-ED.

Jordan, D. R. (1992). *Attention deficit disorder: ADHD and ADD syndromes* (2nd ed.). Austin, TX: PRO-ED.

Jordan, D. R. (1993). Recognizing classroom problems. In *D'Nealian handwriting* (3rd ed., pp. T 33–T 34). Glenview, IL: ScottForesman.

Jordan, D. R. (1995). *Teaching adults with learning disabilities.* Melbourne, FL: Krieger.

Jordan, D. R., & Stephens, H. (1995). The school–marketplace relationship. In R. Rittenhouse & J. Dancer (Eds.), *The full inclusion of persons with disabilities in American society* (pp. 89–94). Levin, New Zealand: National Training Resource Center.

Joseph, R. (1988). The right cerebral hemisphere: Emotion, music, visual-spatial skills, body image, dreams, and awareness. *Journal of Clinical Psychology, 44,* 632–673.

Josephson, M. (1959). *Edison, a biography.* New York: McGraw-Hill.

Kauffman, J. M., & Hallahan, D. P. (1995). *The illusion of full inclusion: A comprehensive critique of a current special education bandwagon.* Austin, TX: PRO-ED.

Kidder, C. B. (1991). Dyslexia and adult illiteracy. Forging the missing link. In *The Lantern* (p. 1). Prides Crossing, VT: Landmark School.

Kirsch, I. W., Jungeblut, A., & Campbell, A. (1992). *Beyond the school doors: The literacy needs of job seekers served by the U.S. Department of Labor.* Princeton, NJ: Educational Testing Service.

Kutchins, H. J., & Kirk, S. (1988). The future of DSM: Scientific and professional issues. *The Harvard Medical School Mental Health Letter,* p. 3.

Latham, P. S., & Latham, P. H. (1993). *Learning disabilities and the law.* Washington, DC: JKL Communications.

Lehmkuhle, S., Garzia, R. P., Turner, L., Hash, T., & Baro, J. A. (1993). A defective visual pathway in children with reading disability. *New England Journal of Medicine, 328,* 989–996.

Lichtheim, L. (1885). On aphasie. *Brain, 7,* 432–484.

Livingstone, M. S., Rosen, G. D., Drislane, F. W., & Galaburda, A. M. (1991). Physiological and anatomical evidence for a magnocellular deficit in developmental dyslexia. *Proceedings of the National Academy of Science, USA, 88,* 7943–7947.

Martin, W. M. (1994, April). Inclusion: Rhetoric and reality. *The Exceptional Parent, 11,* 39–41.

Meynert, T. H. (1868). Die Bedeutung des Gehirns fur das Vorstellungsleben. In T. H. Meynert (Ed.), *Sammlung von popularwissenschaftlichen Vortagen uber den Bau und die Leistungen des Gehirns* (pp. 3–16). Leipzig: Braunmuller.

Missildine, W. H., & Galton, L. (1972). *Your inner child of the past.* New York: Simon and Schuster.

Montgomery, G. (1989). The mind in motion. *Discover, 10*(3), 58–68.

National Joint Committee on Learning Disabilities. (1988). [Letter to NJCLD member organizations].

Opp, G. (1994). Historical roots of the field of learning disabilities: Some nineteenth-century German contributions. *Journal of Learning Disabilities, 27,* 10–19.

Orton, S. T. (1925). "Word-blindness" in school children. *Archives of Neurology and Psychiatry, 14,* 581–615.

Orton, S. T. (1937). *Reading, writing and speech problems in children.* New York: Norton.

Payne, N. (1994). [Learning disabilities in the workplace]. Unpublished raw data.

Pollan, C., & Williams, D. (1992). [Learning disabilities in adolescents and young adult school dropouts]. Unpublished raw data.

Rawson, M. B. (1988). *The many faces of dyslexia.* Baltimore: The Orton Dyslexia Society.

Rourke, B. P., & Finlayson, M. A. J. (1978). Neuropsychological significance of variations in patterns of academic performance: Verbal and visual-spatial abilities. *Journal of Abnormal Child Psychology, 6,* 121–133.

Schachar, R., & Wachsmuth, R. (1990). Oppositional disorder in children: A validation study comparing conduct disorder, oppositional disorder and normal control children. *Journal of Child Psychology and Psychiatry, 31,* 1089–1102.

Semrud-Clikeman, M., & Hynd, G. W. (1990). Right hemispheric dysfunction in nonverbal learning disabilities: Social, academic, and adaptive functioning in adults and children. *Psychological Bulletin, 107,* 196–209.

Siegfried, T. (1995, January 16). What memories are made of. *Dallas Morning News,* pp. D6–D8.

Silver, L. B. (1991). The Regular Education Initiative: A deja vu remembered with sadness and concern. *Journal of Learning Disabilities, 24,* 389–390.

Slingerland, B. (1976). *A multi-sensory approach to language arts for specific learning disability children: A guide for primary teachers.* Cambridge, MA: Educators Publishing Service.

Spalding, R. B., & Spalding, W. T. (1957). *The writing road to reading.* New York: Quill/William Morrow.

Steeves, J. (1987, November). *Computers: Powerful tools for dyslexic children.* Symposium conducted by The Orton Dyslexia Society, San Francisco.

Stolberg, S. (1994, March 6). Science studies nipping violence in the bud. *Tulsa World,* p. 28.

Tallal, P., Miller, S., & Fitch, R. (1993). Neurobiological basis of speech: A case for the preeminence of temporal processing. *Annals of New York Academy of Sciences, 682*(6), 74–81.

Taylor, S. E. (1960). *Eye-movement photography with the reading eye.* Huntington, NY: Educational Developmental Laboratories.

Thurber, D. N. (1993). *D'Nealian handwriting* (3rd ed.). Glenview, IL: ScottForesman.

Tranel, D., Hall, L. E., Olson, S., & Tranel, N. N. (1987). Evidence for a right-hemisphere developmental learning disability. *Developmental Neuropsychology, 3,* 113–127.

Troyer, P. (1986). *Father Bede's misfits.* New York: York.

United States Office of Education. (1977). Definition and criteria for defining students as learning disabled. *Federal Register,* 42:250, p. 65083. Washington, DC: U.S. Government Printing Office.

Voeller, K. K. S. (1986). Right-hemisphere deficit syndrome in children. *American Journal of Psychiatry, 143,* 1004–1009.

Wacker, J. (1975). *The dyslogic syndrome.* Dallas: Texas Association for Children with Learning Disabilities.

Wechsler, D. (1974). *Wechsler Intelligence Scale for Children–Revised.* San Antonio: Psychological Corporation.

Weis, L. (1992). *Attention deficit disorder in adults* (2nd ed.). Dallas: Taylor.

Weisel, L. P. (1992). *POWERPath to adult basic learning.* Columbus: OH: The TLP Group.

Weiss, G., & Hechtman, L. T. (1994). *Hyperactive children grown up* (2nd ed.). New York: Guilford.

Wernicke, C. (1874). *Die aphasische symptomencomplex* [The aphasia syndrome]. Breslau, Germany: Taschen.

Will, M. (1986). *Educating students with learning problems: A shared responsibility.* Washington, DC: U.S. Department of Education, Special Education and Rehabilitative Services.

Wilson, B. C., & Risucci, D. A. (1986). The early identification of developmental language disorders and the prediction of the acquisition of reading skills. In R. L. Masland & M. W. Masland (Eds.), *Prevention of reading failure* (pp. 187–203). Parkton, MD: York.

Wood, F. (1991, February). *Brain, imaging, learning disabilities.* Paper presented at the Learning Disabilities Association national conference, Chicago.

Woodcock, R. W. (1991). *Woodcock-Johnson Psycho-Educational Battery, Revised.* Circle Pines, MN: American Guidance Service.

Zametkin, A. J., Nordahl, T. E., Gross, M., King., A. C., Semple, W. E., Rumsey, J., Hamburger, S., & Cohen, R. M. (1990). Cerebral glucose metabolism in adults with hyperactivity of childhood onset. *New England Journal of Medicine, 323,* 1361–1367.

Author Index

Subject Index

NOTES

NOTES

NOTES

NOTES

NOTES